KU-184-779

DRUG THERAPY IN
Rheumatology
Nursing

Second Edition

Edited by
SARAH RYAN

BICENTENNIAL
1807
WILEY
2007
BICENTENNIAL

John Wiley & Sons, Ltd

Copyright © 2007   John Wiley & Sons Ltd, The Atrium, Southern Gate, Chichester,
West Sussex PO19 8SQ, England

Telephone   (+44) 1243 779777

Email (for orders and customer service enquiries): cs-books@wiley.co.uk
Visit our Home Page on www.wiley.com

All Rights Reserved. No part of this publication may be reproduced, stored in a retrieval system or
transmitted in any form or by any means, electronic, mechanical, photocopying, recording, scanning or
otherwise, except under the terms of the Copyright, Designs and Patents Act 1988 or under the terms of a
licence issued by the Copyright Licensing Agency Ltd, 90 Tottenham Court Road, London W1T 4LP, UK,
without the permission in writing of the Publisher. Requests to the Publisher should be addressed to the
Permissions Department, John Wiley & Sons Ltd, The Atrium, Southern Gate, Chichester, West Sussex PO19
8SQ, England, or emailed to permreq@wiley.co.uk, or faxed to (+44) 1243 770620.

Designations used by companies to distinguish their products are often claimed as trademarks. All brand
names and product names used in this book are trade names, service marks, trademarks or registered
trademarks of their respective owners. The Publisher is not associated with any product or vendor mentioned
in this book.

This publication is designed to provide accurate and authoritative information in regard to the subject matter
covered. It is sold on the understanding that the Publisher is not engaged in rendering professional services. If
professional advice or other expert assistance is required, the services of a competent professional should be
sought.

Other Wiley Editorial Offices

John Wiley & Sons Inc., 111 River Street, Hoboken, NJ 07030, USA

Jossey-Bass, 989 Market Street, San Francisco, CA 94103-1741, USA

Wiley-VCH Verlag GmbH, Boschstr. 12, D-69469 Weinheim, Germany

John Wiley & Sons Australia Ltd, 42 McDougall Street, Milton, Queensland 4064, Australia

John Wiley & Sons (Asia) Pte Ltd, 2 Clementi Loop #02-01, Jin Xing Distripark, Singapore 129809

John Wiley & Sons Canada Ltd, 6045 Freemont Blvd, Mississauga, ONT, L5R 4J3

Wiley also publishes its books in a variety of electronic formats. Some content that appears in print may not
be available in electronic books.

Anniversary Logo Design: Richard J. Pacifico

Library of Congress Cataloging in Publication Data

Drug therapy in rheumatology nursing / edited by Sarah Ryan. — 2nd ed.
    p.   ;   cm.
Rev. ed. of: Rheumatology / Jackie Hill and Sarah Ryan. 2000.
Includes bibliographical references.
ISBN-13: 978-0-470-02766-0 (alk. paper)
ISBN-10: 0-470-02766-5 (alk. paper)
1. Rheumatism—Chemotherapy.   2. Rheumatism—Nursing.
I. Ryan, Sarah.   II. Hill, Jacqueline, 1946– . Rheumatology.
[DNLM: 1. Rheumatic Diseases—nursing.   2. Nursing Assessment.   3. Patient Education.
4. Rheumatic Diseases—drug therapy. WE 544 D7935 2007]
RC927.D78 2007
616.7'23061—dc22
2006029324

Coventry University Library

British Library Cataloguing in Publication Data

A catalogue record for this book is available from the British Library

ISBN-13: 978-0-470-02766-0 (alk. paper)

Typeset in 10/12pt Times by Integra Software Services Pvt. Ltd, Pondicherry, India
Printed and bound in Great Britain by TJ International Ltd, Padstow, Cornwall
This book is printed on acid-free paper responsibly manufactured from sustainable forestry in which
at least two trees are planted for each one used for paper production.

Buchanzeige

Sprachwissenschaft in der Reihe
Beck'sche Elementarbücher

Theodora Bynon
Historische Linguistik
Eine Einführung. Gegenüber dem englischen Original überarbeitete
und erweiterte deutsche Ausgabe
Aus dem Englischen übertragen von Werner und Gerda Abraham
Für den deutschen Leser eingerichtet von Werner Abraham
1981. Etwa 309 Seiten. Paperback

Matthias Hartig / Robert I. Binnick
Grammatik und Sprachgebrauch
Neue Ansätze zur Sprachverhaltensforschung
1978. 171 Seiten. Paperback

John Lyons
Einführung in die moderne Linguistik
Aus dem Englischen von Werner und Gerda Abraham
Für den deutschen Leser eingerichtet von Werner Abraham
5. Auflage. 1980. XXI, 538 Seiten. Paperback

Frank Palmer
Semantik
Eine Einführung. Aus dem Englischen übertragen und für den deutschen
Leser eingerichtet von Christoph Gutknecht.
1977. 160 Seiten mit 6 Textabbildungen. Paperback

Uriel Weinreich
Sprachen in Kontakt
Ergebnisse und Probleme der Zweisprachigkeitsforschung
Mit einem Vorwort von André Martinet
Herausgegeben und mit einem Nachwort von A. de Vincenz
1977. 281 Seiten. Paperback

Verlag C. H. Beck München

Contents

2   Drug Therapy   61

Sarah Ryan, Susan Oliver and Ann Brownfield

4 **Patient Education and Adherence with Drug Therapy**   243
Jackie Hill

List of Contributors

Ann Brownfield, RGN, MSc, BSc (Hons)
Clinical Nurse Specialist, North and South Primary Care Trust, Haywood Hospital, Stoke on Trent

Janet Cushnagan, MSc, MCSP
MRC ERC, Southampton General Hospital, Southampton

Jackie Hill, PhD, MPhil, RN, FRCN
Arc senior lecturer in rheumatology nursing and Co-director ACUMeN, Chapel Allerton Hospital, Leeds

Jackie A McDowell, BSc (Hons), RGN, NDN
Clinical nurse specialist, Hereford Hospitals NHS Trust, Hereford

Susan Oliver, MSc
Nurse Consultant Rheumatology, Litchdon Medical Centre, Devon

Sarah Ryan, RGN, PhD, MSc, FRCN
Nurse Consultant Rheumatology, North and South Primary Care Trust, Haywood Hospital, Stoke on Trent

Margaret Ann Voyce, SRN
Rheumatology Nurse Practitioner, Rheumatology Department, Royal Cornwall Hospital, Truro

List of Figures

List of Tables

Preface

This revised text provides a comprehensive exploration of the drug treatment used in the management of rheumatological and related conditions. It will provide a valuable resource to all nurses and other health professionals in the care of patients with a rheumatological condition, be it in the hospital, community or research setting.

The text has been revised to include the management of patients receiving biologic therapies, my thanks to Susan Oliver who has written this comprehensive section. It is amazing to think that when this book was originally published in 1999, biologic treatments were primarily being used for patients in research studies, whereas now, they have become a mainstream therapy for many patients with an active inflammatory condition. Drugs such as Leflunomide and Mycophenolate are also being used more widely. Also new evidence has altered our use of non steroidal anti-inflammatory drugs (NSAIDs) in practice, this is addressed within this new text and the use of case scenarios will help nurses develop their clinical decision-making skills in the context of the current evidence. There is also a review of community-based provision for patients with a rheumatological condition.

Not only have there been dramatic changes in drug therapy for patients, nurse prescribing has become law and the implications of this for rheumatology nurses are discussed.

Patients will often require a combination of drug therapy to provide symptomatic control and disease suppression. The addition or alteration to a patient's drug treatment will require exploration of the patient's (and their significant others') expectations to ensure that all treatment has meaning and relevance within the patient's contextual framework.

The revised book contains four chapters, each divided into several short sections; each part begins with learning objectives which will guide the reader as to the content of the chapter. The book is based on clinical and research findings to ensure the adoption of evidence-based practice within clinical settings.

The primary aims of this book include:

- An understanding of those rheumatological conditions where drug treatment can be effective.
- The provision of information on different disease processes, so that the utilization of drug therapy can be placed in context.
- Increasing knowledge for nurses and other health professionals on the classification of drugs in common usage, including analgesia, NSAIDs, disease modifying anti-rheumatic drugs (DMARDs), biologic therapies, cytotoxic drugs, steroids, treatments for gout and osteoporosis.

- An exploration of the role of the nurse in the management of drug therapy, focusing on the knowledge and skills required to undertake drug surveillance and assessment of interventions.
- A comprehensive exploration of patient education: theories, principles, content and delivery of education are discussed.
- A review of community based provision for patients with rheumatological conditions.

This book can be used as a reference text for those nurses who seek specific answers regarding an aspect of practice, for example what advice should be given to a patient regarding pregnancy who is taking Leflunomide, as well as providing in-depth information on the principles and components of a wide range of drug therapies for clinicians specializing in this field.

The nurse performs a pivotal role in guiding, supporting and educating the patient and the family to manage their condition effectively. The utilization of this text will enable practitioners to develop and advance their practice to the benefit of the patient.

Sarah Ryan

1 Rheumatological Conditions

JANET CUSHNAGHAN AND JACKIE McDOWELL

Learning objectives

After reading this chapter you should be able to:

- Discuss the anatomy and physiology of the musculoskeletal system in health and illness.
- Describe the process of inflammation and the immune response.
- Develop an understanding of the rheumatic diseases where drug therapy is required.
- Discuss the effects of rheumatic disease on physical, psychological and social well-being.

1.1 INTRODUCTION

The primary objective of this book is to provide the nurse with the knowledge and subsequent understanding of the role drug therapy plays in the management of rheumatological conditions. It is essential therefore that nurses must have a good knowledge and understanding of rheumatological conditions themselves.

Rheumatology is the branch of medicine dealing with disorders of the joints, muscles, tendons and ligaments. Arthritis and the rheumatic diseases in general constitute the major cause of chronic disability in the United Kingdom. It is estimated that musculoskeletal diseases account for one third of the physical disability experienced in the community in the United Kingdom and have an economic cost that exceeds that of heart disease and cancer.

The terms arthritis and rheumatism or rheumatic disease encompass a host of conditions causing much pain and suffering to those affected. The burden of these diseases is felt not only by the sufferer and their family, but also by the community, in terms of the cost of healthcare and the loss of working days. Because of the diversity of rheumatic conditions it is helpful to classify them into groups. This may be undertaken in different ways incorporating:

- clinical and laboratory features;
- disease mechanisms − for example, autoimmunity;
- anatomic structures involved;
- genetic factors;
- involved organ systems and specific abnormalities or deficiencies.

Drug Therapy in Rheumatology Nursing: Second Edition. Edited by Sarah Ryan.
© 2007 John Wiley & Sons, Ltd.

Table 1.1   Classification of rheumatic diseases.

Inflammatory arthritis
    Rheumatoid arthritis
    Juvenile arthritis
    Polymyalgia rheumatica

associated with spondylitis
    Ankylosing spondylitis
    Reiter's syndrome
    Psoriatic arthritis

associated with infectious agents
    Septic arthritis
    Reactive arthritis

associated with crystals
    Gout
    Pseudogout

Non inflammatory
    Osteoarthritis
    Fibromyalgia

Connective tissue disorders
    Systemic lupus erythematosus
    Scleroderma
    Polymyositis

Classification is hampered by the absence of firm aetiological evidence for most diseases but for this chapter we intend to use a simplified classification, which will correspond to the philosophy of drug therapy which is the main purpose of this text. Table 1.1 classifies the rheumatic diseases according to the presence or absence of inflammation and further subclassifies inflammatory arthritis according to associations that may be present.

1.2   FEATURES OF RHEUMATIC CONDITIONS

Symptoms of rheumatic disease can be determined by a clinical history taking and thorough physical examination. Laboratory and radiographic investigations can aid diagnosis and eliminate certain features but nothing can replace the clinician's clinical skills and pattern recognition. Patients with a rheumatological condition often experience symptoms of pain, swelling, stiffness and loss of function. These symptoms give rise to impairments, which in turn may produce handicap or disability, depending on the interaction of environmental, resource and psychological factors.

One of the primary objectives of the clinical history is to ascertain a greater understanding of the pain:

- Is it inflammatory?
- What is the origin of its presentation?
- What are the aggravating factors?
- What is its temporal pattern?
- Are there any constitutional symptoms suggesting a systemic illness, such as fever or weight loss?

PAIN

Arthralgia implies pain originating from or around a joint, but not necessarily from within the joint itself. Periarticular structures may be responsible for the pain or it may be referred from somewhere away from the joint. Pain originating from joint structures should be improved by resting the joint and aggravated by stretching the joint or weight bearing.

STIFFNESS

Stiffness after prolonged immobility suggests inflammatory joint disease or synovitis. Stiffness alone is a non-specific symptom and can be present in other diseases such as Parkinsonism. It is also present in older individuals. Clinically significant stiffness lasts more than 30 minutes, and in inflammatory disease the duration of stiffness is proportional to the severity of inflammation.

SWELLING

Swelling may be due to synovitis, cellulitis or oedema and it is important to distinguish between them. Joint swelling may be due to soft tissue swelling or synovitis or it may be due to bony swelling indicating osteoarthritis (OA).

JOINT INVOLVEMENT

The pattern of joint involvement, including its symmetry, is helpful in making a diagnosis, although it should be noted that there is considerable overlap between the major causes of inflammatory polyarthritis.

FUNCTION

Loss of function is an important consequence to the patient and should be assessed in work, leisure and home activities. Functional ability depends on need, motivation and environmental factors. The assessment of function will be discussed later in this chapter.

1.3 EPIDEMIOLOGY

Epidemiology is the study of the incidence, distribution and determinants of disease in populations in order to identify causes and ultimately lead to prevention (Table 1.2). In studying the epidemiology of rheumatic disease it is important that diagnostic criteria are used to ensure standardization of disease definition and allow comparisons between populations. Criteria that are designed for research purposes or for entry into clinical trials may not be suitable for routine clinical practice. The prevalence estimates for selected rheumatological disorders are shown in Table 1.3.

Mortality from musculoskeletal disorders is low. The major impact in the population is in terms of morbidity and disability. OA is the most common type of arthritis and its frequency increases with age. Back complaints represent a quarter to a third of all musculoskeletal morbidity.

Table 1.2 Epidemiological definitions.

Incidence	The number of new cases of disease per unit time (for example, cases per annum)
Prevalence	Total number of cases of the disease at a given time point in a defined population
Morbidity	Number of cases with a defined outcome of the disease
Mortality	Number of cases dying from the disease per unit time (for example, deaths per annum)

Table 1.3 Prevalence estimates for selected rheumatological disorders.

Rheumatic disorder	Estimated percent prevalence
Arthropathies	
RA	1.0
In children <16 yrs	0.06
Osteoarthritis	
Moderate/severe X-ray changes in hands or feet	23.0
Knee	3.8
Hip	1.3
Ankylosing spondylitis	0.1
Psoriatic arthropathy	0.1
Crystalline arthritis	1.0
Connective tissue disease	
Systemic lupus erythematosus (SLE)	0.006
Systemic sclerosis	0.002
Back troubles	>20.00

1.4 ANATOMY AND PHYSIOLOGY OF THE MUSCULOSKELETAL SYSTEM

Before learning about the pathology of rheumatic diseases it is important to have an understanding of the anatomy and physiology of the musculoskeletal system in health. The musculoskeletal system serves several purposes:

- it provides stable support;
- it facilitates movement
- it protects vital organs
- it allows for growth and renewal over the lifetime of the individual (Simkin, 1994).

Components of the musculoskeletal system are muscle, bone, tendons, ligaments, cartilage and synovial tissue. All musculoskeletal tissues are supplied by the circulation and guided and protected by their innervation.

MUSCLE

Skeletal or striated muscle provides the energy or driving force for musculoskeletal activity. Chemical energy derived from foodstuffs is ultimately converted to the mechanical energy required to do work. Individual striated fibres are bundled in perimysial tissue that transmits the force of muscle contraction through tendons to attachments on bone. Each fibre can only work in the direction of its long axis and it is only the variety of arrangements within muscles and the cooperation between muscles that allow the full range of possible human activities.

BONE

No muscle contraction would be effective unless it could produce directed motion through a skeletal lever. Each effective motion comes about as muscles act on bones to move the limbs, head or torso. In some cases the mechanical advantage of the muscles is poor and they exert substantial transarticular compressive forces in order to generate the desired movement. The bones of the skeleton have evolved to withstand and distribute these forces. Bone is characterized by the deposition of hydroxyapatite crystals in a well organized, collagenous matrix. There are two types of mature bone: compact and trabecular.

Compact bone is predominant and found in the shafts of long bones. The shafts of long bones contain little or no internal osseous structure, but have a marrow cavity filled with fat and loose interstitial tissue. The bone is covered by a sensitive periosteum that is capable of new bone formation.

Trabecular bone refers to the cross-braced architecture found beneath articular surfaces and in the vertebral bodies. All trabeculae undergo remodelling through ongoing processes of osteoclastic resorption and osteoblastic formation of bone.

CARTILAGE

The contact surfaces of bones are covered by a cushion of cartilage. For the most part this is hyaline articular cartilage, which is principally comprised of water. Its structure is of proteoglycan aggregates restrained within a framework of type II collagen fibres. These aggregates are made up of keratan sulfate and chondroitin sulfate. Cartilage is remarkably firm and resilient. It undergoes continuous turnover, the principal players in this being the chondrocytes that are individually active but are relatively sparse in numbers so the overall metabolic activity of cartilage is relatively low. Normal hyaline cartilage lacks blood vessels and nerves and relies on adjacent structures for nutrition, namely the synovial microvessels.

The synovial fluid is the vehicle carrying nutrients to the chondrocytes and returning waste products to the blood stream. The absence of nerves in articular cartilage means that damage to this structure alone cannot be painful but in conjunction with the involvement of adjacent soft tissues or subjacent bone it will cause pain. A second type of cartilage is fibrocartilage, found at sites subject to shearing forces or under tensile stress. Examples include the moon-shaped cartilages called menisci over each tibial plateau and the principal load-bearing region in the roof of the acetabulum. This type of cartilage is more notable for its fibrous component (mainly type I collagen) than for its proteoglycan composition.

SYNOVIUM

This is a living lining and covers all intra-articular surfaces other than the articulating areas of cartilage. It is a thin structure, in health, with a normal depth of $25-35\mu$m. It is comprised of a well-organized matrix of numerous microfibrils and abundant proteoglycan aggregates. Within this matrix lie the synovial cells. The structure has protective and synthetic capabilities.

LIGAMENTS AND TENDONS

Ligaments are strong bundles of parallel type I collagen fibres that serve as 'check-reins' to prevent inappropriate movements. Each hinge joint, for example, is bordered by collateral ligaments to limit movements to flexion and extension. Every ligament runs from bone to bone. Tendons act as active drivers of joint motion as opposed to passive restrainers (ligaments). Tendons and ligaments insert into bone at anatomic sites known as entheses.

TENDON SHEATHS AND BURSAE

Tendons connect muscle bodies to, sometimes distant, insertion sites, and therefore often run through sheaths to avoid adherence to other structures. Similarly, points of potential friction, such as those between ligaments, bony prominences and overlying skin are often protected by lubricating bursae. These flimsy structures are flattened sacks lined by a tissue that is histologically indistinguishable from synovium. They contain a fluid that appears synovial. It is no surprise therefore that tendon sheaths and bursae are the targets of the same inflammatory diseases that affect synovial joints.

SYNOVIAL JOINTS

These are the commonest type of articulation in the body. They are actively driven by muscles and tendons, stabilized by ligaments, cushioned by hyaline cartilage and are both nourished and lubricated by synovial tissue. A film of synovial fluid lubricates the bearing surfaces and the adjacent interfaces of synovium on cartilage and synovium on synovium.

PHYSIOLOGY

Physiology is the study of how living things work. The principal function of almost all joints is movement. Microscopic examination of synovium and cartilage shows them to be composed of metabolically active cells. This implies that they have the same nutritional requirements as other tissues, produce similar waste products and respond to hormonal and other metabolic stimuli in ways analogous to other tissues. Joints age as do other tissues, with subsequent effects on function. Aspects of physiology include circulation, lymphatics, pressure, diffusion, temperature and innervation. Changes in one 'system' can have clinically important effects on another and all are uniquely modified by physical movement.

CIRCULATION

Joints require a blood supply to ensure the health of the cartilage, which lacks blood vessels of its own. The nearest available blood vessels are the capillaries of the synovium. Transport of nutrients is dependent on diffusion. The synovium and synovial space have a major role in facilitating metabolic exchange and in maintaining a normal joint space environment. Large blood vessels of the limbs pass the articular regions, and feeder vessels enter and leave the joint capsule at positions that protect them from mechanical embarrassment during movement.

LYMPHATICS

There is a typical lymphatic system in the synovium but not in the cartilage. Synovial lymphatics carry excess fluid, high molecular weight solutes and protein, tiny particulates and some cells out of the joint. This transfer is powered by normal movement of the joint.

INTRA-ARTICULAR PRESSURE

Normal intra-articular pressure in a resting joint is subatmospheric. In conditions where there is an abnormal volume of fluid in the joint the pressure will rise nonlinearly. The resulting pressure volume curve defines the compliance of the joint space and its surrounding connective tissue.

MOTION

Motion is the function of diarthrodial joints, but motion itself affects the physiology and health of the joint. If a joint is immobilized cartilage thins and loses its mechanical properties. The application and release of weight-bearing forces play a part in joint lubrication and in the diffusion of substances in and out of cartilage. Joint movement is also required to maintain health by:

- Maintaining normal strength and coordination of muscles
- Preserving bone mass
- Maintaining desired weight
- Preserving normal range of joint motion
- Increasing blood flow to the synovial tissues
- Permitting the lymphatic system to clear the joint of particulates and excess fluid.

INNERVATION

There are no nerves in articular hyaline cartilage. Most of the synovium is insensitive but there are small and isolated areas that are painful when stimulated mechanically. Small diameter nerve fibres are present within the confines of the capsule. The capsule, intra-articular fat pads, ligaments, periosteum, muscles and adjacent bone have abundant innervation. The major function of joint innervation appears to be proprioception — the perception of joint position, and the direction and velocity of movement.

TEMPERATURE

The normal intra-articular temperature of peripheral joints is far less than 37°C. Temperature is largely a function of blood flow. Joint movement increases joint temperature.

1.5 ANATOMY AND PHYSIOLOGY OF THE MUSCULOSKELETAL SYSTEM IN INFLAMMATORY ARTHRITIS

The inflammatory arthritides are characterized by inflammation and damage to the joints and their surrounding structures, mediated by the immune system. It is believed that trigger factors (for example, infection) initiate a pathological process in a susceptible individual because of genetic factors. Only a small proportion of susceptible individuals develop disease. Understanding the aetiology of rheumatic diseases requires knowledge of immunopathogenetic mechanisms, determinants of susceptibility and the nature of putative trigger factors.

IMMUNOPATHOGENETIC MECHANISMS

There are four types of immune mechanisms:

- Type I   Allergic

Allergic reactions are mediated by IgE and provoke vasomotor and bronchospastic changes leading to asthma, urticaria or anaphylaxis.

- Type II   Cytotoxic

Cytotoxic reactions involve cellular injury mediated by antibodies (IgG or IgM) and the activation of the complement system.

- Type III   Immune complex

Immune complexes from the circulation deposit in the tissue where they cause activation of the complement system and the generation of proinflammatory mediators.

- Type IV   Cell-mediated

Injury may be mediated by T cells rather than antibodies. T cells may cause tissue injury by direct killing of cells or the elaboration of cytokines which disturb cell growth or function.

Rheumatic diseases are usually the result of type II–IV reactions, although more than one mechanism may operate concomitantly in patients.

In the initiation of the immune response T cells recognize antigen via receptors (T cell receptors). After activation by antigen, T cells can proliferate to serve as helper cells for B-cell antibody production or the generation of cytotoxic T cells. In addition, activated T cells can produce cytokines leading to functional changes, such as synovial cell proliferation in rheumatoid arthritis (Figure 1.1).

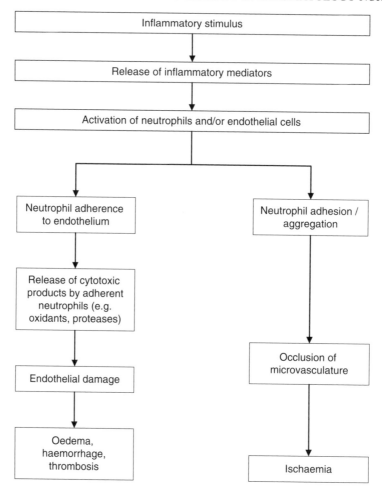

Figure 1.1 The inflammatory cascade.

SUSCEPTIBILITY

Several factors may influence disease susceptibility (Table 1.4).

- Hormones of the neuroendocrine system can modulate immune responses, an action exploited in the use of corticosteroids as anti-inflammatory and immuno-suppressive agents.
- Many rheumatic diseases show an unequal representation of the sexes, with women displaying a generally higher prevalence of inflammatory disease as well as a more serious outcome (Pisetsky, 1994).
- Environmental factors may affect levels of immune cell function and together with inherited factors promote disease pathogenesis.

Table 1.4 Factors influencing disease susceptibility.

Genetic	Environment
MHC	Stress
T-cell receptor	Diet
Immunoglobulins	Drugs
Complement system components	Infection
Cytokines	
Stress responses	
Gender	

- Emotional and physical stress can perturb neuroendocrine function resulting in changes in immune cell function. Rheumatic diseases have long been considered to have a psychosomatic component, indicative of the belief that psychological factors influence disease onset or course (Levine, Goetzl and Basbaum, 1987).
- Diet may have a role in influencing disease susceptibility; in the extreme, malnutrition and serious vitamin or mineral deficiency can impair immune function. The strong influence of environmental factors on disease susceptibility can be observed by comparing disease prevalence in populations that have migrated (Solomon, Robin and Valkenburg, 1975).
- Socioeconomic group and educational level also influence the susceptibility or severity of rheumatic disease, although both are likely markers for other health-related factors which include diet, hygiene, occupation, lifestyle, exposure to infection, use of tobacco and alcohol and access to medical care.

SYNOVITIS

The synovium is the soft connective tissue lining the enclosed spaces of synovial joints, tendon sheaths and bursae. These spaces all contain a small amount of fluid rich in hyaluronic acid (synovial fluid). The functions of the synovium are:

- maintenance of an intact nonadherent tissue surface;
- control of volume and composition of synovial fluid;
- lubrication of cartilage and nutrition of chondrocytes within joints.

Inflammatory arthritides are characterized by synovitis, that is inflammation of the synovium. Acute inflammation begins when an extravascular inflammatory stimulus provokes capillary dilatation, the accumulation of plasma and fluid, and recruits circulating effector cells to the site (Figure 1.1).

There is emerging evidence that the ultimate outcome of the inflammatory response with resulting injury can be ascribed to a complex network involving products of both neutrophils and macrophages (Varani, Mulligan and Ward, 1994).

Inflamed synovium appears dramatically increased in size because of oedema, multiple redundant folds and villae. It takes on a red hue because of a dramatic increase in blood vessels. If the condition becomes chronic, synovial lining hyperplasia becomes prominent. The sublining of the synovium also undergoes dramatic alterations in the degree and content of the cellular infiltrate. The most prominent change is an exuberant infiltration with mononuclear cells, including T cells, B cells, macrophages and plasma cells. Multinucleate giant cells can be seen in granuloma-like lesions in the synovium.

1.6 AN OVERVIEW OF THE RHEUMATOLOGICAL CONDITIONS MOST COMMONLY ENCOUNTERED IN WESTERN EUROPE (SEE TABLE 1.1)

RHEUMATOID ARTHRITIS

Rheumatoid arthritis (RA) is the commonest form of chronic inflammatory joint disease and a common cause of disability. The consensus view, backed up by clinical evidence, is that RA should be treated as early as possible to improve long-term outcome (Maddison and Huey, 2006).

RA is two to three times more common in women compared to men. The current annual incidence is reported as 36/100 000 in women and 14/100 000 in men (Symmons, 2005). The prevalence is 0.8% of the adult population. Symmons (2005) reports that the incidence, prevalence and mortality of RA have fallen in women in the last 50 years. Excess mortality is predominantly due to cardiovascular disease (Symmons, 2005). Sex differences decrease with age as the prevalence of RA appears to increase with age; by the age of 69 years the sex distribution is equal (Dieppe *et al.*, 1985). The peak age of onset varies but is common in the fourth and fifth decades of life. RA imposes a substantial economic burden on both patients and society. This is usually quantified in terms of both direct costs such as treatment and hospitalization and indirect costs resulting from loss of resources due to productivity loss (Cooper, 2000).

RA is a chronic, systemic, inflammatory, autoimmune disease of unknown aetiology. It is hypothesized that viruses, bacterial infection or psychological trauma may be initiating factors. There is a threefold increased risk for first degree relatives of those with RA developing the disease themselves. This risk is approximately sixfold higher in those possessing 'at risk' human leucocyte antigen-DRB1 genotypes (MacGregor and Spector, 2004). Up to 70% of people with rheumatoid arthritis test positive for human leucocyte factor (HLA) DR4 antigen (Le Gallez, 1995). The detection of anticyclic citrullinated peptide (anti-CCP) antibodies in patients has recently been shown to have great specificity for RA (Maddison and Huey, 2006). Anti-CCP antibodies appear early in RA and can predate the clinical onset of disease by years (Rantapaa-Dahlqvist *et al.*, 2003).

Ryan (1997) explains that 'inflammation is usually a self-limiting process – the response of the body to an offending antigen. But for reasons not fully understood, in conditions such as RA the inflammatory response becomes a continual process and can lead to destruction of much of the surrounding tissue'.

Ryan (1997) goes on to to describe 'whereas the complexes created by the immune system are usually ingested by the reticuloendothelial system, and deactivated once their mission is completed, in RA this does not happen. .Instead, the joint lining or synovial lining proliferates, which results in pannus formation. Cartilage, and tissues supporting the joints, are destroyed by enzymes released as a consequence of the inflammatory response. Bone is then also destroyed by the increasing synovial membrane. As the joint space constricts, articular surfaces are reduced and joint movement is restricted.'

It has been suggested that sex hormones may also have a role in the cause of RA (Maini and Feldman, 1993). Whilst their role is not entirely clear, the evidence points to the predominance of RA in females and the increased onset of the disease during the reproductive years and at the menopause (Le Gallez, 1995). Hormones have an important influence in women with RA. In approximately 70% of women the manifestations of RA subside during pregnancy and recur in the early post-partum period (Nicholas and Panayi, 1988).

Areas Affected by RA

RA is characterized by symmetrical small joint polyarthritis involving the hands and feet, particularly the metacarpophalangeal (MCP) and the proximal interphalangeal (PIP) joints in the hands and the metatarsophalangeal (MTP) joints in the feet. RA causes inflammation of the synovium, which lines both the joints and tendon sheaths of the body. In RA as the disease progresses other joints may also be affected, for example the wrists, elbows, shoulders, cervical spine, ribs, jaw (temporomandibular joints), knees and ankles (Figure 1.2).

The course of the disease is variable with exacerbations and remissions over a period of time, and in the majority of patients progressive joint erosions and deformity occurs. Around 30% of people will recover completely within a few years while 5% will deteriorate until they have a significant disability (Ryan, 1997).

The 1987 American Rheumatism Association Revised Criteria for the classification of RA (Table 1.5) currently presents the best definition of the disease in the form of a clinical description (Arnett et al., 1988). However, these criteria were not designed for the diagnosis of early RA and are fairly insensitive in patients with disease duration of less than 12 months (Huizinga et al., 2002).

In practice, therefore, recognition of early RA is usually based on a combination of clinical features and appropriate investigations as well as on the exclusion of other disorders that may mimic RA (Pipitone and Choy, 2003).

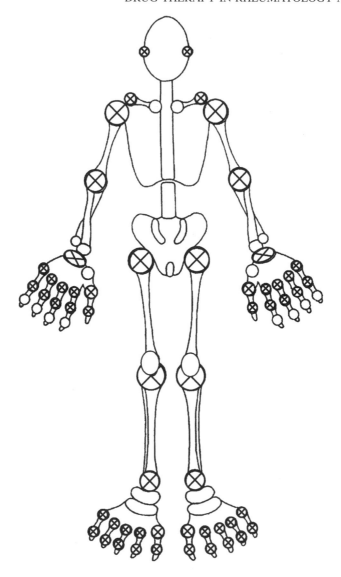

Figure 1.2 Joints affected by rheumatoid arthritis.

Rheumatoid Factor

About 70−80% of patients with RA have circulating rheumatoid factor (an IgM/IgG complex of two immunoglobulins) in the blood (Bird, Le Gallez and Hill, 1985; Ferrari, Cash and Maddison, 1996). These patients are classified as sero-positive; those without a circulating rheumatoid factor are classified as sero-negative.

Table 1.5 1987 American Rheumatism Association Revised Criteria for the classification of RA.

Morning stiffness of at least one hour*
Arthritis in at least three joint areas[†] with swelling or fluid*
Arthritis of hand joints (at least one area swollen in a wrist, MCP, or PIP joint)*
Symmetric joint swelling and involvement*
Subcutaneous nodules
Radiographic changes typical of RA
Positive rheumatoid factor

Notes
*Specified criteria that must be present for at least six weeks
[†]Right or left proximal interphalangeal (PIP), metacarpophalangeal (MCP), wrist, elbow, knee, ankle and metatarsophalangeal (MTP) joint

However, it is important to remember that in 5−15% of healthy subjects rheumatoid factor can be detected. Many patients who test positive for rheumatoid factor (RF) do not have RA. Other diseases commonly associated with rheumatoid factor are:

• Sjogren's syndrome
• systemic lupus erythematosus
• systemic sclerosis
• subacute bacterial endocarditis
• sarcoidosis
• chronic liver disease
• polymyositis
• acute viral infections
• parasitic infections
• tuberculosis
• syphilis (Ferrari, Cash and Maddison, 1996).

Rheumatoid factor can be identified using the sheep cell agglutination test (SCAT), in which serum from a patient containing rheumatoid factor, heavy with immunoglobulin complexes, causes the agglutination of sheep red blood cells that have been previously coated with immunoglobulin (IgG). This test is performed at serial dilutions of the patient's serum. If a large amount of rheumatoid factor is present, flocculation of the sheep cells is likely to be observed with dilutions of the patient's serum as great as 1 in 256. By contrast, if only a small amount of rheumatoid factor is present flocculation will only occur with undiluted serum, perhaps 1 in 8 or 1 in 16 (Bird, Le Gallez and Hill, 1985). A positive SCAT titre of 1 in 80 is normally recognized as significant.

Pain and Stiffness

Widespread symmetrical joint pain and swelling affecting the small peripheral joints are the commonest presenting symptoms. The immediate result of inflammation of the synovial membrane, known as synovitis, is a painful, stiff, hot and swollen joint. During a 'flare' or acute attack of the disease many joints may be involved at the same time. Pain is often the first reported physical symptom, and may vary in intensity and duration from one day to the next. The patient reports early morning stiffness (EMS) of variable duration and tenderness in the affected joints, which because they are swollen and painful are difficult to move, limiting the range of movement of the joints affected. EMS can last from a few minutes to several hours with the duration of EMS being a guide to the level of disease activity. Muscle weakness and spasm are common in the early stages and can be followed by marked muscular atrophy.

Extra-Articular Manifestations

It is important to remember that the disease will have an impact on the patient as a whole by affecting their overall physical condition, psychological well-being and social life. The onset of RA is usually insidious and affects the patient's body as a whole; commonly seen symptoms are general fatigue, fever, depression, weight loss and weakness. Patients may describe extreme mental and physical tiredness that is not relieved by sleep (this is caused by the inflammatory component of RA). Weight loss often occurs early in the disease, but with good disease control weight should be regained and remain stable thereafter. A normochromic or mildly hypochromic anaemia is often found in active RA. The cause seems to be a combination of poor iron intake and absorption, depression of bone marrow function, poor iron utilization and mild haemolysis (Le Gallez, 1995). Iron deficiency anaemia may also be present. People with RA can have any type (or combination) of anaemia; but of those with anaemia, 77% will have anaemia of chronic disorders, and about 23% will have iron deficiency anaemia (Wilson *et al.*, 2004). Tenosynovitis and bursitis commonly accompany the disease.

Many extra-articular features of RA can occur as listed in Table 1.6. The presence of rheumatoid nodules is often associated with a positive rheumatoid factor. They appear principally on extensor surfaces or areas subjected to pressure, including the elbows, finger joints, ischial and sacral prominences, occipital scalp and Achilles tendon. They are not usually painful. Care should be taken to avoid trauma so that nodules do not become ulcerated acting as a possible source of infection. They are composed mainly of fibrinoid material (degenerative tissue cells) and granulation tissue (Judd, 1997). Subcutaneous nodules may regress during treatment with disease-modifying anti-rheumatic drugs (DMARDs), usually as RA improves (Matteson, Cohen and Conn, 1994). Methotrexate treatment may result in an increase in nodules, particularly over finger tendons, despite improvement in the overall disease activity (Segal *et al.*, 1988). In general, higher concentrations of

Table 1.6   Extra-articular manifestations of RA.

Skin	Palmar erythema
	Subcutaneous nodules
	Vasculitis
	Ulceration
Lung	Pleurisy, pleural effusions
	Pneumonitis
	Lung nodules
	Bronchiolitis obliterans
	Fibrosis
Heart	Pericarditis, pericardial effusions
	Valvular disease
	Myocarditis
Neuromuscular	Nerve entrapment
	Cervical cord compression
	Muscle wasting
	Mononeuritis multiplex
	Diffuse peripheral neuropathy
Mouth	Sicca symptoms
Eye	Episcleritis
	Scleritis, scleromalacia perforans
	Melting cornea syndrome
Haematologic	Normocytic, normochromic anaemia
	Felty's syndrome
	Amyloidosis
	Thrombocytosis
Miscellaneous	Sjögren's syndrome
	Pulmonary infections, septic arthritis
	Osteoporosis
	Tenosynovitis
	Bursitis
	Reactive lymphadenopathy
	Splenomegaly

rheumatoid factor, together with the presence of nodules and radiological evidence of erosions, are associated with a poorer prognosis.

Progression

If RA is allowed to continue uncontrolled, inflammation will eventually lead to erosion of the joint, including damage to the tendons and ligaments surrounding the joint. As the disease progresses this damage will cause the joint to become unstable, with corresponding deviation resulting in deformity (Le Gallez, 1995). Such deformities may include:

- radial deviation at the wrist;
- ulnar deviation at the MCP joints;
- palmar subluxation of proximal phalanges;
- swan-neck deformity (hyperextension of PIP with flexion of DIP);
- boutonnière deformity (flexion of PIP, extension of DIP);
- hyperextension of first IP joint with flexion of first MCP (causing loss of thumb mobility and pinch);
- metatarsal prolapse;
- arch collapse;
- hallux valgus;
- atlantoaxial subluxation (Ferrari, Cash and Maddison, 1996).

Judd (1997) describes how instability and irritation of the joint may cause muscle contraction with resulting flexion or extension deformity or subluxation of the joint. Fibrous scar tissue and adhesions develop between the opposing joint surfaces, leading to fibrous ankylosis of the joint. The exposed, roughened ends of bone tissue may eventually proliferate bone cells into the joint cavity, resulting in calcification and bony ankylosis.

Erosions

Erosions can occur in any of the joints involved in RA; they may take many months or even years to develop. Initially, the erosions develop marginally, at the point where the synovium joins the bone, as this is the seat of inflammation (Le Gallez, 1995). Erosions normally occur in the MTP heads of the feet before they are seen in the MCP joints of the hands.

Several conditions that commonly occur with RA adversely affect outcomes and may lead to disability and death. The most important co-morbidities are cardiovascular disease, infection, malignancy, gastrointestinal (GI) disease and osteoporosis. RA is associated with a marked increase in morbidity and mortality and all patients with RA should be screened annually for cardiovascular risk factors (Symmons and Bruce, 2006).

A number of guidelines and standards of care are available to guide practice, and assist and support clinicians in the provision of high quality care and management of RA patients (ARMA, 2004; BSR, 2004; NICE, 2002; SIGN, 2000).

At the present time there is no cure for RA. The management goals include:

- control of the inflammatory process;
- relief of symptoms;
- prevention of joint deformity;
- empowerment of the patient by assisting them to adjust to this chronic condition.

Drug treatment remains one of the major interventions in the relief of symptoms and the prevention of progress. Until the cause of RA becomes known it cannot be precisely defined. Gordon and Hastings (1994) state: 'it may be one disease with more than one cause or more than one disease with a single cause.'

JUVENILE IDIOPATHIC ARTHRITIS

Inflammatory joint disease is common not only in adults but in children also. Juvenile idiopathic arthritis (JIA) is the new term unifying the existing classifications for inflammatory arthritis in children — encompassing juvenile chronic arthritis and juvenile rheumatoid arthritis (Petty et al., 1998).

Juvenile idiopathic arthritis (previously known as juvenile chronic arthritis), and known as juvenile rheumatoid arthritis in the United States, is the most common rheumatic disease of childhood and is often an important cause of disability and blindness (White, 1994). In the United Kingdom the prevalence of JIA is approximately 10 per 100 000 of population (Symmons et al., 1996). The term is used to describe arthritis affecting one or more joints, which occurs in someone under 16 and lasts for more than three months when other forms of arthritis and connective tissue disorders have been excluded (Leach, 1997). It is not a single disease but rather a heterogeneous group of diseases. In patients with a diagnosis of JIA regular assessment by an ophthalmologist and rheumatologist is generally recommended (Ferrari, Cash and Maddison, 1996).

Juvenile arthritis was first described by George Frederick Still, a children's specialist, in 1896. The term 'Still's disease' was used for many years in relation to childhood arthritis. The term 'Still's' tends to be used today only to describe the rash associated with systemic onset arthritis (Leach, 1997).

In very young children who cannot express their pain the first signs may be limping, guarding of joints or even an outright refusal to move (Leach, 1997).

The goals of therapy in juvenile arthritis are pain relief and preservation of joint function, so as to maintain normal growth and psychosocial development (Cassidy, 1994).

The International League of Associations for Rheumatology (ILAR) (Foeldvari and Bidde, 2000) unified the classification of JIA, with clinical criteria as follows:

- age at onset <16;
- minimum duration of arthritis six weeks.

Subtypes:

- Systemic arthritis: arthritis with/preceded by daily fever for at least two weeks and one/more of evanescent non-fixed erythrematous rash, generalized lymphadenopathy, hepato/splenomegaly and serositis.

- Oligoarthritis: arthritis of one to four joints during the first six months.

  persistent: affects no more than four joints throughout the disease course;
  extended: affects more than four joints after the first six months.

- Polyarthritis (rheumatoid factor-negative): affects five or more joints in the first six months of the disease. Tests for rheumatoid factor are negative.
- Polyarthritis (rheumatoid factor-positive): affects five or more joints in the first six months of disease. Tests for rheumatoid factor are positive on two occasions at least two months apart.
- Enthesitis-related arthritis: arthritis and enthesitis, or arthritis or enthesitis with at least two of: sacroiliac tenderness and/or inflammatory spinal pain; HLA B27-positive; family history in a first or second degree relative of medically confirmed HLA B27-associated disease.
- Psoriatic arthritis: arthritis and psoriasis, or arthritis and at least two of dactylitis, nail abnormalities, family history of psoriasis in at least one first degree relative.
- Other: arthritis of unknown cause persisting for at least six weeks that either does not fulfil criteria for any categories or fulfils criteria for more than one category.

Further details about the subtypes are as follows:

Oligoarticular onset (55−75%) arthritis affects fewer than five joints. The knee and ankle are the most commonly affected joints, but the small joints of the hand or the elbow can also be involved (Ansell, 1977). The majority present before the age of five years, approximately twice as many girls are affected than boys (Leach, 1997). Antinuclear antibodies (ANAs) are present in 40−75% of children and are associated with chronic anterior uveitis. Routine eye examination is essential (White, 1994). These children are usually RF-negative (Ferrari, Cash and Maddison, 1996). A subset of children, usually male, are HLA-B27-positive and often develop spondylitis (Leach, 1997).

Polyarticular onset (15−25%): arthritis affects more than five joints. Onset is usually gradual, affecting knees, ankles, wrists, elbows. The smaller joints of the hands and feet may be affected. Most cases are RF-negative, those cases that are RF-positive are similar to adult onset RA and may be titled juvenile-onset adult RA (Leach, 1997). This type is often ANA-positive.

In systemic arthritis (Still's disease, 10−20%) presentation is with systemic features, which may precede the arthritis. These may include:

- remitting fever (more than 39°C);
- adenopathy;
- hepatosplenomegaly;
- pericarditis;
- leucocytosis;
- anaemia (Leach, 1997).

There may be a rash, which coincides with the peaks of fever. The arthritis usually involves multiple joints. Negative RF and ANA are typical (Ferrari, Cash and Maddison, 1996).

Children with arthritis require a multidisciplinary team approach (Hackett *et al.*, 1996). The primary aim is the preservation of joint function and vision. The importance of JIA lies not in its frequency, but in the potential severity of its effects on children, and the misconceptions that surround its treatment (Southwood, 1993). Southwood states that despite their limitations, children with JIA should be able to continue their education in the mainstream schooling system, approximately one third of children will still have uncontrolled arthritis or physical disabilities into adulthood.

POLYMYALGIA RHEUMATICA

Polymyalgia rheumatica (PMR) is a syndrome of older patients characterized by pain and stiffness in the neck, shoulders and pelvic girdle persisting for at least one month (Healey, 1993). It is rare before the age of 50 and becomes more common with increasing age; the cause is unknown. Morning stiffness is very prominent. There are often systemic symptoms such as anorexia, malaise, depression, fever and weight loss. Occasionally there may be synovitis of the large joints. About 10–20% of patients go on to develop temporal (giant cell) arteritis (Bird, Le Gallez and Hill, 1985; Ferrari, Cash and Maddison, 1996). Presentations of temporal arteritis can include scalp pain, pain on chewing, loss of vision in one eye or even stroke (Edwards, 1991).

Diagnosis

There is no diagnostic test for PMR; the diagnosis is based on the clinical presentation. On physical examination there is little to be found other than tenderness and limited motion in the shoulders. Muscle strength is normal. X-rays are unrevealing. The erythrocyte sedimentation rate (ESR) may be very elevated and is an aid to the diagnosis. Other acute phase reactants such as C-reactive protein (CRP) and fibrinogen are also increased. RF and ANAs are not present (Healey, 1993).

The pain of PMR responds dramatically to steroids; patients should expect to be on therapy for at least a year (Ferrari, Cash and Maddison, 1996). The disease is usually self-limiting with a mean duration of two years; during this time patients may need to be on a maintenance dose of prednisolone. In those patients who develop symptoms of temporal arteritis the dose of prednisolone would be increased (Bird, Le Gallez and Hill, 1985).

- The clinical picture of PMR may drift towards RA.
- Here the synovitis is usually more prominent, the arthritis eventually erosive, and the response to low-dose steroids used for PMR usually insufficient (Ferrari, Cash and Maddison, 1996).

INFLAMMATORY ARTHRITIS ASSOCIATED WITH SPONDYLITIS

The sero-negative spondyloarthropathies are characterized by:

- absence of rheumatoid factor;
- a high frequency of HLA-B27 antigen positivity;
- iritis;
- spine and sacroiliac disease;
- a variable extent of peripheral arthritis.

Conditions included in this classification are:

- ankylosing spondylitis;
- psoriatic arthritis;
- reactive arthritis (including Reiter's syndrome);
- bowel associated arthritis (Ferrari, Cash and Maddison, 1996).

ANKYLOSING SPONDYLITIS

Ankylosing spondylitis (AS) is a chronic disorder characterized by inflammation and ensuing ankylosis of the sacroiliac joints and spinal articulations (Judd, 1997). Spondylitis implies inflammation of the spine and is usually used to mean a diffuse inflammation of ligamentous insertions. AS is more frequently seen in males than females, although an increasing number of females who do develop the disease are now recognized (Bird, Le Gallez and Hill, 1985; Judd, 1997).

Symptoms

AS is characterized by stiffness in the back; common sites are the thoracolumbar junction and low cervical region particularly in the early morning or after a period of inactivity. The onset is usually insidious. Stiffness is initially due to inflammation, which can lead to fibrous and eventually bony ankylosis. Spondylitis is associated with sacroiliitis in nearly all cases. Patients with AS generally find their pain improves with exercise and is worst when at rest.

An enthesopathy is responsible for many of the features of AS. It involves inflammation, fibrosis and ossification (reactive bone formation) at the enthesis (site of insertion of ligaments, tendons and joint capsules to the bone) (Ferrari, Cash and Maddison, 1996).

In the early stages of AS attention may be diverted from the back by complaints of aching or sharp pains in the heels, pelvis, buttocks, hips and shoulders. The back may remain silent until years after disease onset. A peripheral arthritis involving usually large joints may occur and the arthritis may precede or follow spine disease by years.

Assessment

Examination of the spine may reveal restriction of movement. Objective assessments and spinal measurements may be undertaken to confirm and monitor this by performing a Schober's test (this assessment has been shown to correlate well with radiological movement of the lumbar spine), tragus to wall test, lateral flexion measurements and chest expansion measurements (Bird, Le Gallez and Hill, 1985; Ferrari, Cash and Maddison, 1996). More recently developed assessments are now in common use, especially when deciding whether patients are eligible for anti-tumour necrosis factor (anti-TNF) therapy or not. These are divided into scales for metrology, disease activity, functional ability and global score. The metrology index incorporates measurements of cervical rotation, lumbar side flexion, lumbar flexion, tragus to wall distance and intermalleolar distance (BASMI Jenkinson *et al.*, 1994, BASDAI Garrett *et al.*, 1994, BASFI Calin *et al.*, 1994 and BAS-G Jones *et al.*, 1996).

Iritis occurs in 20–40% of cases and has little correlation with spine disease. Uveitis (inflammation of the iris, ciliary body and choroid of the eye) responds well to local steroid therapy. Prompt recognition and treatment is important; an ophthalmological opinion is therefore worthwhile (Bird, Le Gallez and Hill, 1985; Ferrari, Cash and Maddison, 1996; Judd, 1997).

Other complications that may occur for patients with AS include:

- lung fibrosis;
- aortitis with aortic valve regurgitation;
- psoriasis;
- inflammatory bowel disease.

Management

Treatment consists of anti-inflammatory medication for pain relief and exercises to maintain mobility. Management has been revolutionized by the introduction of intensive exercise programmes, with close involvement from a physiotherapist, the importance of which cannot be overemphasized.

Some AS patients may require disease-modifying treatments such as sulfasalazine or methotrexate as used in rheumatoid arthritis.

Anti-TNF therapy has been shown to be effective in AS (Van den Bosch *et al.*, 2002; Brandt *et al.*, 2003; Braun *et al.*, 2002). There are guidelines for its use that are similar to those for rheumatoid arthritis. That is they define the requirements for starting a patient on therapy and suggest criteria for assessing response to therapy and whether or not to continue it (Braun *et al.*, 2003).

REITER'S SYNDROME

Reiter's syndrome is a type of reactive arthritis in which certain classic extra-articular features are present. These are typically not seen in the other sero-negative spondylarthropathies. There are two variants of Reiter's syndrome. One is venereally acquired, the initial event being a urethritis, which is caused by *Chlamydia*. The other is acquired from food poisoning and starts with diarrhoea, the episode following infection with *Shigella flexneri*, *Salmonella* species, *Yersinia* species or *Campylobacter* species (Bird, Le Gallez and Hill, 1985; Ferrari, Cash and Maddison, 1996). Commonly the infectious process subsides before the onset of the arthritis. Approximately 50% of patients with Reiter's syndrome will be HLA-B27 antigen-positive (Bird, Le Gallez and Hill, 1985).

Symptoms

The classic triad of Reiter's syndrome refers to the presence of arthritis, urethritis and conjunctivitis, and is observed in 33% of patients (Cush and Lipsky, 1993), although the majority of cases do not have all three features (Ferrari, Cash and Maddison, 1996). The diagnosis of these individuals may be identified on the basis of an acute, additive, lower extremity oligoarthritis accompanied by one or more of the following extra-articular features: diarrhoea, urethritis, cervicitis, ocular inflammation, low back pain, enthesitis, keratoderma blennorrhagica or other mucocutaneous lesions (Cush and Lipsky, 1993).

The arthropathy of Reiter's syndrome is typically an acute, asymmetric, additive and ascending inflammatory oligoarthritis. At onset involvement of the first metatarsophalangeals, ankles, knees and toes is most common (Cush and Lipsky, 1993). This is a disease of young people, males being more commonly affected than females. Involvement of the digits is sometimes accompanied by the presence of dactylitis; inflammatory swelling of a whole digit, resulting in the so-called 'sausage digit'.

Management

The aims of management of Reiter's syndrome are:

* to maintain function
* to achieve optimum joint protection
* pain relief
* suppression of inflammation
* when appropriate, eradicate infection.

For the majority of patients the initial episode of arthritis is of between two and three months' duration, but may last up to a year. About 20–50% of patients demonstrate a chronic course of peripheral arthritis with the potential for progressive spondylitic changes (Cush and Lipsky, 1993).

PSORIATIC ARTHRITIS

Psoriatic arthritis (PsA) is an inflammatory erosive arthritis associated with psoriasis, a negative rheumatoid factor and the absence of rheumatoid nodules. Dactylitis, iritis, unilateral oedema and enthesopathy (particularly around the heel) may occur. The skin manifestations may precede or follow the arthritis by many years; when arthritis antedates the skin lesions the definitive diagnosis cannot be made and only becomes apparent with time. A family history of psoriasis should be sought. Familial aggregation suggests there is a genetic susceptibility to PsA. There is poor correlation between the severity of skin lesions and the arthritis. The sex ratio in PsA is close to unity.

Psoriasis is a papulosquamous, coarse scaling lesion. It may be localized (scalp, chest, periumbilicus, perianal, and extensor limb surfaces), and may have accompanying pustular lesions, diffuse erythroderma and generalized exfoliative dermatitis (Ferrari, Cash and Maddison, 1996).

Five clinical patterns of PsA have been recognized:

Group 1

Predominant involvement of the distal interphalangeal joints (DIP), almost always associated with psoriatic nail changes (nail pitting, onycholysis, subungual hyperkeratosis and transverse ridges − the presence of 20 pits in total suggests PsA, more than 60 being diagnostic).

Group 2

Arthritis mutilans. This is rare. Dissolution of the bones produces shortening of the digits with redundant folds of skin, the so called main-en-lorgnette deformity (opera-glass hands).

Group 3

Symmetric polyarthritis. This is similar to RA, but with a higher frequency of DIP involvement, association with psoriasis, persistent sero-negativity, associated sacroiliitis, and distinctive radiographic changes.

Group 4

Oligoarthritis. This affects large joints such as knee or hip, together with one or two DIP, PIP, MCP and MTP joints, and a dactylitic or 'sausage' digit or toe.

Group 5

Axial involvement. Both sacroiliitis and spondylitis can be associated with PsA. Spine symptoms are seldom the presenting complaint (Bennet, 1993; Helliwell and Wright, 1994).

Patients with PsA have to bear the burden of two chronic and currently incurable diseases and have a dual disability in terms of employment since certain industries have self-imposed limitations on patients with any form of skin disease (Helliwell and Wright, 1994). These patients require a multidisciplinary approach to give support in the emotional adjustment to the presence of arthritis and skin rash.

Methotrexate can be useful in the treatment of PsA as it is particularly effective in managing the skin disease as well. The use of systemic corticosteroids is avoided where possible as tapering can cause an exacerbation of the skin disease. Anti-tumour necrosis factor therapy has been shown to be effective for treating both the joints and the skin (Antoni et al., 2005; Brandt and Braun, 2006; Kavanaugh et al., 2006; Mease et al., 2005).

SEPTIC ARTHRITIS

Definition

Septic arthritis is defined as joint inflammation caused by the presence of live intra-articular micro-organisms and must be distinguished from reactive arthritis in which synovitis is triggered by a primary infection at a site distant from the joint (Hughes, 1996). Hughes states that septic arthritis arises as a result of infection with bacteria, viruses, fungi and, more rarely, other obscure micro-organisms such as protozoa.

Septic arthritis is uncommon but early diagnosis is vital to ensure that effective antimicrobial treatment may commence as delay may cause joint destruction.

Presentation

Characteristically septic arthritis has a monoarticular presentation. Typical onset would be acute, with an infected joint that is warm, painful and effused. Erythema — superficial redness of the skin — may be present. The affected joint will have a restricted range of movement. The patient may have a fever with chills from haematogenous bacterial entry into the joint.

Atypical onset also occurs, where infection may not be obvious in joints previously damaged by prior disease that are chronically painful and swollen. Patients undergoing treatment with immunosuppressive or corticosteroid therapy are more vulnerable and may show less evidence of inflammation than other patients (Schmid, 1993). Prosthetic joints are more susceptible to infection; in these joints pain that is dull, is present at night, and is described as deep and gnawing could indicate infection (Ross, 1990). The appearance of sinuses or fistula and tissue necrosis surrounding prosthetic joints also suggests joint infection (Hughes, 1996).

Atypical onset may be seen in children; for example, when sepsis of the hip is present it will be held immobile in flexion and abduction with little pain or swelling apparent.

Other conditions can mimic septic arthritis and should be excluded:

- crystal arthritis (gout, pseudogout);
- acute inflammatory arthritis or palindromic arthritis;
- post-traumatic arthritis;

- extra-articular inflammation (e.g. olecranon bursitis);
- haemarthrosis (an effusion of blood into a joint);
- rheumatic fever;
- oligoarticular syndromes associated with the spondylarthropathies or juvenile RA.

Routes of Infection

Hughes (1996) describes the five main routes by which infection of the joint in septic arthritis can occur:

- Haematogenous spread, for example, following septicaemia from wound infection, abscesses, mouth sepsis following dental procedures, recent respiratory or urogenital infection.
- Direct trauma, for example, penetrating trauma with a sharp object or during a traumatic injury.
- Diagnostic and therapeutic procedures to a joint, for example, joint aspiration/injection/surgical procedure for example, joint replacement.
- Osteomyelitis.
- Inflamed extra-articular structures, for example, inflamed bursae or tendon sheaths.

Micro-Organisms Responsible for Arthritis

Almost any micro-organism can cause infectious arthritis and the aetiology will vary according to the age of the patient and other concomitant diseases present, the route of spread of infection and the distribution of joints affected. The main micro-organisms causing bacterial septic arthritis are:

- Gram-positive cocci: *Staphylococcus aureus* (the most common cause in all ages and clinical situations), *Streptococcus pyogenes*, *Streptococcus pneumoniae*, viridans-group streptococci.
- Gram-negative cocci: *Haemophilus influenzae*, *Neisseria gonorrhea* and meningitidis.
- Gram-negative bacilli: *Escherichia coli*, *Salmonella* species, Pseudomonas, Coliforms, *Bacteroides fragilis*, *Brucella* species, Fusiform bacteria.
- Acid-fast bacilli: *Mycobacterium tuberculosis*, atypical mycobacteria.
- Spirochaetes: *Leptospira icterohaemorrhagica* (Hughes, 1996; Schmid, 1993).

Investigation and Diagnosis

The history obtained should include evidence of prior or current infection elsewhere in the body; exposure to recent antibiotic treatment could mask ongoing joint infection.

Where sepsis is suspected in a joint, aspiration carried out under aseptic technique is essential so that fluid analysis can be undertaken and the diagnosis confirmed. The presence of crystals should be excluded. A high neutrophil and total white cell count in the synovial fluid raises the probability of infection. Blood cultures should be taken. Swabs should be taken, if appropriate after examination, from the ears and throat especially of children. If gonococcal infection is a possibility in adults, genital, throat and anal swabs are required.

Treatment

Patients with a definitive diagnosis of septic arthritis should be admitted to hospital for intravenous antibiotics, even before an exact identification of the infecting micro-organism is made. When culture and sensitivity results are available treatment can be changed. The duration of intravenous antibiotics will vary and long-term oral antibiotics may be needed particularly for patients with prosthetic joints.

Non-steroidal anti-inflammatory drug (NSAID) therapy may not significantly affect septic arthritis. Corticosteroid injection is not recommended since it may significantly improve the symptoms of septic arthritis only to have joint destruction continue, and symptoms recur (Ferrari, Cash and Maddison, 1996).

Joint aspiration and surgical joint washout is sometimes performed. It may be necessary to surgically remove a prosthetic joint and all associated foreign material if a joint replacement is confirmed as being infected.

It is vital that, as soon as the patient's pain and infection are improved, mobilization and the involvement of the physiotherapist is commenced to begin mobilizing the joint and to prevent joint contractures.

REACTIVE ARTHRITIS

Reactive arthritis refers to the occurrence of an acute, non-suppurative, sterile, sero-negative inflammatory arthropathy that is thought to occur after exposure to an infectious agent. The infectious agent is thought to initiate an immunologic response in the body, initiating a train of incompletely understood events, which result in the development of synovitis at a distant site, without viable micro-organisms travelling to the joint – that is, the infection is not active within the joints (Ferrari, Cash and Maddison, 1996; Keat, 1995). There is an association with the antigen HLA-B27 in patients with reactive arthritis. Reactive arthritis is the commonest form of inflammatory arthritis in young men (Keat, 1995).

Reiter's syndrome, already discussed, is a common type of reactive arthritis in which certain classic extra-articular features are seen. Reactive arthritis is diagnosed in the absence of the classic findings of Reiter's syndrome, the absence of psoriasis and a clear history of antecedent infection (Ferrari, Cash and Maddison, 1996).

The onset of reactive arthritis may be insidious or acute, with associated fatigue, fever or weight loss. In a substantial number of cases, an identifiable infectious event 1–4 weeks beforehand precedes the onset of an asymmetric oligoarthritis involving the large joints. About 50% of patients present with synovitis and effusion in one or both knees (Keat, 1995). Other joints less commonly affected at onset are the metatarsophalangeals (MTPJs), ankle joints or symptoms resulting from extensor tendinitis or enthesopathy. The infectious process subsides before the onset of the arthritis. In some patients, an identifiable infectious trigger is not apparent. Extra-articular features may include inflammatory symptoms affecting the eye, mucosal surfaces and entheses. Although reactive arthritis is frequently self-limiting it does have the potential for chronicity and articular damage (Cush and Lipsky, 1993).

TRIGGERING FACTORS

Commonly associated and well documented with reactive arthritis are:

- gastrointestinal infections (salmonella, shigella, yersinia, campylobacter)
- genital tract infections (chlamydia).

Other infections less commonly reported are:
Bacterial:

- streptococcal (group A,G)
- *clostridium difficile*
- propionibacterium acne
- *staphylococcus aureus* (toxic shock arthritis).

Spirochetal:

- *borrelia burgdorferi* (lyme disease).

Viral:

- human immunodeficiency virus (HIV)
- parvovirus.

Mycobacterial:

- mycoplasma pneumoniae.

Parasitic:

- cryptosporidium (Cush and Lipsky, 1993; Keat, 1995).

Information obtained during the history taking which may assist the clinician in reaching a diagnosis of reactive arthritis may be a recent viral or gastrointestinal infection, recent overseas travel (this may be associated with gastrointestinal infection) or a new sexual partner within three months of onset of the arthritis (associated with genital tract infection).

Management

Some patients whose disease is minor and short-lived may require no more than an accurate diagnosis and observation. However, the majority of patients will require treatment with a NSAID. Treatment of the original infection, where possible, with antibiotics is believed by some to be important (Ferrari, Cash and Maddison, 1996) but is of unproven efficacy (Hughes, 1996).

Local steroid injections are useful if only one or two joints are affected and joint infection has been excluded. Steroid injection may also relieve painful enthesopathies.

Associated Urethritis or Cervicitis

Antibiotic therapy with tetracycline may be given; treatment is advisable for both patient and sex partner, however this may not influence either the duration of the arthritis or the likelihood of recurrence (Keat, 1995).

Associated bacterial diarrhoea is usually managed without antibiotics.

Those patients with progressive disabling arthritis may require treatment with a disease-modifying anti-rheumatic drug (DMARD) such as methotrexate or azathioprine.

OSTEOARTHRITIS

OA is the commonest form of arthritis and accounts for a major amount of disability in the community (Felson, 2000). OA is primarily a disease of articular cartilage and subchondral bone. Focal loss of articular cartilage in part of a synovial joint is accompanied by a hypertrophic reaction in the subchondral bone and margin of the joint. There is a variable, patchy synovitis, and fibrotic thickening of the joint capsule (Figure 1.3). Radiographic changes include joint space narrowing, subchondral sclerosis and cyst formation, and marginal osteophytosis. It is an extremely common condition, which is age-related, the peak age of onset being between 50 and 60 years. Common sites which are affected include the knees, hips, distal interphalangeal and thumb base joints of the hands and facet joints of the spine. In all joint sites except for the hips it is commoner in women than men. There are marked racial differences in its prevalence and distribution. Clinical manifestations are use-related joint pain, stiffness of joints after a period of inactivity and loss of range of joint movement. Although age-related it is not simply an inevitable consequence of ageing but a dynamic reaction pattern of a joint responding to insult or injury. It can occur without any obvious predisposition, or it can result from a previous injury or disease of a joint (secondary OA); hence there is great heterogeneity in the spectrum of disease covered by this term (Table 1.7). There is a lack of correlation between radiographic, pathologic and clinical manifestations and therefore attempts at strict definition have failed. The exact aetiology

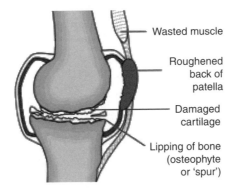

Wasted muscle

Roughened
back of
patella

Damaged
cartilage

Lipping of bone
(osteophyte
or 'spur')

Figure 1.3 An osteoarthritic knee joint. Reproduced by permission of The Arthritis Research Campaign.

Table 1.7 Classification of OA.

Classification by the joints involved

Monoarticular, oligoarticular or polyarticular (generalized)

Chief joint site and localization within the joint

    Hip (superior pole, medial pole, concentric)

    Knee (medial, lateral, patellofemoral compartments)

    Hand (IP joints and/or thumb base)

    Spine (facet joints or intervertebral disc disease)

    Others

Classification into primary and secondary forms of OA

Primary = idiopathic

Secondary = a likely cause can be identified

    Causes of secondary OA:

    1. Metabolic

    – for example, Ochronosis, Acromegaly, Haemachromatosis, Calcium crystal deposition

    2. Anatomic

    – for example, slipped femoral epiphysis, Epiphyseal dysplasias, Perthe's disease, congenital dislocation of the hip, leg length inequality, hypermobility syndromes

    3. Traumatic

    – for example, major joint trauma, fracture through a joint, joint surgery (e.g. meniscectomy), chronic injury (occupational arthropathies)

    4. Inflammatory

    – for example, any inflammatory arthropathy, septic arthritis

Classification by the presence of specific features

Inflammatory OA

Erosive OA

Atrophic or destructive OA

OA with chondrocalcinosis

Others

and pathogenesis are unknown, but are thought to involve a complex interaction of intrinsic abnormalities in connective tissue integrity and extrinsic physical insults to joints. OA is currently viewed as a heterogeneous disease process rather than a disease entity.

FIBROMYALGIA SYNDROME

This is a common but often overlooked condition. It occurs predominantly in women and is associated with marked disability and handicap.

Diagnosis

It presents with a variable symptom complex of widespread musculoskeletal pain (in all four quadrants), severe fatigue and multisystem 'functional' disturbance. Diagnosis is based on typical symptoms, the presence of multiple tender trigger sites (11 out of 18) and the exclusion of any inflammatory or endocrine disease. There is no specific treatment and the prognosis is often poor. Nevertheless, some patients may be helped by an explanation of the condition, limited tricyclic treatment, an increase in aerobic exercise and various coping strategies that shift the 'control' back to the patient. Medicine has a bias towards a pathological explanation of disease and fibromyalgia has often been considered an expression of psychological disturbance. The symptoms and disability, however, are real, not fabricated or imagined, and reflect 'functional' rather than 'pathological' abnormality. Figure 1.4 attempts to show a possible mechanism of induction and perpetuation of fibromyalgia syndrome. Fibromyalgia may be superimposed upon pre-existing painful conditions such as OA or cancer, although it is usually

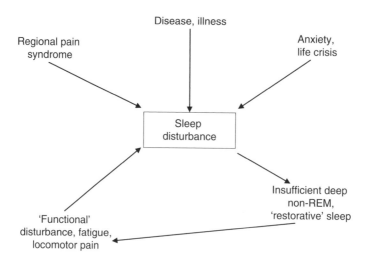

Figure 1.4 A possible mechanism of induction and perpetuation of fibromyalgia syndrome.

primary in nature. There is overlap in symptoms and impaired function between fibromyalgia, anxiety and depression, and fibromyalgia patients score highly on anxiety and depression questionnaires. Evidence for triggering viral infections in the vast majority of patients is lacking. Most patients are women, often in their forties and fifties; the condition is rare in children. Pain and fatigue are often associated with severe disability. Patients may not be able to cope with their jobs or household activities.

Symptoms

The pain is predominantly axial and diffuse but may affect any region and at times be felt 'all over'. Characteristically the pain is not relieved by analgesics or NSAIDs. There is often a poor sleep pattern, with patients waking unrefreshed and feeling more tired in the morning than later in the day. It is important to take a full history and examination but clinical findings are usually unremarkable with no objective weakness, synovitis or neurological abnormality. The important and sometimes the only positive examination finding is the presence of multiple hyperalgesic tender sites (Figure 1.5). These sites are tender to pressure in the normal individual but in fibromyalgia patients similar pressure elicits marked tenderness and a wince/withdrawal response. Tender sites should be found axially, in upper and lower limbs and on both sides — i.e. widespread and symmetrical. In addition hyperalgesia should be absent at control sites such as the forehead, distal forearm and fibular head.

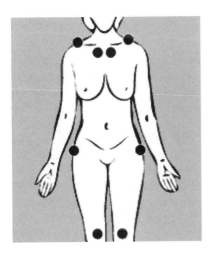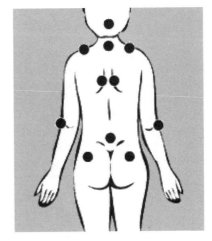

Figure 1.5 Common hyperalgesic tender sites. Reproduced by permission of The Arthritis Research Campaign.

Management

Aspects of management include:

- patient and family education about the condition;
- trial of tricyclics;
- cessation of other ineffective drugs;
- graded aerobic exercise regime;
- coping strategies — for example, yoga.

The prognosis is poor with less than 1 in 10 patients in a study in Nottingham losing their symptoms over a 5-year period. With suitable advice patients, although not 'cured', can learn to live better with their condition and more importantly avoid further unnecessary investigations and drug treatments (Doherty, 1993).

CONNECTIVE TISSUE DISEASE

The connective tissue diseases are a group of multisystem diseases frequently characterized by pathologic changes in blood vessels and connective tissues. These diseases often have overlapping clinical features and share immunologic abnormalities; these include:

- general systemic features (malaise, weight loss, fever);
- musculoskeletal involvement varying from inflammatory polyarthritis to generalized arthralgia and myalgia;
- immune aberration leading to immune-mediated inflammation as an underlying pathogenic mechanism (Kimberly and Urowitz, 1994).

SYSTEMIC LUPUS ERYTHEMATOSUS

SLE is an inflammatory, multisystem disease of unknown aetiology with diverse clinical and laboratory manifestations and a variable course and prognosis. Immunologic aberrations give rise to excessive autoantibody production, some of which cause cytotoxic damage, while others participate in immune complex formation resulting in immune inflammation.

Clinical manifestations may be constitutional or result from inflammation in various organ systems including skin and mucous membranes, joints, kidney, brain, serous membranes, lung, heart and occasionally gastrointestinal tract. Organ systems may be involved individually or in any combination. Involvement of vital organs (particularly kidneys and central nervous system) accounts for significant morbidity and mortality. Morbidity and mortality result from tissue damage due to the disease process or its therapy. SLE is recognized worldwide; its prevalence varies in different geographic areas. It is more prevalent in women, particularly in their reproductive years. In the United States it has been noted that SLE is three times more common among Blacks than Whites.

Symptoms

Clinical features of the disease include:

- General constitutional complaints (weight loss, fever, malaise, overwhelming fatigue);
- Skin manifestations (lupus-specific or lupus-nonspecific):
  - Lupus-specific lesions:
    (1) Acute (malar rash, generalized erythema, bullous LE).
    (2) Subacute.
    (3) Chronic lupus changes (localized discoid, generalized discoid, lupus profundus).
    (4) Photosensitivity (over 50% of patients).
    (5) Alopecia (patchy or diffuse).
  - Mucous membrane lesions (ulcers of the mouth or vagina or nasal septal erosions).
    (1) musculoskeletal features (arthralgias and/or arthritis), often the presenting manifestation. The acute arthritis typically involves the small joints of the hands, wrists and knees. Most cases are symmetrical. Nodules are found in 10% of cases. Unlike RA the arthritis of SLE is typically not erosive or destructive of bone. However, clinical deforming arthritis does occur and may take a number of different forms; there may be mild synovial thickening about PIP joints or over tendon sheaths, ulnar deviation of the fingers and subluxations and contractures. Patients with SLE may complain of muscle pain and weakness. This may be due to arthritis, be drug-induced (corticosteroids, antimalarials) or due to true muscle inflammation (polymyositis).
- Renal disease (urinalysis and serum creatinine assessments must be made regularly). A renal biopsy may be needed to assess the lupus nephritis accurately.
- Neuropsychiatric manifestations (patients often present with a mixture of neurologic and psychiatric manifestations).
- Neurologic manifestations (seizures, headache, transverse myelitis, cranial or peripheral neuropathy).
- Psychiatric manifestations (psychosis, psychoneurosis and neurocognitive dysfunction).
- Serositis (pleurisy, pericarditis, peritonitis).
- Pulmonary involvement (lupus pleuritis, lupus pneumonitis, pulmonary haemorrhage, pulmonary embolism, pulmonary hypertension).
- Cardiac involvement (pericarditis, myocarditis, endocarditis, coronary artery disease).
- Gastrointestinal involvement (oesophageal disease, mesenteric vasculitis, inflammatory bowel disease, pancreatitis, liver disease).

- Haematologic abnormalities (anaemia, leucopenia or lymphopenia and thrombo-cytopenia). The most significant anaemia is the autoimmune haemolytic anaemia due to autoantibodies directed against red blood cell antigens. The lupus antico-agulant is the commonest haemostatic abnormality. The serology of lupus shows evidence for complement consumption by immune complexes. Antibodies seen in SLE include ANA, anti-smooth muscle, anti-Ro, anti-La and antibodies to double-stranded DNA (dsDNA).

There is a greater incidence of spontaneous abortion, prematurity and interuterine death, although SLE does not interfere with conception. Survival rates of SLE have improved over the last four decades from less than 50% at 5 years in 1955 to over 90% survival at 5 years in 1990. Reasons for this improvement include earlier diagnosis, better therapeutic modalities, improved antibiotics and antihypertensive drugs and the availability of renal dialysis and transplantation (Gladman and Urowitz, 1994).

SCLERODERMA (SYSTEMIC SCLEROSIS)

This is a generalized disorder of connective tissue affecting skin and internal organs. It is characterized by fibrotic arteriosclerosis of peripheral and visceral vasculature. Variable degrees of extracellular matrix accumulation occur (mainly collagen), both in skin and viscera. It is associated with specific autoantibodies, most notably anticentromere and Scl-70.

Clinical Features

- Raynaud's phenomenon;
- tightening and thickening of skin (scleroderma);
- involvement of internal organs, including gastrointestinal tract, lungs, heart and kidneys, accounts for increased morbidity and mortality;
- risk of internal organ involvement strongly linked to extent and progression of skin thickening.

The first convincing description of scleroderma was of a 17-year-old woman in Naples in 1753 (Rodnan and Benedek, 1962). The relationship of scleroderma to Raynaud's phenomenon was first described by Maurice Raynaud himself in 1865. In 1945 Goetz proposed the term *progressive systemic sclerosis* based on his detailed review of the visceral lesions (Goetz, 1945). The aetiology and pathogenesis remain unknown and no effective therapies for the basic disorder have been developed. Breakthroughs in treatment of specific clinical features have derived from agents developed for other purposes and include angiotensin-converting enzyme (ACE) inhibitors for the hypertension associated with renal involvement and histamine-2 (H2) receptor antagonists for chronic acid reflux.

Epidemiology

Studies based on hospital records and death registries suggest occurrence in between 4 and 12 individuals per million of population per year. It is likely that many cases of systemic sclerosis are unrecognized, particularly in limited disease. Onset is highest in the fourth and fifth decade of life and is three to four times more common in women than men (Medsger and Masi, 1971). Disease is not linked to race, season, geography, occupation or socioeconomic status. Environmental aetiologies are possible and include silica dust, silicone surgical implants and epoxy resins as implicated vectors. Familial occurrence is quite rare and convincing genetic associations are lacking.

Clinical Features

Systemic sclerosis is a remarkably heterogeneous disorder with diverse initial presentations and variable disease course. Periodic waxing and waning of symptoms is unusual (unlike RA or SLE).

Vascular Abnormalities

Raynaud's Phenomenon

This is defined as episodic colour changes (pallor, cyanosis, erythema) occurring in response to environmental cold and/or emotional stress. Although most typically noted in the fingers, the circulation of the toes, ears, nose and tongue is also frequently affected. Subjects complain of symptoms of numbness and pain associated with the phases of pallor and cyanosis and of tingling and burning during the hyperaemic recovery phase. The impact on hand function in cold environments can be substantial. Raynaud's phenomenon is the initial complaint in around three quarters of patients with systemic sclerosis. The potential importance of Raynaud's phenomenon in systemic sclerosis cannot be understated. Taken alone it has considerable clinical impact; however, abnormalities similar to those of the peripheral circulation are widely distributed in the visceral vasculature as well and have major effects on morbidity and mortality. In systemic sclerosis structural narrowing of the digital arteries causes severe (>75%) attenuation of the arterial lumen. The principal lesion is one of intimal hyperplasia consisting of collagen. Lesser degrees of fibrosis are noted in the adventitia but the media (smooth muscle) is little affected. Normal peripheral vasoconstriction in response to cold superimposed on the narrowed vessel would cause occlusion of the lumen. Similarly, treatment of Raynaud's phenomenon with smooth muscle relaxants is less likely to work in the presence of a fixed obstructive lesion. The hallmark of severity of Raynaud's phenomenon in systemic sclerosis is the frequency of digital ischaemic injury. Around one third of patients experience at least one digital ulceration per year, and patients are at risk of catastrophic peripheral digital gangrene. Modern clinical studies suggest that the internal organs (heart, lungs) sustain Raynaud-like intermittent ischaemia during cold exposure.

Microvascular Abnormalities

There are characteristic architectural abnormalities of the microvasculature in systemic sclerosis, which are easily appreciated by widefield microscopy of the nailfold capillary bed (Maricq, 1981). These changes include enlargement and tortuosity of individual capillary loops interspersed with areas of capillary loop dropout. At later stages of clinical disease, punctate telangiectasias develop with typical locations including fingers, face, lips and oral mucosa.

Skin Involvement

The early tissue lesion features ingress of immigrant inflammatory cell populations. The net effect of this array of cells and signals is an accumulation of extracellular matrix including collagen glycosaminoglycan, fibronectin, adherence molecules and tissue water. The patient and clinician recognize the result as the tightened and thickened skin (scleroderma), which is the hallmark of disease.

Oedematous Change

An intrinsic feature of early systemic sclerosis is the painless swelling of the fingers and hands. Symptoms include early morning stiffness and arthralgia. Carpal tunnel syndrome is a frequent occurrence. Pitting oedema of the fingers and dorsum of the hand is present on examination.

Scleroderma

Scleroderma skin thickening begins on the fingers and hands in virtually all cases. The skin initially appears shiny and taut and may be erythematous. Pruritus is common and may be intense. Digital skin creases are obscured and hair growth is reduced. The skin of the face and neck is usually involved next. Facial scleroderma causes an immobile and pinched facies. The lips become thin and pursed. Local skin thickening limits the ability to fully open the mouth impairing effective dental hygiene. Skin thickening may stay limited to hands and face; in some patients there is rapid spread to the upper arms, shoulders, chest, back, abdomen and legs. Prominent localized areas of hyperpigmentation and hypopigmentation may develop.

Skin Thickening and Disease Classification

The diagnosis of systemic sclerosis is clinically obvious once skin thickening has developed. Accurate and early classification is the paramount clinical issue because the relative risk of accruing new internal organ involvement closely parallels the pace, progression and extent of skin involvement (Table 1.8).

Table 1.8 Classification of systemic sclerosis.

1. Diffuse scleroderma − skin thickening present on the trunk in addition to the face, proximal and distal extremities.
2. Limited scleroderma − skin thickening restricted to sites distal to the elbow and knee, but also involving the face and neck Synonym − CREST syndrome (calcinosis, Raynaud's, esophageal dysmotility, sclerodactyly, telangiectasias).
3. Sine scleroderma − no clinically apparent skin thickening but with characteristic internal organ changes, vascular and serologic features.
4. In overlap − criteria fulfilling systemic sclerosis occurring concomitantly with criteria fulfilling diagnoses of SLE, RA or inflammatory muscle disease.
5. Undifferentiated connective tissue disease − Raynaud's phenomenon with clinical and/or laboratory features of systemic sclerosis.

Skin, Visceral Involvement and Disease Outcome

Skin involvement alone is symptomatic and by virtue of local tethering contributes to loss of motion, impaired hand function, cosmetic problems and lessened sense of well-being (McClosky, Patella and Seibold, 1990). The importance of skin involvement stems from its linkage with visceral changes.

Systemic Features

General Manifestations

Fever is uncommon; its presence should prompt a search for infection. Weight loss is universal even in the absence of gastrointestinal involvement. Profound fatigue occurs frequently and is often a limiting factor in daily activities. Both the unrelenting persistence of symptoms and concern over the cosmetic impact of the disease lead to frequent reactive depression. Systemic sclerosis is uncommon; many patients have not heard of the disease prior to their diagnosis.

Gastrointestinal Involvement

This is the third most common feature following Raynaud's phenomenon and scleroderma. Incompetence of the lower oesophageal sphincter is suggested by symptoms of heartburn and associated bitter regurgitation. Impaired contractility of the smooth muscle of the oesophagus presents as dysphagia and odynophagia for solid foods. Complaints of a 'sticking' sensation are typical. Small intestine involvement is a major source of morbidity. Symptoms include intermittent bloating with abdominal cramps, intermittent or chronic diarrhoea and presentations of intestinal obstruction. Malabsorption can be shown by an increased quantitative faecal fat elimination. Bacterial overgrowth in areas of intestinal stasis is well documented.

Musculoskeletal Features

The majority of patients experience arthralgia and morning stiffness. Overt arthritis is uncommon; erosive arthropathy is demonstrable on radiograph in 20–30% of patients (Blocka *et al.*, 1981). Inflammatory and fibrinous involvement of tendon sheaths may mimic arthritis. Muscle weakness occurs both from disuse atrophy and from a disease-related myopathy. Resorption of bone of the digital tufts occurs in long-standing disease. Subcutaneous calcinosis can occur; common locations include the fingers, preolecranon area, olecranon and prepatellar bursae. These areas become intermittently inflamed and a source of discomfort. Spontaneous extrusion through the skin is a frequent occurrence and a source of local infection.

Pulmonary Involvement

Pulmonary involvement is the leading cause of mortality and morbidity in later stages of systemic sclerosis. Any combination of vascular obliteration, fibrosis and inflammation may be present. Clinical presentations are insidious and include exertional dyspnoea, diminished exercise tolerance and nonproductive cough. Pulmonary function testing is the mainstay of clinical diagnosis and serial assessment.

Myocardial Involvement

Patchy fibrosis of the myocardium is present at autopsy in as many as 81% of patients with systemic sclerosis. Myocardial involvement is a principal determinant of survival. Many patients complain of diminished exercise tolerance, palpitations and dyspnoea and therefore separating myocardial from pulmonary involvement in clinical assessment is difficult.

Renal Involvement

The syndrome of 'scleroderma renal crisis' is due to the sudden onset of accelerated hypertension, rapidly progressive renal insufficiency, microangiopathic haemolysis and consumptive thrombocytopenia in the presence of hyperreninaemia.

Pregnancy

Menstrual irregularities and amenorrhoea occur in relation to the severity of illness. Difficulty with conception is frequent. Pregnancy is not associated with worsening of scleroderma.

Immunologic Features

Systemic sclerosis occurs in overlap with other connective tissue disorders including SLE, polymyositis, RA and Sjögren's syndrome. Antinuclear antibodies are present in the sera of over 90% of patients with systemic sclerosis.

INFLAMMATORY MUSCLE DISEASE (POLYMYOSITIS)

Definition

- A member of the connective tissue disease family (autoimmune disease associations, other immunologic features).
- Characterized by chronic inflammation of striated muscle (polymyositis) and sometimes the skin (dermatomyositis).
- Autoantibody associations define clinical subsets of the disease.

Signs and Symptoms

- Painless proximal muscle weakness with or without rash
- Elevation of serum muscle enzymes (creatine kinase)
- Other organ systems affected (joints, lungs, heart, gastrointestinal tract)
- Probable association with malignancy (elderly).

Epidemiology

Classification of these diseases is being refined as new insights into aetiology and pathogenesis emerge. These disorders are recognized as part of a single disease spectrum. Certain features are used to separate subsets:

- childhood versus adult onset
- polymyositis versus dermatomyositis
- presence or absence of other connective tissue diseases or malignancy.

In the future it is likely that disease subsets will be identified according to serum autoantibodies and/or other immunologic characteristics.

Incidence

The annual incidence of polymyositis/dermatomyositis ranges from 2−10 new cases per million persons at risk in various populations. Published rates are likely to be underestimates as not all possible sources of ascertainment are examined.

Inflammatory myopathy can occur at any age but the observed pattern of incidence includes childhood and adult peaks. The incidence sex ratio is 2.5:1 female to male. This ratio is 1:1 in childhood disease and associated malignancy but 10:1 when there is an associated connective tissue disease. Polymyositis/dermatomyositis has a 3-4:1 Black to White incidence ratio.

Environmental Factors

- No striking associations with environmental factors.
- Onset more frequent in winter and spring months (precipitation by viral and bacterial infections).
- D-penicillamine (drug-induced myositis).

Genetic Factors

At least in some families there seems to be a genetic predisposition. It is not uncommon to find close relatives suffer from other autoimmune diseases (Walker *et al.*, 1982). The reported associations of certain HLA types with clinical subsets of disease are weak.

Presentations

- Insidious, progressive, painless proximal muscle weakness over three to six months.
- Acute onset muscle pain and weakness developing over several weeks (associated with fever and fatigue).
- Proximal myalgias only.
- Slowly evolving weakness over 5−10 years (inclusion body myositis).

Clinical Features

- Constitutional

Fatigue, fever and weight loss.

- Skeletal muscle

Patients complain of difficulty performing activities of daily living requiring normal muscle strength. Walking may become clumsy with a 'waddling' gait. Bulbar weakness results in hoarseness or dysphonia, difficulty in initiating swallowing with regurgitation of liquids and episodic coughing immediately after swallowing. Physical examination is necessary to confirm weakness of individual muscles or groups of muscles. The distribution of weakness is usually symmetric, affecting all proximal muscles. Distal muscles are only weak in 10−20% of cases. Ocular and facial muscles are rarely involved. Swelling of muscle is usual. Firmness to touch and incomplete passive stretching suggest fibrous replacement of muscle and contractures respectively.

- Skin

Dermatomyositis.

- Erythematous or violaceous
- Scaling
- Oedema
- Cuticular hypertrophy and haemorrhage, periungual erythema and telangiectasia
- Ulceration

Polymyositis/dermatomyositis.

- Panniculitis
- Cutaneous mucinosis
- Vitiligo
- Multifocal lipoatrophy.

Other Features

- Joints
  Polyarthralgias and/or polyarthritis which are rheumatoid-like in distribution. Wrists, knees and small joints of the hands most frequently affected. Arthritis tends to occur early in the disease and is mild and transient.
- Calcinosis
  Can be a late problem in polymyositis/dermatomyositis. Intracutaneous, subcutaneous and fascial sites are affected, as well as the connective tissue surrounding muscle bundles.
- Respiratory
  Dyspnoea on exertion may be due to respiratory muscle (diaphragm, intercostal) weakness. It may be due to congestive heart failure or cardiac arrythmia from myocardial or conduction system involvement. Intrinsic causes of dyspnoea include interstitial alveolitis or fibrosis, aspiration pneumonia (from pharyngeal dysmotility), bacterial infection and methotrexate pulmonary toxicity (Dickey and Myers, 1984). Cough is frequent. There are three common presentations of lung disease:

  (a) aggressive form of diffuse alveolitis (myositis often overlooked);
  (b) slowly progressive lung disease (disability from myopathy may mask severity of lung disease);
  (c) asymptomatic but with radiographic and/or physiologic manifestations of interstitial lung disease.

- Cardiac involvement
  Common but seldom symptomatic until it is very advanced. The most frequent abnormality is a rhythm disturbance. Less common is congestive heart failure due to myocarditis or fibrous replacement of the myocardium.
- Gastrointestinal tract
  Pharyngeal dysphagia can occur. Involvement of the smooth muscle of the intestinal tract is uncommon unless there is overlap with systemic sclerosis. Lower oesophageal dysphagia results in the sensation of food 'sticking' in the retrosternal area during the act of swallowing. A weak lower oesophageal sphincter leads to reflux of gastric acid causing heartburn. Chronic distal oesophagitis predisposes to stricture formation. Constipation is the most common symptom of colonic hypomotility.
- Peripheral vasculature
  Raynaud's phenomenon is a frequent accompanying complaint.

- Association with malignancy
  The relationship between myositis and malignancy is controversial. Cancer in myositis patients is most frequently obvious rather than occult.

Investigations

- General
  Low-grade anaemia is present in polymyositis (anaemia of chronic disease). ESR may be mildly elevated.
- Musculoskeletal

  (a) Enzymes from injured skeletal muscle
      Creatine kinase, aldolase, the transaminases (ALT and AST) and lactate dehydrogenase
  (b) Electromyogram (EMG)
      A sensitive but nonspecific method of evaluating inflammatory myopathy. Typical findings include irritability of myofibrils on needle insertion and at rest and short duration, low amplitude, complex potentials on contraction. The EMG is a useful method for following disease activity.
  (c) Biopsy
      Muscle biopsy should be performed in all cases to confirm the diagnosis of inflammatory myopathy. The presence of chronic inflammatory cells in the perivascular and interstitial areas surrounding myofibrils is pathognomonic. More common than inflammation are degeneration and necrosis of myofibrils, phagocytosis of necrotic cells and myofibril regeneration. In long-standing myositis, fibrous connective tissue replaces necrotic myofibres and separates bundles of myofibres.

- Lung
  Reduced respiratory muscle strength is determined by measuring inspiratory pressures at the mouth. The chest radiograph in interstitial lung disease shows bilateral basilar thickening. Thin section computerized axial tomography reveals evidence of interstitial fibrosis. Ventilation-perfusion studies are abnormal and pulmonary function tests show a restrictive physiologic pattern with reduced forced vital capacity.
- Heart
  The most common alterations are conduction defects and atrial and ventricular dysrhythmias, which are due to involvement of working myocardium and/or the conducting system.
- Intestine
  Barium studies are used to demonstrate pharyngeal dysphagia, delayed gastric emptying and small bowel dilatation and hypomotility.
- Serum autoantibodies
  In polymyositis/dermatomyositis, more than 80% of patients have autoantibodies to nuclear and/or cytoplasmic antigens (ANA, ANCA). About 50% of patients have

myositis-specific antibodies. Myositis-specific antibodies may be important in the pathogenesis of the inflammatory myopathies (association with subsets, selective response against antigens, variation of antibody titre with disease activity).

Natural History

The majority of patients have multiple exacerbations and remissions or persistent disease activity. With each episode of myositis there is the potential for absolute loss of muscle mass.

Prognosis

Assessment of prognosis is difficult as the disease is relatively rare, a classification system based on meaningful pathophysiologic and serologic data has not been developed and objective criteria for improvement (or deterioration) are not standardized.

Survival

Since the availability of corticosteroids there has been improved survival, although there have been no double blind placebo-controlled studies. Currently the expected survival in incident cases of polymyositis/dermatomyositis is over 90% at five years after initial diagnosis. Factors associated with poor survival include:

- older age
- malignancy
- delayed initiation of corticosteroid therapy
- pharyngeal dysphagia with aspiration pneumonia
- myocardial involvement
- complications of corticosteroid/immunosuppressive drugs.

Disability

Each major exacerbation results in a reduction in muscle strength, but therapy almost never returns the patient to the preceding level of total body muscle mass or strength. Fortunately a minor amount of atrophy and weakness in one or more muscle groups most often does not translate into functional impairment.

1.7 THE IMPACT OF RHEUMATOLOGICAL CONDITIONS ON PHYSICAL, PSYCHOLOGICAL, SOCIAL AND OCCUPATIONAL FUNCTION

Over 200 conditions affecting joints, bones, soft tissues and muscles are covered by the term arthritis, often referred to as 'rheumatic disease' or 'musculoskeletal disease' (Symmons and Bankhead, 1994). Arthritis is the biggest cause of physical disability in the United Kingdom (Martin, Meltzer and Elliot, 1988).

The two main types of arthritis in terms of diagnosis are:

- non-inflammatory − for example, OA
- inflammatory − for example, RA.

RA is characterized by progressive disability over time. Using the Stanford Health Assessment Questionnaire (HAQ) it has been clearly demonstrated that functional status deteriorates over time (Doyle, 1996). Research has shown that disability occurs early in the course of the disease (Wolfe and Cathey, 1991; Wolfe, Hawley and Cathey, 1991).

The impact and personal costs of rheumatological conditions on the individual and their family − in terms of pain, loss of physical movement, loss of independence, self-esteem, employment, education, disruption to relationships, reduced quality of family and social life − is incalculable (Ashcroft, 1997).

The current aim of medical care, in the absence of a cure, is a reduction in the impact of RA. Although some accept that there is a need to consider and take into account the impact of the disease on the individual's social functioning (Long and Scott, 1994), health professionals tend to work within the medical model of disability and aim to establish 'what works on whom, and why' (Ashcroft, 1996). However, the impact of a chronic rheumatological condition on the quality of life for both individuals and their families should not be ignored. Carr (1996) states that quality of life measures are required to identify and assess the disabling consequences of RA and the effectiveness of medical attempts to prevent or postpone them.

The International Classification of Functioning, Disability and Health (WHO, 2001), known more commonly as ICF, has moved away from being a 'consequences of disease classification' (1980 version) to become a 'components of health classification' and provides a standard language and framework for the description of health and health-related states. The ICF is WHO's framework for health and disability. In ICF disability and functioning are viewed as outcomes of interactions between health conditions (diseases, disorders and injuries) and contextual factors, among which are external environmental factors and internal personal factors that influence how disability is experienced by the individual. Measurement tools to assess impairment and disability are well established in the field of rheumatology; quality of life measurement tools to assess the consequences suffered by an individual as a result of a disease or handicap are not.

Carr (1996) tells us that 'handicap is the social consequence of disease, is specific to individuals and depends not only on the severity of the disease, but also on his or her life role'. She goes on to say that 'the degree to which an individual is handicapped depends on the perception of the importance of the role that can no longer be filled'. Discrepancies between the views of society (employers, healthcare professionals) and individuals with regard to handicaps can be considerable.

PERSONAL IMPACT OF ARTHRITIS

It must be remembered that RA affects the patient's body as a whole, not just the articular system, and invariably has an impact on every aspect of the patient's physical and psychosocial life (Gordon and Hastings, 1994).

The impact of a rheumatological condition can be felt even before a diagnosis has been made when, due to pain and stiffness in the joints, performing everyday activities of daily living such as washing, dressing and cooking are both painful and difficult.

From a patient's perspective Ashcroft (1996) describes how 'an early diagnosis brings with it a never ending stream of appointments with consultants, doctors, occupational therapists, physiotherapists, blood tests, X-rays, trips to the general practitioner (GP) and chemist etc. This, coupled with the extreme fatigue that accompanies RA, leads to your entire life being absorbed within the medical world.' She goes on to describe how this 'represents the insidious nature of RA, sucking you very quickly into an "illness mode" – the medical model of disability, and like most things held in by suction, it is very difficult, if not impossible to get back out'.

It is vital that health professionals ensure adequate information is given to every patient either newly diagnosed or who have established disease to enable them to understand what type of arthritis they have, its course and how it may progress and how they can learn to manage their condition themselves.

Diagnosis can bring about many emotions – denial, relief or disbelief to name but a few.

It might be assumed that anxiety and depression would correlate with continuing disease activity, but it appears that socioeconomic factors may be greater determinants of depression than physical factors (Hawley and Wolfe, 1988; McFarlane and Brooks, 1988).

The impact of the diagnosis will affect not only the individual but family and friends also, and being diagnosed with arthritis at various age groups will have different implications (Ashcroft, 1997).

The Young Child

Children may become withdrawn, isolated and depressed if they are not able to join their friends in normal childhood school, playground and recreational activities. Schooling may be disrupted. Friction may develop with other siblings if they perceive more attention is given to the 'disabled' child by parents.

Teenagers

Although nearing independence they may require assistance due to physical limitations and may need help with personal care, which is difficult to come to terms with both for parent and child. The attainment of independence, physical maturity, social and sexual identity may all be delayed. Depression and anxiety may become problems. Parents can then become overprotective.

Young Adults

May no longer be able to pursue their chosen career ambition.

Middle Aged Adults

Can curtail a successful career or prompt an unwanted change of direction. A reduction of income may result. Taking time off work may be necessary and can affect relationships with workmates.

For any age group the impact on long-term relationships can be the greatest. Ashcroft (1997) explains 'the spontaneity of a hug can cause excruciating pain and the reaction to being the cause of that pain is often guilt'. Tensions can easily develop within a relationship.

The fluctuating nature of arthritis can be a contributory factor to stress within the family and workplace as people find it difficult to understand the ability to do a thing one day and not the next.

FINANCIAL IMPACT OF ARTHRITIS

To the individual person and their family, living with arthritis can be expensive. Extra expenses incurred can include:

- additional heating and hot water;
- personal assistance and care;
- domestic help;
- household and garden maintenance;
- home adaptations;
- specialist equipment – lever taps, lever door handles, electric tin openers, bottle and jar openers, aids to assist with washing and dressing, aids to assist with preparing and cooking food;
- mobility – taxi or bus fares, car adaptations – power-assisted steering, automatic transmission, electric windows, central locking, hand brake adaption;
- prescription and non-prescription medicines.

IMPACT ON EDUCATION

Two important principles are at stake in the education of a child with arthritis (Southwood, 1993):

- The child should be made to feel as independent and normal as possible.
- Keeping the child in mainstream schooling is crucial.

The child with arthritis may have a decreased attention span, irritability, increased sleepiness and altered mood secondary to the disease itself or its treatment (Southwood, 1993).

It should be possible for children who need to spend time in hospital or at home to continue their education. Liaison between parents, school and hospital teachers and individual tutors is important to ensure a work plan is formulated. Minimal disruption is desirable to ensure career choices are not prejudiced at a later date.

Children with arthritis may have pain and stiffness in their hands, which may cause slowness and difficulty in writing. They should be allowed extra time to complete work and consideration for the use of a word processor, electric typewriter or tape recorder may be useful.

Mobility and movement in general may be a problem and extra time should be allocated, if necessary, for carrying books from one classroom to another.

It may not be possible to fully participate in physical education lessons but close liaison with a physiotherapist who can suggest appropriate exercises is useful. Swimming is excellent provided the pool is not too cold. Contact sports, which may cause direct injury to a joint, are not usually advisable; non-contact sports are preferred.

A patient's educational background and occupation may affect management and outcome. Notwithstanding genetic and sex factors, patients with more years of education seem to develop less severe disease (Leigh and Fries, 1991).

Hilliquin and Menkes (1994) describe how relationships between education and outcome in RA are not well understood. They go on to explain how low formal education appears to be a marker identifying behavioural risk factors that may be associated with a poor outcome in RA. These factors include the patient's sense of self-efficacy, problem-solving capacity, sense of personal responsibility and capacity to cope with life stress. Patients with less schooling may not know where to turn for help, may seek medical care less promptly and report to physicians later in the course of the disease. Compliance with treatments could also be reduced.

IMPACT ON EMPLOYMENT

Employment is known to be of benefit to health psychologically as it provides a source of identity, status and self-esteem (Gignac et al., 2004), giving purpose, structure and social contact to each day (Barrett, 1998).

The onset of arthritis, particularly inflammatory arthritis, may result in a change of a chosen career path. Some people who developed their arthritis at a young age may have difficulty gaining employment, whilst some people with arthritis may have to stop work altogether. For some the pain and fatigue associated with arthritis, which may be exacerbated by stress, affects the hours of work they can manage. Thus 40% of people with rheumatoid arthritis stop working within five years of being diagnosed with the condition (NICE, 2002).

Gordon and Hastings (1994) claim that people whose occupations are associated with less physical stress show a better functional outcome.

Mancuso et al. (2000) found individuals with RA made major adaptations to maintain employment and still perceived their employment to be at risk. Work changes made include use of holidays, sick days, reducing hours, reducing responsibilities, changing jobs or forgoing promotion (Gignac *et al.*, 2004).

Individuals should be encouraged to discuss at an early stage with their employers modifications or adjustments that could reasonably be made to make it easier for them to carry out their work. Practical help and support is available to employers through the government's Access to Work scheme. This scheme is administered by the employment service through local placing, assessment, and counselling teams (PACTs).

Being able to gain and retain employment is not easy at the best of times and for people with arthritis it can be more difficult. However, it is important to remember that everyone, regardless of whether they have arthritis or not, is an individual and will bring their own skills, strengths and weaknesses to their work.

THE ROLE OF SOCIAL SUPPORT

As has already been mentioned, coping with rheumatic disease involves facing a number of stresses and challenges. In addition to coming to terms with the meaning of the illness for one's life, and the more emotive issues of disease progression and deformity, individuals must cope with pain, stiffness and activity restrictions on a daily basis. Many of these adaptive challenges require help from others. Thus, for patients with rheumatic disease an available and satisfying network of interpersonal relations is essential, on which they can count for both emotional support and more practical assistance during periods of pain and disability.

Rheumatic disease has an inevitable impact on the patient's family. The emotional reactions of patients to their illness spill over into feelings of helplessness and distress among family members. The fluctuating nature of many of the rheumatic conditions means family members must learn when to give and when to withhold help, as providing too much support or providing it at the wrong time may produce negative outcomes (Revenson, 1990).

IMPACT ON FAMILY RELATIONSHIPS

Rheumatic disease can affect the family in many ways. Some patients report that their arthritis brings them closer as a family; some say it makes no difference and others feel it has a negative effect on family life.

The Spouse and the Marriage

There is conflicting evidence as to whether the divorce rate is higher in patients with rheumatic disease, whether illness precipitates divorce or whether the lower rate of remarriage is associated with disease course (Medsger and Robinson, 1972). There is no dispute that rheumatic disease causes stress for the healthy spouse and on the marriage. Stressors caused by the conditions create demands for increased emotional support and tangible assistance from the healthy partner. Responsibilities may move outside traditional gender roles (Staines, 1986). As well as the patient possibly feeling more anxious and depressed, the spouses of ill individuals often experience depression and anxiety, marriage communication difficulties and problems at work (Flor, Turk and Scholz, 1987).

Effects of Parent's Disease on Children

In one study, adolescents with a parent who had arthritis had poorer self-esteem than the comparison group (no parental disorder) (Hirsch, Moos and Reischl, 1985). It has been suggested that for adolescents whose parents have arthritis, involvement of friends with their families presents more opportunities for friends to 'see the disability', and consequently evaluate the parent and, by extension, the adolescent negatively. Thus, the parent's physical disability might have a negative impact on the adolescent's ability to draw on friendships for support (Hirsch and Reischl, 1985).

Benefits of Social Support

Arthritis patients receiving more support from friends and family exhibit greater self-esteem (Fitzpatrick *et al.*, 1988), psychological adjustment (Affleck *et al.*, 1988) and life satisfaction (Burckhardt, 1985). They cope more effectively with the illness (Manne and Zautra, 1989) and show less depression (Fitzpatrick *et al.*, 1988). Support from family members may also enhance compliance with treatment interventions (Radojevic, Nicassio and Weisman, 1992).

The Costs of Receiving Social Support

Receiving, using or requesting social support has its costs as well as its benefits (Revenson and Majerovitz, 1990). The costs of asking for or receiving help involve threats to self-esteem, loss of autonomy and decreased psychological well-being. In one study common types of unhelpful support were:

- minimizing illness severity;
- pessimistic comments;
- pity or overly solicitous attitudes (Affleck *et al.*, 1988).

Support needs to change over time in response to changing treatment regime demands, disability, pain and symptomatology. What may be useful one day may be perceived as inappropriate the next.

Implications for Clinical Practice

Social support is amenable to change through psychosocial intervention. Goals for practitioners to work towards are:

- teaching patients how to develop and maintain family ties;
- teaching patients how to recognize and accept the help and emotional encouragement provided by family members;
- improving family members' skills for determining the patients' support needs, and offering help;
- facilitating positive appraisals of support.

The key is to promote open communication among family members including feedback, and not criticism, when the help that was offered was not the help that was desired (Revenson, 1990).

Spouses of chronically ill patients should be encouraged to build support networks outside the marriage, both within their existing social milieu and through more formal support groups of others facing similar stresses. These networks become critically important as the patient's health declines and disability increases; however, network building should be encouraged in the early stages of the illness so that networks are in place later on, when the patient is more limited and social activities with the support network may be restricted.

DEPRESSION

The onset of symptoms and eventual diagnosis of a chronic disease typically cause emotional distress. Anxiety, depression, shock and anger can persist throughout the duration of the condition (Treharne *et al.*, 2004) A significant minority of people, however, will develop less transient and more severe psychological distress that can result in additional disability and suffering. Depression is the most common psychological disturbance associated with medical illness and can significantly increase the disability associated with the medical condition (Wells *et al.*, 1989). Depression in the medically ill frequently goes undetected and untreated; if this is so the depression can become progressively debilitating and interfere with the optimal treatment for the medical condition. The presence of depression in rheumatic disease is particularly problematic as it is often associated with somatic symptoms that overlap or resemble symptoms of arthritis. To further complicate the picture, depression can lead to the amplification of somatic symptoms of arthritis, causing physician and patient mistakenly to attribute worsening symptoms and disability to worsening of the medical condition. This in turn can result in unwarranted treatment changes and overmedication (Katon and Sullivan, 1990). Depression is a debilitating and often life-threatening disorder and rheumatologists must be on the alert for depressive co-morbidity among their patients and be prepared to provide appropriate treatment or referral. A diagnosis of major depression, according to DSM-III-R criteria, requires the occurrence of one or more major depressive episodes. A major depressive episode requires the presence of at least five of the following symptoms for at least two weeks:

- depressed mood;
- diminished interest and pleasure in activities;
- significant weight loss or gain;
- sleep disturbance;
- agitation or retardation;
- fatigue or loss of energy;
- feelings of worthlessness or guilt;
- poor concentration;
- recurrent thoughts of death or suicide.

One of the first two symptoms *must* be included in the five required to diagnose a depressive episode. Symptoms clearly due to a physical condition do not satisfy the diagnostic criteria — for example, fatigue. Most of the research efforts have focused on psychological sequelae in five rheumatological conditions (RA, juvenile RA, SLE, fibromyalgia and OA) (Baum, 1982). The majority of studies suggest that there is a greater prevalence of depressive symptoms and depressive disorders among clinical samples of people with rheumatological diseases than in the general population. Dickens and Creed (2001) found individuals with rheumatoid arthritis were twice as likely to experience depression as members of the general population. The level of disturbance, however, is comparable to that found among clinical samples of people with other chronic medical conditions. Rheumatological disease severity and status have, at most, a very weak direct relation to the presence of depressive disorders and level of depressive symptoms. Depressive disorders and symptoms among people with rheumatological diseases are influenced more by pain, socioeconomic factors and social and other psychological resources, such as social support, a sense of control, illness intrusiveness and coping than by disease severity itself. Depressive disorders and even depressive symptoms have devastating effects on social, family and vocational functioning; when added to a chronic medical condition such as arthritis functional declines are additive. Compared to the general population, the prevalence of depressive disorders and symptoms appears to be higher among people with rheumatological diseases. Rheumatologists therefore must be alert to depressive co-morbidity and must guard against mistakenly attributing the additive effects of these co-morbid conditions to worsening primary medical illness (DeVellis, 1993).

REFERENCES

Affleck, G., Pfeiffer, C., Tennen, H. and Fifield, J. (1988) Social support and psychosocial adjustment to rheumatoid arthritis. *Arthritis Care and Research*, **1**, 71–7.

Ansell, B.M. (1977) Joint manifestations in children with juvenile chronic arthritis. *Arthritis and Rheumatism*, **20**, 204–6.

Antoni, C., Krueger, G.G., de Vlam, K. *et al.* IMPACT 2 Trial Investigators. (2005) Infliximab improves signs and symptoms of psoriatic arthritis: results of the IMPACT 2 Trial. *Annals of Rheumatic Disease*, **64** (8), 1150−7.

ARMA. (2004) Standards of Care for people with Inflammatory Arthritis. Arthritis and Musculoskeletal Alliance (ARMA), www.arma.net.uk

Arnett, F.C., Edworthy, S.M., Bloch, D.A. *et al.* (1988) American rheumatism association 1987 revised criteria for the classification of rheumatoid arthritis. *Arthritis and Rheumatism*, **31**, 315−24.

Ashcroft, J. (1996) A patient's perspective, in *Measuring Outcomes in Rheumatoid Arthritis* (eds A.F. Long and D.L. Scott), Royal College of Physicians, London, Chapter 5, pp. 29−34.

Ashcroft, J. (1997) Understanding people's everyday needs. Arthritis − getting it right − a guide for planners. *Arthritis Care.*

Barrett, E.M. (1998) Arthritis and employment, in *Rheumatology for Nurses: Patient Care* (ed. P. Le Gallez), Whurr Publishers, London Chapter 11, pp. 272−89.

Baum, J. (1982) A review of the psychological aspects of rheumatic diseases. *Seminars in Arthritis and Rheumatism*, **11**, 352−61.

Bennet, R.M. (1993) Psoriatic arthritis, in *Arthritis and Allied Conditions − A Textbook of Rheumatology*, 12th edn (eds D.J. McCarty and W.J. Koopman), Lea & Febiger, Pennsylvania, Chapter 61, pp. 1079−94.

Bird, H.A., Le Gallez, P. and Hill, J. (1985) *Combined Care of the Rheumatic Patient*, Springer-Verlag Berlin Heidelberg, Great Britain.

Blocka, K.L.N., Bassett, L.W., Furst, D.E. *et al.* (1981) The arthropathy of advanced progressive systemic sclerosis: a radiographic survey. *Arthritis and Rheumatism*, **24**, 874−84.

Brandt, J. and Braun, J. (2006) Anti-TNF-alpha agents in the treatment of psoriatic arthritis. *Expert Opinion on Biological Therapy*, **6** (2), 99−107.

Brandt, J., Kariouzov, A., Listing, J. *et al.* (2003) Six months results of a German double-blind placebo controlled, phase-III clinical trial of etanercept in active ankylosing spondylitis. *Arthritis and Rheumatism*, **48**, 1667−75.

Braun, J., Brandt, J., Listing, J. *et al.* (2002) Treatment of active ankylosing spondylitis with infliximab: a randomised controlled multicentre trial. *Lancet*, **359**, 1187−93.

Braun, J., Pham, T., Sieper, J. *et al.* (2003) International ASAS consensus statement for the use of anti-tumour necrosis factor agents in patients with ankylosing spondylitis. *Annals of Rheumatic Disease*, **62**, 817−24.

BSR. (2004) BSR guidelines on standards of care for persons with rheumatoid arthritis. BSR. London.

Burckhardt, C. (1985) The impact of arthritis on quality of life. *Nursing Research*, **34**, 11−6.

Calin, A., Garrett, S. Whitelock, H. *et al.* (1994) A new approach to defining functional ability in ankylosing spondylitis: the development of the Bath Ankylosing Spondylitis Functional Index (BASFI). *Journal of Rheumatology*, **21**, 2281−5.

Carr, A.J. (1996) Measuring handicap, in *Measuring Outcomes in Rheumatoid Arthritis* (eds A.F. Long and D.L. Scott), Royal College of Physicians, London, Chapter 9, pp. 61−70.

Cassidy, J.T. (1994) Juvenile chronic arthritis, in *Rheumatology*, Vol 3 (eds J.H. Klippel and P. Dieppe), Mosby-Year Book Europe Limited, London, pp. 20.1−20.10.

Cooper, N.J. (2000) Economic burden of rheumatoid arthritis: a systematic review. *Rheumatology. Oxford*, **39**, 28−33.

Cush, J.J. and Lipsky, P.E. (1993) Reiter's syndrome and reactive arthritis, in *Arthritis and Allied Conditions − A Textbook of Rheumatology*, 12th edn (eds D.J. McCarty and W.J. Koopman), Lea & Febiger, Pennsylvania, Chapter 60, pp. 1061−78.

DeVellis, B.M. (1993) Depression in rheumatological diseases, in *Psychological Aspects of Rheumatic Diseases. Clinical Rheumatology* (eds S. Newman and M. Shipley), WB Saunders (Bailliere Tindall), London, pp. 241–57.

Dickens, C. and Creed, F. (2001) The burden of depression in rheumatoid arthritis. *Rheumatology*, **40**, 1327–330.

Dickey, B.F. and Myers, A.R. (1984) Pulmonary disease in polymyositis/dermatomyositis. *Seminars in Arthritis and Rheumatism*, **14**, 60–76.

Dieppe, P., Doherty, M., Macfarlane, D.G. and Maddison, P.J. (1985) *Rheumatological Medicine*, Churchill Livingstone, Edinburgh.

Doherty, M. (1993) Fibromyalgia syndrome. Reports on rheumatic diseases Series 2 No 23, Chesterfield: Arthritis and Rheumatism Council.

Doyle, D.V. (1996) The rheumatologist's perspective, in *Measuring Outcomes in Rheumatoid Arthritis* (eds A.F. Long and D.L. Scott), Royal College of Physicians, London, Chapter 4, pp. 23–7.

Edwards, J. (1991) *UCL Notes on Rheumatology, Sponsored by Roche Products Ltd. Broadwater Press, Herts.*

Felson, D.T. (2000) Osteoarthritis: new insights. Part 1: the disease and its risk factors. *Annals of Internal Medicine*, **133**, 637–46.

Ferrari, R., Cash, J. and Maddison, P. (1996) *Rheumatology Guidebook – A Step-by-Step Guide to Diagnosis and Treatment*, BIOS, Oxford.

Fitzpatrick, R., Newman, S., Lamb, R. and Shipley, M. (1988) Social relationships and psychological well-being in rheumatoid arthritis. *Social Science and Medicine*, **27**, 399–403.

Flor, H., Turk, D.C. and Scholz, O.B. (1987) Impact of chronic pain on the spouse: marital, emotional and physical consequences. *Journal of Psychosomatic Research*, **31**, 63–71.

Foeldvari, I. and Bidde, M. (2000) Validation of the proposed ILAR classification criteria for juvenile idiopathic arthritis. International league of associations for rheumatology. *Journal of Rheumatology*, **27**, 1069–72.

Garrett, S., Jenkinson, T., Kennedy, L.G. *et al.* (1994) A new approach to defining disease status in ankylosing spondylitis: The Bath Ankylosing Spondylitis disease activity index (BASDAI). *Journal of Rheumatology*, **21**, 2286–91.

Gignac, M.A.M., Badley, E.M., Lacaille, D. *et al.* (2004) Managing arthritis and employment: making arthritis related work changes as a means of adaptation. *Arthritis and Rheumatism*, **51**, 909–16.

Gladman, D.D. and Urowitz, M.B. (1994) Systemic lupus erythematosus: clinical features, in *Rheumatology*, Vol **6** (eds J.H. Klippel and P. Dieppe), Mosby-Year Book Europe Limited, London, pp. 2.1–18.

Goetz, R.H. (1945) Pathology of progressive systemic sclerosis (generalized scleroderma) with special reference to changes in the viscera. *Clinical Procedures (S Africa)*, **4**, 337–42.

Gordon, D.A. and Hastings, D.E. (1994) Rheumatoid arthritis – clinical features: early, progressive and late disease, in *Rheumatology*, Vol **3** (eds J.H. Klippel and P. Dieppe), Mosby-Year Book Europe Limited, London, pp. 4.1–14.

Hackett, J., Johnson, B., Parkin, A. and Southwood, T.R. (1996) Physiotherapy and occupational therapy for juvenile chronic arthritis: custom and practice in five centres in the UK, USA and Canada. *British Journal Rheum*, **35**, 695–9.

Hawley, D.J. and Wolfe, F. (1988) Anxiety and depression in patients with rheumatoid arthritis: a prospective study of 400 patients. *Journal of Rheumatology*, **15**, 932–41.

Healey, L.A. (1993) Polymyalgia and giant cell arteritis, in *Arthritis and Allied conditions — A Textbook of Rheumatology*, 12th edn (eds D.J. McCarty and W.J. Koopman), Lea & Febiger, Pennsylvania, Chapter 81, pp. 1377–80.

Helliwell, P.S. and Wright, V. (1994) Psoriatic arthritis: clinical features, in *Rheumatology* (eds J.H. Klippel and P. Dieppe), Mosby-Year Book Europe Limited, London, pp. 31.1–8.

Hilliquin, P. and Menkes, C.-J. (1994) Rheumatoid arthritis — evaluation and management early and established disease, in *Rheumatology*, Section 3 (eds J.H. Klippel and P. Dieppe), Mosby-Year Book Europe Limited, London, pp. 13.1–14.

Hirsch, B.J., Moos, R.H. and Reischl, T.M. (1985) Psychosocial adjustment of adolescent children of a depressed, arthritic or normal parent. *Journal of Abnormal Psychology*, **94**, 154–64.

Hirsch, B.J. and Reischl, T.M. (1985) Social networks and developmental psychopathology: a comparison of adolescent children of a depressed, arthritic or normal parent. *Journal of Abnormal Psychology*, **94**, 272–81.

Hughes, R.A. (1996) Practical problems — septic arthritis, reports on rheumatic diseases. Arthritis and Rheumatism Council for Research. *Series* 3: No 7.

Huizinga, T.W., Machold, K.P., Breedveld, F.C. *et al.* (2002) Criteria for early rheumatoid arthritis: from Bayes' law revisited to new thoughts on pathogenesis. *Arthritis and Rheumatism*, **46**, 1155–9.

Jenkinson, T.R., Mallorie, P.A., Whitelock, H.C. *et al.* (1994) Defining spinal mobility in ankylosing spondylitis (AS): the bath AS metrology index. *Journal of Rheumatology*, **21**, 1694–8.

Jones, S.D., Steiner, A., Garrett, S.L. and Calin, A. (1996) The bath ankylosing spondylitis patient global score (BAS-G). *British Journal of Rheumatology*, **35**, 66–71.

Judd, M. (1997) Caring for the patient with bone and joint disease, in *Watson's Clinical Nursing and Related Sciences*, 5th edn (ed. M. Walsh), Bailliere Tindall, London, Chapter 22, pp. 873–98.

Katon, W. and Sullivan, M.D. (1990) Depression and chronic medical illness. *Journal of Clinical Psychiatry*, **51** (Suppl.), 3–14.

Kavanaugh, A., Antoni, C., Krueger, G.G. *et al.* (2006) Infliximab improves health related quality of life and physical function in patients with psoriatic arthritis. *Annals of Rheumatic Disease*, **65** (4), 471–7.

Keat, A. (1995) Reiter's syndrome and reactive arthritis. Collected reports on the rheumatic diseases. *Arthritis and Rheumatism Council for Research*, 61–4.

Kimberly, R.P. and Urowitz, M.B. (1994) Connective tissue disorders, in *Rheumatology*, Vol **6** (eds J.H. Klippel and P. Dieppe), Mosby-Year Book Europe Limited, London, p. 1.1.

Le Gallez (1995) Rheumatoid arthritis. *Primary Health Care*, **5** (7), 31–8.

Leach, M. (1997) Juvenile chronic arthritis: epidemiology and genetics. *Nursing Times*, **93** (18), 46–8.

Leigh, J.P. and Fries, J.F. (1991) Education level and rheumatoid arthritis: evidence from five data centers. *Journal of Rheumatology*, **18**, 24–34.

Levine, J.D., Goetzl, E.J. and Basbaum, A.I. (1987) Contribution of the nervous system to the pathophysiology of rheumatoid arthritis and other polyarthritides. *Rheumatic Disease Clinics of North America*, **13**, 369–83.

Long, A.F. and Scott, D.L. (1994) Measuring health status and outcomes in rheumatoid arthritis within routine clinical practice. *British Journal of Rheumatology*, **33**, 682–5.

MacGregor, A.J. and Spector, T.D. (2004) Epidemiology of rheumatic diseases, in *ABC of Rheumatology*, 3rd edn (ed. M.L. Snaith), BMJ Books, London, pp. 114–20.

Maddison, P. and Huey, P. (2006) Rheumatic Diseases – Seriological Aids to Early Diagnosis. Reports of the Rheumatic Diseases series 5 – Topical Reviews. ARC. Chesterfield. Feb 2006 no: 8.

Maini, R.N., Feldman, M. (1993) Immunopathogenesis of rheumatoid arthritis, in *Oxford Textbook of Rheumatology*, Vol 11 (eds P.J. Maddison, D.A. Isenberg, P. Woo, D.N. Glass *et al.*), Oxford University Press, Oxford, pp. 621–38.

Mancuso, C.A., Paget, S.A. and Charlson, M.E. (2000) Adaptations made by rheumatoid arthritis patients to continue working: a pilot study of workplace challenges and successful adaptations. *Arthritis Care and Research*, **13**, 89–97.

Manne, S.L. and Zautra, A.J. (1989) Spouse criticism and support: their association with coping and psychological adjustment among women with rheumatoid arthritis. *Journal of Personality and Social Psychology*, **56**, 608–17.

Maricq, H.R. (1981) Widefield capillary microscopy. Technique and rating scale for abnormalities seen in scleroderma and related disorders. *Arthritis and Rheumatism*, **24**, 1159–63.

Martin, J., Meltzer, H. and Elliot, D. (1988) The prevalence of disability among adults. OPCS surveys of disability in Great Britain. Report 1, HMSO.

Matteson, E.L., Cohen, M.D. and Conn, D.L. (1994) Rheumatoid arthritis clinical features – systemic involvement, in *Rheumatology*, Vol 3 (eds J.H. Klippel and P. Dieppe), Mosby-Year Book Europe Limited, London, p. 5.1.

McClosky, D.A., Patella, S.J. and Seibold, J.R. (1990) Health assessment questionnaire in systemic sclerosis. *Procedures of Allied Health Profession 25th Meeting*, **182**.

McFarlane, A.C. and Brooks, P.M. (1988) Determinants of disability in rheumatoid arthritis. *British Journal of Rheumatology*, **27**, 7–14.

Mease, P.J., Gladman, D.D., Ritchlin, C.T. *et al.* (2005) Adalimumab for the treatment of patients with moderately to severely active psoriatic arthritis: results of a double-blind, randomised, placebo-controlled trial. *Arthritis and Rheumatism*, **52** (10), 3279–89.

Medsger, A.R. and Robinson, H. (1972) A comparative study of divorce in rheumatoid arthritis and other rheumatic diseases. *Journal of Chronic Disease*, **25**, 269–75.

Medsger, T.A. and Masi, A.T. (1971) Epidemiology of systemic sclerosis (scleroderma). *Annals of Internal Medicine*, **74**, 714–21.

NICE. (2002) Technology appraisal no 36. Guidance on the use of Etanercept and Infliximab for the treatment of Rheumatoid Arthritis. *NICE*, London.

Nicholas, N.S. and Panayi, G.S. (1988) Rheumatoid arthritis in pregnancy. *Clinical Experimental Rheumatology*, **6**, 179–82.

Petty, R.E., Southwood, T.R., Baum, J. *et al.* (1998) Revision of the proposed classification criteria for juvenile idiopathic arthritis: Durban, 97, *Journal of Rheumatology*, **25**, 1991–4.

Pipitone, N. and Choy, E.H.S. (2003) Treatment of rheumatoid arthritis. *Rheumatic Disease – Topical Reviews*, ARC, Chesterfield, Jan 2003 no: 10.

Pisetsky, D.S. (1994) Rheumatic disease etiology: immune-mediated inflammation, in *Rheumatology*, Vol 1 (eds J.H. Klippel and P. Dieppe), Mosby-Year Book Europe Limited, London, pp. 131–6.

Radojevic, V., Nicassio, P.M. and Weisman, M.H. (1992) Behavioral intervention with and without family support for rheumatoid arthritis. *Behavior Therapy*, **23**, 13–30.

Rantapaa-Dahlqvist, S., de Jong, B.A., Berglin, E. *et al.* (2003) Anti-bodies against cyclic citrullinated peptide and IgA rheumatoid factor predict the development of rheumatoid arthritis. *Arthritis and Rheumatism*, **48** (10), 2741–9.

Revenson, T.A. (1990) Social support processes among chronically ill elders: patient and provider perspectives, in *Communication, Health and the Elderly* (eds H. Giles, N. Coupland and J. Wiemann), University of Manchester Press, Manchester, England, pp. 92–113.

Revenson, T.A. and Majerovitz, S.D. (1990) Spouses' support provision to chronically ill patients. *Journal of Social and Personal Relationships*, **7**, 575–86.

Rodnan, G.P. and Benedek, T.G. (1962) An historical account of the study of progressive systemic sclerosis (diffuse scleroderma). *Annals of Internal Medicine*, **57**, 305–19.

Ross, A.C. (1990) Infection complicating orthopedic procedures and arthroplasties. *Current Opinion in Rheumatology*, **2**, 628–34.

Ryan, S. (1997) Rheumatology – knowledge for practice. *Nursing Times Learning Curve*, **1** (2), 5–8.

Schmid, F.R. (1993) Principles of diagnosis and treatment of bone and joint infections, in *Arthritis and Allied Conditions – A Textbook of Rheumatology*, 12th edn (eds D.J. McCarty and W.J. Koopman), Lea & Febiger, Pennsylvania, Chapter 115, pp. 1975–2001.

Segal, R., Caspi, D., Tisher, M. *et al.* (1988) Accelerated nodulosis and vasculitis during methotrexate therapy for RA. *Arthritis and Rheumatism*, **31**, 1182.

SIGN. (2000) Management of early rheumatoid arthritis – A National Clinical Guideline. No 48. Scottish Intercollegiate Guidelines Network.

Simkin, P.A. (1994) The musculoskeletal system, in *Rheumatology* (eds J.H. Klippel and P. Dieppe), Mosby-Year Book Europe Limited, London, pp. 2.1–2.10.

Solomon, L., Robin, G. and Valkenburg, H.A. (1975) Rheumatoid arthritis in an urban South African Negro population. *Annals of Rheumatic Disease*, **34**, 128–33.

Southwood, T. (1993) School children with arthritis. *Head Teachers Review*, **Winter**, 20–2.

Staines, G.L. (1986) Men and women in role relationships, in *The Social Psychology of Female-Male Relations* (eds R.D. Ashmore and F.K. Del Boca), Academic Press, New York, pp. 211–58.

Symmons, D. and Bankhead, C. (1994) Health care needs assessment for musculoskeletal diseases. *Arthritis and Rheumatism Council for Research*.

Symmons, D. and Bruce, I. (2006) Management of cardiovascular risk in RA and SLE. Reports of the rheumatic diseases series 5 – Hands on – practical advice on management of rheumatic disease. ARC. Chesterfield. Feb 2006 no: 8.

Symmons, D.P.M. (2005) Looking back: rheumatoid arthritis – aetiology, occurrence and mortality. *Rheumatology. Oxford*, **44**, 4 pg iv14.

Symmons, D.P.M., Jones, M., Osborn, J. *et al.* (1996) Paediatric rheumatology in the United Kingdom: data from the British Paediatric Rheumatology Group Register. *British Journal of Rheumatology*, **23** (11), 1975–80.

Treharne, G.J., Lyons, A.C., Booth, D.A. *et al.* (2004) Reactions to disability in patients with early versus established rheumatoid arthritis. *Scandinavian Journal of Rheumatology*, **33**, 30–8.

Van den Bosch, F., Kruithof, E., Baeten, D. *et al.* (2002) Randomized double-blind comparison of chimeric monoclonal antibody to tumour necrosis factor α (infliximab) versus placebo in active spondylarthropathy. *Arthritis and Rheumatism*, **46**, 755–65.

Varani, J., Mulligan, M.S. and Ward, P.A. (1994) The vascular endothelium and acute inflammation, in *Rheumatology*, Vol 3 (eds J.H. Klippel and P. Dieppe), Mosby-Year Book Europe Limited, London, pp. 11.1–11.12.

Walker, G.L., Mastalgia, F.L. and Roberts, D.F. (1982) A search for genetic influence in idiopathic inflammatory myopathy. *Acta Neurologica Scandinavica*, **66**, 432–3.

Wells, K.B., Stewart, A., Hays, R.D. *et al.* (1989) The functioning and well-being of depressed patients: results from the medical outcomes study. *Journal of the American Medical Association*, **262** (7), 914—19.

White, P. (1994) Juvenile chronic arthritis — clinical features, in *Rheumatology*, Vol **3** (eds J.H. Klippel and P. Dieppe), Mosby-Year Book Europe Limited, London, pp. 17.1—17.10.

Wilson, A., Yu, H.T., Goodnough, L.T. and Nissenson, A.R. (2004) Prevalence and outcomes of anemia in rheumatoid arthritis: a systemic review of the literature. *American Journal of Medicine*, **116** (Suppl. 7A), S50—7.

Wolfe, F. and Cathey, M.A. (1991) The assessment and predication of functional disability in rheumatoid arthritis. *Journal of Rheumatology*, **18**, 1298—306.

Wolfe, F., Hawley, D.J. and Cathey, M.A. (1991) Clinical and health status measures over time: prognosis and outcome assessment in rheumatoid arthritis. *Journal of Rheumatology*, **18**, 1290—7.

World Health Organisation. (1997) *International Classification of Impairments, Activities, and Participation. (ICIDH-2). A Manual of Dimensions of Disablement and Functioning. Beta-1 Draft for Field Trials*, WHO, Geneva.

WHO (World Health Organization). (2001) *International Classification of Functioning, Disability and Health*, World Health Organization, Geneva. http://www.who.int/classification/icf

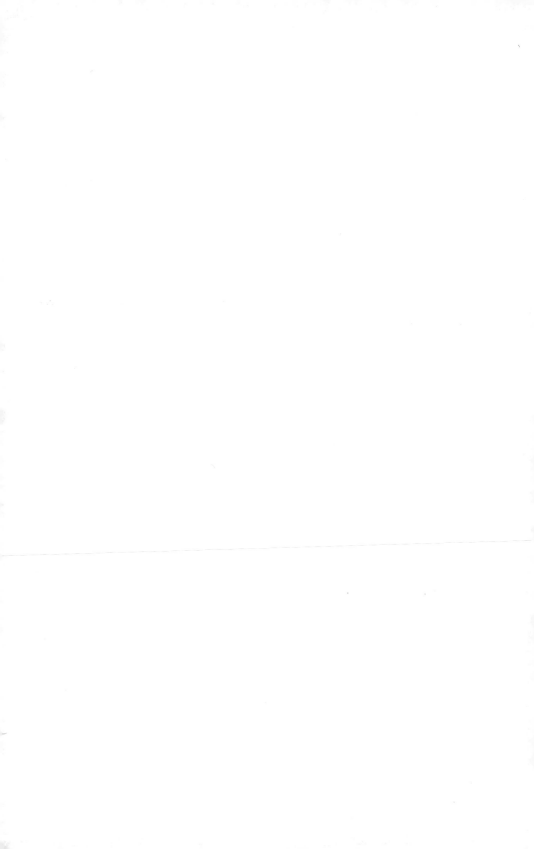

2 Drug Therapy

SARAH RYAN, SUSAN OLIVER AND ANN BROWNFIELD

Objectives

After reading this chapter you should be able to:

- Explain the mechanism of pain.
- Describe the purpose and mode of action of analgesia, NSAIDs, DMARDs, biologic therapies and steroids.
- Discuss the drug management of a patient with inflammatory arthritis.
- Debate the advantages and disadvantages of introducing a self-medication programme in the clinical area.
- Discuss the role of complementary therapies in the management of arthritis.

The treatment of rheumatological disorders will involve many components including education, exercise, adaptation and drug therapy. The main objectives of drug intervention will be to:

- Reduce or alleviate symptoms such as pain and stiffness.
- Suppress disease activity in chronic disorders such as RA.

2.1 PAIN

The experience of pain can only be defined in terms of human consciousness. As with all sensory experience there is no way of being certain that one person's experience of pain is the same as another's (Jones, 1997). Pain is a paradox while being an accepted phenomenon experienced by everyone at some time during their life. It is also a unique, subjective and unverifiable personal experience (Turk and Melzack, 1992). Pain is one of the cardial symptoms of rheumatoid arthritis and will affect both physical and psychological aspects of functioning. It is the major contributor to the morbidity, disability and socioeconomic cost of musculoskeletal disorders (Cohen, 1994).

There are a number of evidence-based guidelines which can support the clinician in the managment of pain (ARMA, 2005; Australian Acute Musculoskeletal Pain Guidelines Group, 2004; Koes, Van Tulder and Osteso, 2001; Pain Society, 2005; Turk, Dworkin and Allan, 2003).

Acute pain is a transient experience where the source of pain is usually identifiable. Here pharmacological interventions are able to suppress the pain stimuli (Pearce and Wardle, 1989). In comparison chronic pain is an ongoing experience; often patients may demonstrate an array of associated disorders such as anxiety, depression and insomnia.

Drug Therapy in Rheumatology Nursing: Second Edition. Edited by Sarah Ryan.
© 2007 John Wiley & Sons, Ltd.

The successful pharmacological control of pain dictates that nurses possess a comprehensive pharmacological knowledge and effective interpersonal skills to enable the assessment, planning, implementation and evaluation of pharmacological interventions in the management of pain (Lubkin, 1990).

PHYSIOLOGY OF PAIN

The Gate Control Theory of Pain

The gate control theory originates from Melzack and Wall (1982). It has been most influential in developing our present understanding of the mechanism of pain. Occasionally viewed as oversimplified or too rigid it has provided a framework which demonstrates the complexity of the pain response (Jackson, 1995).

The theory is founded on two main concepts (see Figure 2.1).

- The transmission of pain messages can be modulated within the spinal cord. This occurs via descending messages from the brain, which inhibit sensations from peripheral and internal sources being experienced as pain. Two neurotransmitters appear to be involved in this process. The release of enkephalin at the spinal cord inhibits the uptake of calcium ions by the spinal cord neurones. This prevents further transmission of the pain message. Serotonin (the second neurotransmitter) is involved in the transmission of pain messages between the raphe magnus and the cord.

- The transmission of pain messages to the brain can be altered by activating another source of sensory receptor.

When pain impulses enter the dorsal horn of the spinal cord the gate control mechanism is either opened or closed. A number of laminae within the dorsal horn

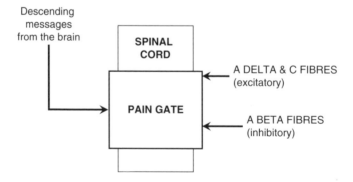

Figure 2.1   Influences on the pain gate.

form the gate control mechanism and this specialized area enabled the pain impulses to be modulated (Jackson, 1995).

The primary sensory neurones involved in pain transmission are:

- Type A delta fibres. These are small myelinated fibres capable of transporting messages at speeds of 6–30 metres per second.
- Type C fibres. These are very small and have no myelin insulation. Therefore messages are transmitted a lot slower at speeds of 0.5–2 metres per second (Guyton, 1991). Type C fibres transmit slower chronic pain.

Impulses from A delta and C fibres are excitary in nature and promote the release of an exitory neurotransmitter Substance P, which opens the gate facilitating the perception of pain.

The opening of the gate allows the transmission of pain impulses along the spinoreticular and reticular thalamic tracts through various junctions into the sensory cortex (Fordham, 1986).

Studies of the thalamus and somatosensory cortex show that in arthritis some cells have an abnormally large response to joint stimulation causing changes in the way impulses are transmitted (Newman et al., 1996).

- Type A beta fibres. These are larger fibres than other sensory neurones and electrical impulses travel along them at a greater speed. Therefore, the pain stimulus conducted along type A beta fibres will be quicker and faster than transmission along the other fibres. If activated, type A beta fibres will occupy the secondary neurones first thereby blocking other pain messages. These fibres can be activated by rubbing or vibration of the skin and their activation will close the 'pain gate'. This theory has been instrumental in the development of treatment interventations such as transcutaneous electrical nerve stimulation machines (TENS).

PAIN RECEPTORS

Sensory receptors are situated in the tissues of the body, especially in the skin, synovium of joints and in the walls of arteries. These receptors are referred to as nociceptors as they respond to noxious stimuli. Such receptors can be divided into three categories.

- Mechanical changes in the receptor. In active inflammatory conditions such as RA, increased synovial fluid in the joint cavity and proliferation of the inflamed synovial tissues causes pain by distention and stretching of the capsule.
- Temperature changes. Exposure of the tissues to extremes of temperature can cause stimulation of the receptors.
- Inflammatory changes. The inflammatory response initiated by tissue damage will cause the release of prostaglandin, bradykinin, histamine and serotonin. This will stimulate a reaction in the receptors.

Some nociceptor receptors will respond to all the above stimulants. They terminate in the dorsal horn of the spinal cord and transmit their pain messages to secondary neurones. The destination for secondary neurones is the thalamus.

THE ROLE OF THE BRAIN

Pain signals terminate in the brain. Fast pain signals are relayed via the brain stem and the thalamus to areas of the cortex, especially the somatosensory area. This region of the cortex can differentiate the area of the origin of the pain message.

Slow pain messages are relayed over a wide area of the brain stem and thalamus. The reticuloactivitating system is situated in the brain stem; when it is stimulated it increases the excitability of the brain. This is why people with chronic pain conditions such as fibromyalgia report difficulty in sleeping, resting and relaxing. Also it provides us with a reason why chronic pain is difficult to locate because the pain messages are not relayed to the somatosensory areas.

Once stimulation of the receptor ceases so should the pain but pain pathways cannot explain all pain experiences and patients can continue to experience pain after the original cause of the pain has been removed.

Woolf (1994) offers a theory for the development of chronic pain states. He proposes that neurones in the dorsal horn of the spinal cord become hypersensitive and develop alternative synapses with neighbouring neurones. This causes pain messages to go astray.

Also, other substances released within the spinal cord can mediate the transmission of pain signals. N-Methyl-D aspartate (NMDA) and neurokinin (NK) cause the spinal cord neurones to become hypersensitive. This can cause the reproduction of *hyperalgesia* (severe pain to a stimulus that would normally only produce mild pain) and *allodynia* (pain in response to a stimulus that would not normally be painful — for example, stroking the skin — Woolf, 1994).

Additionally, many aspects of higher levels of processing will have a considerable effect on how unpleasant a pain stimulus is. The experience of pain is influenced by anxiety, cultural factors, the environment and past experiences (Gibson, 1994). Reassurances that a stimulus will be brief considerably reduces the unpleasantness rating (Jones, 1997). This assumes that there is an inevitable behavioural sequence that is initiated by a noxious stimulant referred to as the 'bottom up approach' (Jones, 1997). However the brain is quite capable of simply ignoring noxious stimuli altogether under conditions of severe stress (Melzack and Wall, 1982) and it is capable of selecting what sensory information is acted on; this is known as the 'top down approach'. It is the balance between these ascending and decending processes that determines our perception of pain (Jones, 1997).

PHYSIOLOGICAL EFFECTS OF ACUTE PAIN

Once the acute pain impulse has passed the gate control mechanism it enters the reticular activating system, and sympathetic nervous system activity increases aiding the body's flight of fight mechanism (Jordan, 1992).

This activity includes:

- An increase in hormonal activity. The anti-diuretic hormone increases the reabsorption from the renal tubules retaining water within the body (this can elevate blood pressure).

Aldosterone increases the reasorption of sodium from the renal tubules;
Adrenaline causes increased consciousness and emotion;
  Cortisol increases blood glucose levels and the secretion of hydrochloric acid and pepsinogen.

- An increase in cardiovascular activity. Tachycardia and increased cardiac output.
- An increase in gastric activity. This leads to a reduction in gastric emptying.

2.2 PHARMACOLOGICAL INTERVENTIONS IN RHEUMATOLOGY

The major pharmacological interventions for the management of pain include the following categories of drug therapy:

- Non-opioid analgesia
- Compound analgesia
- Opioid analgesia
- Antidepressant drugs
- Non-steroidal anti-inflammatory drugs (NSAIDs).

NON-OPIOID ANALGESIA

These medications are administered to treat mild—moderate pain.

Acetaminophen – Paracetamol

Paracetamol is an undervalued effective analgesic agent (Cohen, 1994). Its mechanism of action remains poorly understood although there is evidence of direct effect on the central nervous system (CNS) rather than on peripheral tissue. It blocks the synthesis and secretion of prostaglandin preventing nociceptor sensitization (Speight, 1987). It has both analgesic and anti-pyretic properties.

Pharmacokinetics

Taken orally paracetamol is well absorbed from the gastrointestinal tract and inactivated in the liver. A major advantage is the lack of upper gastrointestinal toxicity, especially ulceration and bleeding.

Adverse Effects

The well-known hazard of hepatoxicity is virtually only seen in conjunction with a drug overdose and is increased with liver disease and alcoholism. The daily dose should be closely monitored in these situations. The risk of nephrotoxicity with chronic dosing remains uncertain but is probably very small (Cohen, 1994).

COMPOUND ANALGESIA

Compound analgesia are fixed ratio combinations of non-opioid (aspirin or paracetamol) and opioid analgesia (dextropropoxyphene or codeine) preparations.

Compound analgesia contain either a low dose or full dose of opioid analgesic. Thus this range of analgesia is able to bridge the therapeutic gap between non-opioid and opioid analgesia. However it is worth noting that the compound or combined analgesic effect may also result in a combination of the side effects of both analgesia. Examples of these drugs include Co-Codamol and Codydramol. Adverse effects are shown in Table 2.1.

OPIOIDS

This group of drugs is classified in terms of its efficacy into two categories — low and high efficacy opioids (See Table 2.2). Their role in the management of moderate to severe musculoskeletal pain is controversial (Cohen, 1994). Although certain patients may benefit without experiencing adverse effects and addiction, the question of true efficacy has not yet been answered (Davis, 2000; Jamison, 1996).

Opioid analgesies work by fitting into the opioid receptors of the brain and spinal cord. These receptors are also used by endorphins, the body's own opioid. Opioid analgesia inhibits the transmission of nociceptive messages to the higher centres

Table 2.1   Adverse effects of compound analgesia.

Dizziness
Sedation
Nausea/vomiting
Constipation
Abdominal pain
Rashes
Headaches
Weakness
Euphoria
Dysphoria
Hallucinations
Minor visual disturbances
Abnormal liver function tests

Table 2.2   Opioids.

Low efficacy
    Codeine
    Dihydrocoedeine
    Dextropropoxyphene
    Nalbuphine
    Pentazocine
High efficacy
    Buprenorphine
    Dextromaramide
    Diamorphine
    Dipipanone
    Meptazinal
    Morphine
    Papaveretum
    Pethidine
    Tramadol

or through activation of the decending anti-nociceptive pathways (Ferrante, 1983). Evidence from Stein (1991) highlights the peripheral analgesic action of these medications in conditions characterized by inflammatory hyperalgesia.

Low Efficacy Opioids

Codeine Phosphate

Primarily prescribed as an analgesic but also used as an antidiarrhoeal drug and a cough suppressant, codeine has been in use for nearly 100 years. Although codeine's analgesic properties are similar to morphine its analgesic action is equal to approximately only 10% of morphine.

Pharmacokinetics

Taken orally codeine is quickly absorbed within the gastrointestinal tract and metabolized within the liver. It has a half life of approximately two to three hours. Excretion of codeine is via the kidneys into the urine. The analgesic effect of 30 mg of codeine is suggested to equal 300−600 mg of aspirin.

Dihydrocodeine tartrate − this medication possesses a similar analgesic effect to codeine.

Dextropropoxyphene Hydrochloride

The analgesic effect of dextropropoxyphene is considerably less than that of codeine. Chemically it is structurally related to methadone but it possesses less analgesic, antitussive and dependency properties. The main use of dextropropoxyphene is as a compound analgesia with aspirin (doloxene).

Pharmacokinetics

Dextropropoxyphene is rapidly absorbed in the gastrointestinal tract and metabolized within the liver. In the event of an overdose the rapid absorption of dextropropoxyphene is able to produce respiratory arrest, hypotension and cardiac dysrhythmia within one hour.

High Efficacy Opioids

Buprenorphine (Temgesic)

This opioid can be useful because of the length (six hours) and strength of its analgesic properties. It also possesses both opioid agonist and antagonist qualities. It is therefore less likely to produce addiction, respiratory depression or affect cardiovascular function than other opioid analgesics.

Pharmacokinetics

Administered sublingually; if swallowed buprenorphine is metabolized within the liver and possesses a half life of five hours.

Dextromoramide (Palfium)

A derivative of the opium poppy, dextromoramide is a powerful quick acting analgesia which has been prescribed in Britain since the 1950s for severe and intractable pain. In relation to morphine it has a shorter duration of action and is less sedating. Therefore it is able to produce pain relief without affecting consciousness, mental activity or inducing constipation unlike other opioids.

   Concomitant administration of tranquillizers such as clopromazine produces a synergistic analgesic effect.

Pharmacokinetics

Taken orally dextromoromide is quickly absorbed and metabolized within the liver. It is short acting with a duration of approximately three hours.

Diamorphine Hydrochloride

Introduced 100 years ago diamorphine is indicated for both severe and chronic pain. It is a powerful opioid analgesia and is a derivative of the unripe seed pod of the opium poppy. Although diamorphine mirrors morphine in both its actions and uses it is able to produce enhanced pain relief with less adverse effects such as nausea or hypotension.

Pharmacokinetics

Following administration diamorphine is rapidly converted into monoacetyl morphine and more slowly metabolized into its main active metabolite morphine. Within 24 hours approximately 80% of the dose is excreted via the urine.

Fentanyl

Fentanyl is more efficacious than morphine. It is normally administered as an intra-operative analgesic. Fentanyl can also be used for chronic pain in the form of a patch for transdermal drug delivery (Durogesic). This mode of administration possesses the ability to maintain its efficacy for 72 hours.

Morphine

Derived from opium and in use since the last century morphine is prescribed for moderate to severe pain in both acute and chronic conditions. Morphine acts on the CNS to eliminate pain and it also possesses the ability to transform the unpleasant sensation of pain into a sense of euphoria. Morphine therefore has two major effects, one depressing, the other stimulating (Trouce and Gould, 1990).

The 'depressing' effects of morphine can include:

- Reduction of the appreciation of pain
- Suppression of respirations and the cough reflex
- Reduction of anxiety and inducing the feeling of euphoria
- Some levels of sedation (due to its mildly hypnotic properties)
- Reduction of the peristaltic activities of the bowel
- Urinary retention.

The stimulant effects of morphine can include:

- Increased arousal of the chemoreceptor trigger zone within the brain stem including nausea and vomiting.
- Increased arousal of the vagus nerve which may produce such effects as brady-cardia and hypotension, owing to a parasympathic action in the cardiovascular system (Trouce and Gould, 1990)

Morphine works on specific opioid receptors situated throughout the body. Such receptors are divided into categories and include delta, kappa and mu receptors. It is the mu receptor on which morphine has its main effects. Mu receptors are associated with analgesia, respiratory depression, euphoria and dependance (Walker, 1994). The pharmacological effects of morphine on each individual will differ considerably (Rowbotham, 1993).

Pharmacokinetics

Following oral administration morphine is absorbed from the gastrointestinal tract where is undergoes conjugation in the gut wall and liver with approximately 20% of the dose actually reaching the systemic circulation. Elimination of the majority of morphine is via the kidneys in the urine. Subcutaneous and intramuscular administration is quicker than oral administration. Drug interactions and adverse effects are shown in Tables 2.3 and 2.4.

Pethidine Hydrochloride

Akin to morphine, pethidine provides rapid pain relief for short durations of time. Prescribed inappropriately it can be addictive.

Tramadol Hydrochloride (Zydol)

Tramadol can enhance both serotonenergic and adrenergic pathways. It is considered equal to morphine regarding its efficacy when prescribed for moderate chronic pain but is less likely to cause respiratory depression, addiction or constipation than

Table 2.3   Drug interactions of opioids.

Alcohol: enhances the sedative and hypotensive efects
Antidepressants: may result in CNS excitement or depression
Antipsychotics: enhance the sedative and hypotensive effects
Anxiolytics and hypnotics: enhance the sedative effect
Antihistamines; enhance the sedative effects
Cisparide: may antagonize the effect of gastrointestinal motility
Ulcer healing drugs: may increase plasma concentrations of opiods
Antiemetics: antagonize the effects of gastrointestinal activity

Table 2.4   Adverse effects of opioids.

Nausea and vomiting
Constipation
Respiratory depression
Hypotension
Dry mouth
Micturition difficulties
Bradycardia/tachycardia
Hallucinations
Mood changes
Addition
Reduced libido

morphine. Tramadol has been shown to reduce NSAID consumption and relieve pain in osteoarthritis of the knee (Brant, 2004). It is also available in combination with paracetamol.

Pharmacokinetics

Administered orally tramadol is quickly absorbed from the gastrointestinal tract. It possesses a half life of six hours. Tramadol is excreted in the urine and approximately a third of the dose is excreted unchanged.

ANTIDEPRESSANT DRUGS

Antidepressant therapy may enhance the analgesic effect induced by other drugs. The presumed site of action is at the spinal cord level. Although there is a beneficial effect on sleep and mood, suggesting action elsewhere in the neuroaxis, debate continues over possible modes of action and whether or not these drugs induce analgesia in the absence of depression in chronic pain generally (Watson, 1994).

Serotonin uptake inhibitors: These drugs block the reuptake of serotonin. The commonest ones used in clinical practice are fluoxetine, paroxetine and sertraline. They should be avoided in patients with epilepsy, cardiac disease, diabetes mellitus and glaucoma. They may cause drowsiness and abrupt withdrawal can cause a variety of side effects (Bird, 2004).

Tricyclic drugs: The increased incidence of anxiety and depression amongst chronic pain sufferers is not the only justification put forward for the use of tricyclic drugs. They also appear to have a synergistic effect with centrally acting analgesia and the stimulation of endorphine production (Brown and Bottomley, 1990).

Amitriptyline is of proven efficacy (Carrette *et al.*, 1994). It is taken in small incremental doses of 10−50 mg, two hours prior to settling at night to avoid the hypnotic effect. Sleep usually improves within two weeks whilst pain relief may take many months. Common side effects include dry mouth and palpitations. Dothiepin has been shown to be of comparable effect in controlled studies (Caruso, Sarzi Puttini and Bocassini, 1987).

Venlafaxine, an inhibitor of both serotonin and noradrenaline re-uptake, has been shown to be useful in the treatment of fibromyalgia (Dwight *et al.*, 1998).

Pregabalin is of proven benefit in the treatment of neuropathic pain (Mease *et al.*, 2003) and has also been shown to improve sleep quality and diminish fatigue.

NON-STEROIDAL ANTI-INFLAMMATORY DRUGS

NSAIDs have become an integral part of the management of inflammatory conditions. The ultimate goal of NSAIDs therapy is to reduce the inflammation that is occurring. The decision to commence therapy will include consideration of the risks weighted against the potential for therapeutic benefit for the patient and will take into account the nature of the underlying condition and the severity of the patient's symptoms.

The objective of commencing NSAIDs is to decrease the cardinal symptoms of inflammation which include pain, stiffness, swelling and warmth. These symptoms are not only unpleasant for the patient but also affect physical and psychological functioning. In addition to reducing inflammation this group of drugs also possesses analgesic and anti-pyretic properties, which are necessary to treat the associated features of inflammation. The effectiveness of NSAIDs should be evident within a few days and make an almost immediate impression on the patient's symptoms. The therapy will continue to be effective as long as blood levels of the drug are maintained. If a patient stops taking this therapy for any reason, this action could result in a reoccurrence of the symptoms of inflammation. Although the patient will start to feel better once the features of inflammation are reduced this therapy will not influence the progression of conditions such as RA.

Classification of NSAIDs

The NSAIDs can be classified on the basis of their chemical structure. The older NSAIDs – for example, Indomethian – have excellent anti-inflammatory properties but commonly produce adverse side effects especially on the gastrointestinal system, whereas agents such as the propionic acid derivatives have less likelihood of causing side effects and are generally better tolerated. The chemical classification of the NSAIDs is shown in Table 2.5.

Which NSAIDs to Use?

The choice between the various NSAIDs is largely empirical (Schlegal, 1987). There is a wide individual variability of response (Thompson and Dunne, 1995). The cause for this variability is not known. If a patient experiences a poor response to one NSAID another agent should be tried. There can be a variation in response even when the NSAID is from the same chemical family. Once a NSAID is commenced the patient should be maintained on it for two weeks before an assessment of its efficacy is made, unless the patient experiences an adverse reaction. The ultimate goal of NSAIDs intervention is to choose a preparation that combines the greatest

Table 2.5 Chemical classification of NSAIDs.

Types of NSAID	Examples
Carboxylic acids	aspirin, choline, salicylate, diflunisal
Acetic acids	indometacin, diclofenac, etodaloc
Propionoc acids	brufen, fluribiprofen, fenbrufen, fenoprofen, ketoprofen, tiaprofenic acid
Fenamic acids	piroxicam, phenylbutazone, azapropazone, tenoxicam
Non-acidic compounds	nabumetone
COX 2 inhibitors	rofecoxib, celecoxib

effectiveness with the least toxicity for each individual patient (Schlegal, 1987). There is significant co-morbidity associated with NSAID use (Moore, 2003) and the clinician needs to balance the benefits against the risks proir to prescribing NSAID therapy.

NSAIDs can be divided into two groups according to their half life. Those drugs with a half life of greater than 12 hours – for example, piroxicam, tenoxicam and azapropazone – need only to be administered once or twice daily, which should aid concordance; although it should be noted that these medications with a long half life may build up excessively in the plasma of older patients increasing the potential for the occurrence of side effects. The majority of other NSAIDs are referred to as short half life drugs as their half life is usually less than six hours.

The Administration of NSAIDs

NSAIDs can be administered in many different ways, including by slow release compounds, topically, intramuscularly and in suppository form.

Topical preparations – These are only available for a few NSAIDs. They are more efficacious than placebo (Thompson and Dunne, 1995). Local skin sensitivity may occur and there is some absorption into the circulation leading to the rare occurrence of systemic side effects.

Suppositories are rarely used but do reduce the risk of gastric irritation by the direct effect of the drug on the mucosa. However, there is still a risk (although reduced) of gastric ulceration mediated via the circulation. NSAIDs given in suppository form can also cause local irritation in the rectum. Patients can also find them difficult to administer especially if they have reduced manual dexterity.

Patients at Risk from Gastrointestinal Problems

In patients with peptic ulcers disease NSAIDs are contraindicated. If a patient is at risk from GI symptoms the clinician will often prescribing gastric cytoprotection in the form of proton pump inhibitors for example, omeprazole and lansoprazole. These drugs inhibit the gastric acid by blocking the hydrogen–potassium adenosine triphosphatase enzyme system (the proton pump) of the gastric parietal cell. They are the treatment of choice for stricturing and erosive oesophagititis and are effective in the short-term treatments of gastric and duodenal ulcers.

Indicators for the Use of NSAIDs

In chronic inflammatory rheumatology conditions such as RA, ankylosing spondylitis, psoriatic arthritis and connective tissue disorders (with polyarthritis), patients may well have to take NSAIDs on a regular basis to provide symptomatic relief from the effects of ongoing inflammation. If the patient experiences a reduction in disease activity they may no longer need regular administration of the NSAID therapy and a trial will establish whether this is the case.

Patients with OA are better managed on simple analgesia. In the older patient the risk of side effects can outweigh the potential therapeutic effects of a NSAID, although their use may be considered if they experience a flare of inflammatory symptoms. Here the use of NSAID would be considered short term for symptom relief. Other conditions where it may be appropriate to use NSAIDs on a short-term basis include: gout, pseudogout and certain sport injuries.

Mode of Action of NSAIDs

NSAIDs appear to be involved in many of the pathways that are influential in the production of inflammatory mediators as well as actively involved in the interactions between inflammatory cells. NSAIDs are known to play a role in the suppression of prostaglandin synthesis partly by inhibiting the enzyme prostaglandin synthetase H (also known as cyclo-oxygenase). Prostaglandins are synthesized from membrane phospholipids; when induced they act to produce many of the features of inflammation including warmth, erythema and oedema. NSAIDs have effects on various other aspects of the inflammatory response including leukotriene synthesis, superoxide production and cytokine production (see Figure 2.2).

The suppression of prostaglandins by NSAIDs may help relieve the symptoms of inflammation but this suppression is also responsible for the major adverse effects of NSAIDs including gastrointestinal disturbances and effects on kidney functioning (Brooks, 1994; Flowers, 1996).

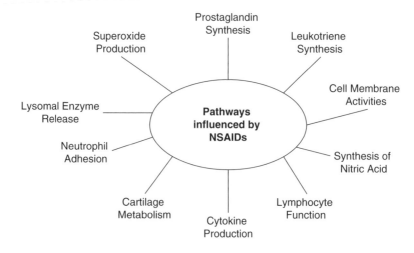

Figure 2.2 Pathways influenced by NSAIDs.

Pharmacokinetics

Most NSAIDs are completely absorbed from the gastrointestinal tract. They bind strongly to plasma proteins and are predominately cleared by the liver. The metabolites are excreted in the urine. Some NSAIDs are absorbed in the active form whilst others, referred to as pro-drugs, are converted by hepatic metabolism to active drugs.

Cyclo-Oxygenase 2 Inhibitors

Cyclo-oxygenase-2 (COX-2) inhibitors are a selective type of non-steroidal anti-inflammatory drug (NSAID). They were developed to reduce the gastrointestinal side effects of traditional NSAIDs. Although COX-2 inhibitors are as effective as traditional NSAIDs in relieving pain (Bombardier et al., 2000) serious concerns about their cardiovascular safety have arisen. COX-2 plays a beneficial role in vascular health and its inhibition may create an imbalance between thromboxane and prostacyclin. Thromboxane is critical for platelet aggregation and vasoconstriction, and prostacyclin dampens the effects of thromboxane through fibrinolysis and vasodilation (Solomon, 2005). Other mechanisms linking coxibs (or NSAIDs) to cardiovascular events include hypertension from inhibition of prostagalandin-dependent counterregulatory mechanisms and COX-independent oxidative stress.

Concerns with trials regarding the safety of COX-2 inhibitors:

- Most trials have excluded patients with coronary heart disease (Topol and Falk 2004), and patients taking aspirin, and there has been no consensus regarding cardiovascular outcomes/endpoints.
- Trials have been of short duration and not included enough people to observe the incident of cardiovascular events and consequently studies have been unable to demonstrate whether the risk of cardiovascular events associated with coxibs is concentrated in certain subgroups of patients (Solomon, 2005).

Research Findings

- The Adenomatous Polyp Prevention on Vioxx trial examined rofecoxib 25 mg daily against placebo among 2586 patients with a prior adenomatous polyp (Bresalier et al., 2005). Seventeen per cent were taking daily aspirin at the commencement of the study. Patients taking rofecoxib experienced a 4.61 increase in the risk of congestive cardiac failure. Severe thrombotic cardiovascular events including acute myocardial infarction, peripheral arterial thrombosis, peripheral venous thromboisis and pulmonary embolus occurred twice as often in patients taking rofecoxib compared to patients on placebo. In 2005 rofecoxib was withdrawn because of its adverse cardiovascualar profile.
- The Adenoma Prevention with Celecoxib trial demonstrated that high dose long-term celecoxib use was associated with an increase in the risk of thrombotic

events. The aspirin user subgroup did not experience a lower risk of cardiovascular events than those not using aspirin. Also patients taking aspirin do not experience a reduced risk of GI toxicity while taking coxibs compared with nonselective NSAIDs (Farkouh *et al.*, 2004). The FDA has requested that the manufacturers of all NSAIDs including celecoxib include a warning highlighting the potential cardiovascular risks of these agents.

- Trials of patients receiving valdecoxib undergoing coronary artery bypass grafting (Nussmeier *et al.*, 2005; Ott *et al.*, 2003) have shown an increased risk of cardiovascular events. The risk ratio for confirmed cardiovascular events was 3.7 when the valdecoxib group was compared with the double placebo group (Nussmeier *et al.*, 2005). In April 2005 the FDA requested that valdecoxib's manufacturer withdraw the drug from the US market based on insufficient long-term cardiovascular safety data, evidence of an increased cardiovascular risk in short-term studies amongst patients undergoing heart surgery, the risk of life-threatening skin reactions and no proven advantages over other NSAIDs (Solomon, 2005).

Prescribing Advice Regarding the Use of COX-2 Inhibitors

- COX-2 inhibitors must not be used in patients with established ischaemic heart disease and /or cerebrovascular disease (stroke) or in patients with peripheral arterial disease.
- Healthcare professionals should exercise caution when presecribing COX-2 inhibitors to patients with risk factors for heart disease such as hypertension, hyperlipidaemia, diabetes and smoking.
- Given the association between cardiovascular risk and exposure to COX-2 inhibitors, prescribers are advised to use the lowest effective dose for the shortest possible duration of treatment.
- Skin reactions can occur with all COX-2 inhibitors. In the majority of cases these occur in the first month of use and patients with a history of drug allergies may be at greatest risk.

Side Effects of NSAIDs

In general the NSAIDs share a common spectrum of side effects although the frequency of particular side effects varies between different compounds. Mild adverse effects are relatively common, occurring in approximately 10−15% of users. Due to the fact that these drugs are prescribed in large numbers worldwide, a significant number of people will experience more serious side effects. The major side effects occur in several organ systems. These include:

- the gastrointestinal tract
- the central nervous system
- cardiovascular

- the haematopoetic system
- the kidney
- the skin
- the liver.

Gastrointestinal Tract

The gastrointestinal tract is the system most commonly affected by NSAIDs and often necessitates discontinuation of therapy. Symptoms patients may experience include dyspepsia, epigastric pain, indigestion, nausea and vomiting. Gastrointestinal lesions may range from hypermia to diffuse gastritis, erosions or ulcers.

Factors associated with increased risk of ulceration include:

- Age (over 65 years)
- Previous peptic ulcer disease
- Concomitant steroid therapy
- Heart failure
- High dose NSAIDs.

Low dose ibuprofen appears to be associated with a low risk of upper gastrointestinal symptoms. Diclofenac, naproxen and indomethacin are associated with intermediate risk of adverse events and azapropazone is associated with the highest risk. If patients are experiencing adverse reactions it will be necessary to carry out an endoscopy to assess any irritation or ulceration in the tract. All patients are advised to take NSAIDs with food.

Kidney

The synthesis of renal prostaglandins is simulated by vasoconstrictor substances involved in circulating haemostasis such as angiotensin II, norepinephrine and vasopressin. By modulating the effects of these vasoconstrictor substances on the kidney, vasodilatory prostoglandin — especially prostaglandin E2 and prostacyclin — helps to maintain adequate renal blood flow and glomeruler filtration rate. This modulatory effect plays a minor role in controlling renal function in healthy individuals but under circumstances of circulating stress the prostaglandins become essential to the maintenance of adaquate renal function. In this situation treatment with cyclo-oxygenase inhibitors such as NSAIDs may precipitate acute renal failure.

Patients at risk from NSAID-induced renal insufficiency include those with:

- congestive heart failure
- cirrhosis with ascites
- neprotic syndrome
- age (over 60 yrs)
- concurrent diuretic therapy (that causes potassium retension).

Renal side effects from NSAIDs appear to be dose-related and occur more often in older people (Thompson and Dunne, 1995). NSAIDs can also affect the salt and water balance causing sodium retension which may result in hypertension, oedema or heart failure in predisposed individuals.

Drugs such as tiaprofenic acid have also been associated with cystitis. Acute interstial nephritis and nephrotic syndrome have been linked with naproxen, indomethacin, phenylbutazone, fenoprofen and diflunisal. The pathogenesis is unknown.

Hypersensitivity phenomena may also be present with nephrotic syndrome including fever, skin rash and eosinophilia.

Central Nervous System

Cognitive dysfunction, memory loss, inability to concentrate, confusion, personality change, forgetfulness, depression, sleeplessness and paranoid thoughts have all been reported in older patients treated with naproxen and ibuprofen (Goodwin and Regan, 1982).

Headaches and dizziness may occur with indomethacin. Aspirin can affect hearing and cause tinnitus.

Several of the NSAIDs have been associated with aseptic meningitis − for example, ibuprofen and sulindec (Schlegal, 1987). Patients with collagen diseases seem to be at the highest risk from the complication.

Cardiovascular

An increased risk of myocardial infarction was found in patients taking diclofenac and ibuprofen in an observational study (Hippisley-Cox and Coupland, 2005). For ibuprofen, one additional myocardial infarction would happen for every 1005 patients aged 65 and over, and for diclofenac one additional myocardial infarction for every 521 treated patients (Hippisley-Cox and Coupland, 2005). Ray *et al.* (2002) reported an increased risk of acute myocardial infarction associated with the use of ibuprofen in a high risk population over the age of 50. Patients taking diclofenac had a 55% increased risk of myocardial infarction, which is similar to that reported in a much smaller study of non-selective NSAIDs in patients with RA from the general practice database (Watson *et al.*, 2002). There have been suggestions that naproxen has a protective cardiovascular effect but this has not been shown in a meta analysis (Juni *et al.*, 2004). The potential for NSAIDs to cause other cardiovascular events including hypertension is well recognized (Solomon, 2005). At present the Committee on the Safety of Medicines has concluded that there is insufficient evidence to change practice on non-selective non-steroid anti-inflammatory drugs. It advises that prescribing should be based on the overall safety profiles of NSAIDs and individual risk factors. Patients should take the lowest effective dose of NSAIDs or COX-2 inhibitors for the shortest time necessary.

Haematological Reactions

The most common reaction is iron deficiency anaemia as a result of gastrointestinal blood loss that occurs secondary to erosion or ulceration. Blood dyscracies associated with NSAIDs therapy are rare but among the major causes of death with this therapy. Agranulocytosis, thrombocytopenia, neutropenia and aplastic anaemia have all been reported. The latter is very rare except with phenylbutazone, the administration of which is limited to hospital prescriptions in the United Kingdom.

Inhibitors of platelet aggregation by NSAIDs may cause a mild prolongation of the bleeding time in patients. This becomes a particular concern for those patients receiving anticoagulation therapy or those who have hereditory clotting factor deficiencies.

Liver

NSAIDs can cause a transient rise in liver enzymes and more rarely a hepatic illness such as hepatitis. Older patients with a reduced renal function and receiving high dose NSAID therapy are at greatest risk of adverse liver reactions.

Respiratory System

NSAIDs may precipitate asthmatic attacks in predisposed individuals. In some patients with bronchial asthma the inhibitor of cyclo-oxygenase may reduce bronchodilatory prostaglandins. This diverts arachidonic acid metabolism towards lipoxygenase products (leukotrienes). This activity may precipitate bronchospasm.

Pulmonary effects including effusions have been reported with ibuprofen, naproxen and phenylbutazone therapy.

Skin

All NSAIDs can provoke skin reactions including photosensitivity, vesiculobullous eruptions, serum sickness and exfoliative erythroderma. Urticaria has been reported with aspirin, ibuprofen and indomethacin.

Phenylbutazone and oxyphenbutazone are the NSAIDs that have the highest incidence of serious or fatal skin reactions including erythema multiforme, exofoliative dermatitis, Stevens–Johnson syndrome and toxic epidermal reaction.

Cultaneous vasculitis is a rare occurrence but has been related to the use of indomethacin, fenbrufen and naproxen.

Pregnancy

The inhibitor of prostaglandins synthesis by NSAIDs during pregnancy may cause prolongation of gestation and increase post-partum and neonatal bleeding. NSAIDs should be avoided during pregnancy especially as they may promote premature closure of the ductus arteriosus and impair fetal circulation.

Drug Interactions

The major interactions that occur with the administration of NSAIDs are shown below. For safe practice, consult the manufacturer's guidelines before advocating usage.

- Anticoagulant therapy may be enhanced.
- Antidepressant therapy − for example, moclobemide − can acclerate the absorption of NSAIDs.
- Cardioglycosides. The plasma concentration of cardiac glycoside can be increased, exacerbating heart failure.
- Diuretics. There is an increased risk of nephrotoxicity and a possible risk of hyperkalaemia associated with potassium sparing diuretics.
- Lithium. There is an increased risk of toxicity.
- Muscle relaxants − for example, baclofen. There is an increased risk of toxicity.
- ACE inhibitors. There is an increased risk of renal damage and an antagonistic hypotensive effect.
- Beta blockers. NSAIDS are antagonistic of hypotensive effects.
- Cytotoxic agents. There is a reduction in the excretion of these agents. The potential interaction between NSAIDs and low dose methotrexate is not a problem at the dose used in patients with RA (Thompson and Dunne, 1995).
- Uricosurics − for example, probenecid. These drugs increase the plasma concentration of many NSAIDs and delay their excretion.
- Anti-epileptic drugs may be enhanced.

Interactions with Specific NSAIDs

- Brufen − can increase digoxin levels.
- Fenoprofen − its half life may be reduced following the co-administration of barbiturates − for example, phenobarbitone.
- Ketoprofen − this may increase the level of sulfonamides in the blood.
- Indomethacin − increases the bioavailability of biophosphates.
- Diclofenac − the plasma concentration can be increased if taken with ciclosporin.
- Azapropazone − this may interfere with the action of oral hypoglycaemic drugs. Also the plasma concentration of azapropazone may increase with the administration of cimetidine.

The administration of two or more NSAIDs will increase the risk of adverse effects occurring.

Appendix 2.A entitled 'What happens next' contains case scenarios of patients in whom it may or may not be appropriate to prescribe a NSAID. What would your decision be?

2.3   DISEASE-MODIFYING ANTI-RHEUMATIC DRUGS (DMARDs)

USE OF DMARDs

A number of agents can be used to control rheumatological disorders, particularly RA. Their terminology can be confusing as they are known as either slow-acting anti-rheumatic drugs (SAARDs), second line therapies or disease-modifying anti-rheumatic drugs (DMARDs). In this chapter they will be known as DMARDs.

EARLY TREATMENT OF RA

Historically the pharmacological interventions for patients with early RA were guided by the pyramidal approach.

This approach dictated that initial drug interventions were limited to NSAIDs and analgesics which aimed to modify the symptoms of the disease process; hence these drugs were referred to as either symptom modifying drugs or first line therapies, and only when radiological evidence of erosions had been confirmed were DMARDs introduced in the therapeutic regime.

However, within the past decade, a consensus of opinion has existed which challenges the traditional pyramidal approach and advocates that DMARDs should be prescribed earlier in the disease process and prior to, rather than following, any structural damage; thus minimizing the disease activity quickly and effectively. The following factors suggest therefore that the pyramidal approach should be inverted:

- There is evidence that joint destruction and concurrent functional disability occurs within the first 12 months of the disease process (Van de Heij de *et al.*, 1992). Therefore it is suggested that irreversible destruction of both cartilage and bone, resulting in functional disability, rapidly occurs within the early stages of the disease process, despite the fact that RA is a chronic progressive disease. Consequently it is suggested that the optimum time to introduce DMARDs to gain control or modify the disease process is when the patient initially presents (Donnelly, Scott and Emery, 1992). Also, functional deterioration will occur if patients remain untreated (Deodhar *et al.*, 1995; Gough *et al.*, 1994).
- In comparison with the general population, patients with RA experience increased morbidity and reduced life-expectancy, which has implications not only for the individual patient (pain, disability and loss of self-esteem), but also on society in general relating to loss of earnings, state payments and healthcare costs.

The efficacy of DMARDs in RA proves difficult to validate due to:

- the inconsistency of the disease process;
- the individual response to DMARDs;
- the potential for concurrent toxic side effects.

The limited effectiveness of DMARDs may be attributed to the discontinuation of DMARD therapies because adverse effects are experienced by the patient, rather than inefficacy of the DMARD themselves.

COMBINATION THERAPY

Combination therapy (i.e. the use of more than one DMARD) has evolved due to several factors:

- The long-term efficacy of a single DMARD regimen has revealed disappointing results.
- The change in philosophy entailing a more aggressive treatment regimen in an attempt to gain disease remission as early as possible.

The aim of combination therapy is to achieve a synergistic effect using two or more DMARDs in order to arrest the disease process and to achieve disease remission with minimal adverse reactions. Combination therapy can be implemented either by:

- a step up regimen where one DMARD is initially prescribed and a second DMARD added if disease remission is not achieved;
- a step down approach may be prescribed; this entails the initial treatment regimen of multiple DMARDs until disease suppression is achieved, then the number of DMARDs can be reduced.

Initially combination therapy research studies have targeted patients with established aggressive uncontrolled RA. However, in order to achieve maximum benefits for the maximum of patients, research studies have been extended to include early RA patients (Haagsma, van de Putte and van Riel, 1995).

MODE OF ACTION AND PHARMACOKINETICES OF DMARDs

Although DMARDs have different chemical structures, they all possess common properties:

- To control the signs and symptoms of RA, which include certain blood parameters denoting inflammation, painful swollen inflamed joints and sometimes slowing down the progression of radiological damage (Donnelly, Scott and Emery, 1992).
- Their effectiveness is delayed, thus a therapeutic response tends to occur for approximately two to four months.
- All DMARDs (excluding the antimalarials) have the potential to cause adverse effects, which include serious haematological toxicity. Consequently the incidence of adverse effects, which may be major or minor, presents a major constraint on the continual use of these agents, so much so that approximately 20–50% of patients will have to stop their DMARD within one year of

commencement. The safety monitoring required in the surveillance of DMARDs is discussed in depth in Chapter 3.
Their mechanism of action is poorly understood.

THE ANTI-MALARIALS

Chloroquine Sulfate/Hydroxychloroquine Sulfate

Hydroxychloroquine and chloroquine are two drugs that were principally prescribed for both the treatment and prophylaxis of malaria. However, since the 1950s, research studies have revealed the efficacy of both hydroxychloroquine and chloroquine as disease-modifying anti-rheumatic drugs (DMARDs) in the treatment of rheumatoid arthritis and systemic lupus erythematosus (Brooks, 1990). Because of their low toxicity profiles, hydroxychloroquine sulfate and chloroquine sulfate are rated as milder DMARDs, which may be prescribed independently or in combination with other DMARDs when only partial efficacy is achieved. An interesting property of hydroxychloroquine, when used in combination with methotrexate, is its protective mechanism against methotrexate-induced hepatotoxicity.

Indications for Use

- active RA;
- juvenile arthritis;
- systemic and discoid lupus erythematosus.

Treatment Regime

Hydroxychloroquine orally 200–400 mg daily with food. The dosage may be reduced to 200 mg daily depending on the clinical response. Maximum dose should not exceed 6.5 mg/kg body weight per day.
Chloroquine orally 250 mg daily with food.

Cautions

- patients with renal and liver impairment;
- it may reduce the threshold for convulsions in patients with epilepsy;
- it may exacerbate psoriasis;
- avoid antacids within four hours of administration.

Contraindications

- breastfeeding;
- pre-existing maculopathy.

Retinal Effect

It is generally agreed that retinal toxicity is due not to the cumulative dose but to the daily dose. Therefore, the maximum prescription limit for adults should be 4 mg/kg/day for chloroquine and 6 mg/kg/day for hydroxychloroquine(Day, 1994).

To prevent potential toxicity, individual physicians' regimen may differ; therefore patients may be prescribed hydroxychloroquine or chloroquine for 5 days of the week or for 7 days a week for 11 months of the year with a 1-month 'drug holiday'. The 'drug holiday' will also allow the clinician to test the efficacy of the drug.

Before commencing treatment the patient should be asked about visual impairment that is not corrected by glasses. The visual acuity of each eye should be recorded using a reading chart. Treatment should only be commenced if there is no abnormality.

The Royal College of Ophthamologists recommends annual review either by an optometrist or enquiring about visual symptoms, rechecking visual acuity and assessing for blurred vision using the reading chart. Patients should be advised to report any visual disturbance. The treatment should be stopped if there is any development of blurred visison or changes in visual acuity. If patients are requiring long-term treatment (more than five years) it should be discussed with an ophthalmologist.

Mode of Action

The mode of action of both hydroxychloroquine and chloroquine remains unknown, although research studies have suggested that antimalarials affect subcellular organelles such as polymorphs, lymphocytes and macrophages, which produce an anti-rheumatic and immunosuppressive reaction (Brooks, 1990).

Pharmacokinetics

To avoid gastrointestinal disturbances, hydroxychloroquine and chloroquine should be administered with food. Food is not thought to affect bioavailability.

Hydroxychloroquine and chloroquine accumulate extensively in tissues, and both white and red blood cells.

These medications possess above average half lives (approximately six weeks); steady concentrations are not achieved for approximately three to four months.

Metabolized primarily by dealkylation and thus high renal clearance, approximately 40% of chloroquine and 25% of hydroxychloroquine are excreted unchanged in the urine; therefore therapeutic regimens should be adjusted to accommodate those patients with renal impairment.

Adverse Effects

- nausea;
- diarrhoea;

- abdominal pain;
- headaches;
- dizziness;
- convulsions;
- blurred vision;
- irreversible retinal damage;
- skin reactions (rashes, pruritis);
- depigmentation or loss of hair;
- ECG changes;
- rarely blood disorders (thrombocytopenia, agranulocytosis, aplastic anaemia) (Brooks, 1990).

Contraindications

Psoriatic arthritis (may exacerbate psoriasis).

SULFASALAZINE

Prescribed for patients with early RA, and in combination with other DMARDs, sulfasalazine has also been found to have some efficacy when treating sero-negative spondyloarthropathies, juvenile arthritis and psoriatic arthritis (Day, 1994). Developed in the 1930s when RA was thought to possess an infective aetiology (Porter and Capell, 1990), sulfasalazine contains the combination of an anti-inflammatory agent (5-aminosalicylic acid) and an antibiotic (sulfapyridine). However, as a result of early conflicting reports regarding the efficacy of sulfasalazine, the drug was originally dismissed by rheumatologists until the 1970s when further studies revealed its efficacy.

Mode of Action

The precise mode of action of sulfasalazine is unknown but it is thought that sulfasalazine in some way suppresses relevant immunological processes in the large bowel and, in addition, sulfasalazine possesses the ability to scavenge pro-inflammatory oxygen species released from activated phagocytes (Day, 1994).

Pharmacokinetics

Following oral administration the majority of the dose is absorbed in the large bowel where it reacts with colonic bacteria and separates into 5-aminosalicylic acid and sulfapyridine. Elimination is via the kidneys in the urine.

D-PENICILLAMINE

Used in the treatment of RA for 25 years, D-penicillamine has also been useful in treating progressive systemic sclerosis as well as unrelated rheumatological conditions such as Wilson's disease, heavy metal poisoning and cystinuria.

Studies have revealed D-penicillamine to be effective in the reduction of joint inflammation, joint pain, early morning stiffness, laboratory inflammation indices and the improvements of rheumatoid nodules (Joyce, 1990). However, due to a lack of controlled studies, it has not been possible to determine if D-penicillamine is able to slow progressive radiological damage (Joyce, 1990).

Mode of Action

For the past 25 years the precise mode of action and toxicilogy of D-penicillamine has remained elusive, although it is thought to suppress the immune system (Joyce, 1990).

Pharmacokinetics

D-penicillamine is taken orally one to two hours before food; following absorption, peak plasma levels are present within one to four hours.

MYOCRISIN

Initially introduced and prescribed earlier in the twentieth century for the treatment of tuberculosis, gold salts were found to be of little value but were found to be efficacious for the treatment of RA. In the treatment of RA, myocrisin (injectable gold) has been shown to impede progressive radiological damage and concomitant fuctional impairment in both short- and medium-term treatment.

Mode of Action

To date there is no consensus regarding the precise mode of action of intramuscular gold although it is known to regulate gene transcription and affect polymorphonuclear and synovial cells, monocytes, lymphocytes and immunoglobins (Champion, Graham and Ziegler, 1990; Day, 1994).

Pharmacokinetics

Intramuscular gold is polymeric and water soluble and therefore not absorbed orally. Following intramuscular injection, absorption takes place quickly and gold travels to synovial tissue where it binds to inflamed synovial tissues; consequently the majority of gold is located in the synovial lining cells. Elimination of gold is initially rapid and largely in the urine. However, gold has been detected in tissues some 20 years after therapy.

AURANOFIN

Introduced in the last decade auranofin is a gold-based drug that can be taken orally. Although considered less efficacious than sodium aurothiomalate, auranofin possesses fewer serious side effects. The same is true when auranofin has been compared with D-penicillamine and methotrexate (Champion, Graham and Ziegler, 1990).

Mode of Action

Akin to sodium aurothiomalate, precise mode of action remains elusive.

Pharmacokinetics

Following oral administration of auranofin absorption is rapid but incomplete as only 20–25% of the gold is absorbed (Blocka *et al.* 1982), approximately 15% is then excreted via the kidneys but the majority of gold is excreted in the faeces and consists of both unabsorbed gold and gold that has been absorbed in the gastrointestinal tract and bound to gastric epithelium (Champion, Graham and Ziegler, 1990, Day, 1994).

METHOTREXATE

Initially introduced 50 years ago for the treatment of acute leukaemia, methotrexate is classed as one of the first antimetabolites. The introduction of methotrexate as a treatment for RA took place in the 1950s. However, it was to be some 30 years later, in the 1980s, before methotrexate was used widely by rheumatologists for the treatment of RA and psoriatic arthritis. It is now the commonest DMARD used in the treatment of RA (Cronstein, 1996). It is prescribed as monotherapy and in combination with other DMARDs and biological agents.

Mode of Action

Methotrexate is a cytotoxic drug which acts as a folate antagonist to cause cell death by affecting the synthesis of DNA. However, its precise mode of action in the treatment RA is not entirely understood.

Pharmacokinetics

Following administration (oral or intramuscular), methotrexate is absorbed rapidly and almost entirely, taking one to two hours before a peak concentration is achieved. The majority of methotrexate is excreted via the kidneys, and biliary elimination is suggested to account for approximately 10–30% of methotrexate (Songsiridej and Furst, 1990).

LEFLUNOMIDE

Leflunomide is one of the newer DMARDs that has proven efficacy and safety in randomized controlled trials (Smolen *et al.*, 1999). It appears as effective as sulfasalazine and methotrexate as a monotherapy and can also be used as combination therapy usually with methotrexate or infliximab (Flendrie *et al.*, 2005). It may have a faster onset of action in reducing synovial vascularity (Maddison *et al.*, 2005).

Mode of Action

It is an isoxazole derivate and its active metabolite inhibits *de novo* pyrimidine synthesis, resulting in inhibition of T cell proliferation.

Pharmacokinetics

Leflunomide has a long elimination half life of 15−18 days, which results from low hepatic clearance and enterohepatic cycling (Flendrie *et al.*, 2005). Its active metabolite is detectable in plasma up to two years after discontinuation of the drug. If a severe adverse event occurs a washout of the drug may need to be considered using oral cholestyramine, 8 mg three times daily for 11 days.

AZATHIOPRINE

Azathioprine is a cytotoxic immunosuppressant drug, originally prescribed to prevent the rejection of transplanted organs. It has also proved to be efficacious in the treatment of RA, vasculitis, systemic lupus erythematosus, polymyalgia rheumatica/giant cell arteritis, Behçet's disease, polymyositis, dermatomyositis, myasthenia gravis and chronic inflammatory bowel disease.

Mode of Action

The precise mode of action of azathioprine is unclear but, as an immunosuppressant, azathioprine interferes with DNA synthesis by either inhibiting cell division or causing cell death in relation to RA. This results in fewer circulating B and T lymphocytes (Furst and Clements, 1994, Luqmani, Palmer and Bacon, 1990). Azathioprine is also administered as a steroid sparing agent.

Pharmacokinetics

Following oral administration, azathioprine remains inactive until it is metabolized in the liver into 6-thioinosinic acid and 6-thioguanylic acid. Elimination is via the kidneys.

CYCLOPHOSPHAMIDE

Cyclophosphamide, a derivative of nitrogen mustard, is an alkylating agent which was developed 50 years ago as an anticancer drug. Cyclophosphamide has been shown to possess both immunosuppressive and immunostimulatory effects (Miller and North, 1981; Turk and Parker, 1979). Its use by rheumatologists for the treatment of RA began in the late 1960s even though research studies revealed conflicting results regarding its efficacy in controlling or slowing down radiographic changes. Cyclophosphamide has proved to be an effective in the treatment of the systemic complications of RA, such as vasculitis, and it has also proved to be effective treatment of systemic lupus erythematosus (Austin *et al.*, 1986).

Mode of Action

The mode of action of cyclophosphamide is not entirely understood. It is known to cross link DNA and possess properties that act to stop DNA replication and halt cell division. Additionally, it has a toxic effect on resting cells. This is said to account for its quick action, which is accompanied with increased toxicity in comparison with azathioprine (Brooks, 1990, Furst and Clements, 1994).

Pharmacokinetics

Cyclophosphamide may be administered orally or intravenously. Although metabolized to some extent in both the kidneys and lungs, cyclophosphamide is predominately metabolized in the liver (Bagley, Bostick and De Vita, 1973). Cyclophosphamide is excreted via the faeces, expiration, spinal fluid, perspiration, breast milk, saliva and synovial fluid (Furst and Clements, 1994). The majority however is excreted by the kidneys unchanged (less than 20%) and as metabolites in the urine (65%), the dominant metabolite of cyclophosphamide (acrolein) having been highlighted as the major source of bladder toxicity (Mouridsen and Jacobsen, 1975). Hence an increased fluid intake is essential when administering this drug.

CICLOSPORIN

Ciclosporin is an immunosuppressant initially developed to suppress the rejection of organ transplantation. Its anti-arthritis properties were initially identified in the mid-1970s (Borel *et al.*, 1976). Further studies have demonstrated that it is able to reduce bone and cartilage destruction (Del Pozo *et al.*, 1990) and also to restore T-helper and T-suppressor subsets (Bersani-Amado *et al.*, 1990; Yocum *et al.*, 1986). Ciclosporin has been used in the treatment of RA and retinal vasculitis including that witnessed in Behçet's syndrome.

Mode of Action

Ciclosporin is able to inhibit T cell response and interaction by blocking IL-2 and other pro-inflammatory cytokines.

Pharmacokinetics

Taken orally, absorption is noted to be both incomplete and erratic (Kowal, Carstens and Schinitzer, 1990) with distribution taking place outside rather than inside the blood volume; hence ciclosporin has been detected in the body fat, liver, lungs, kidneys, adrenal glands, spleen and lymph nodes. Consequently elimination is mainly via the biliary system and, to a much lesser extent, via the urine (Furst and Clements, 1994).

CHLORAMBUCIL

Although generally out of vogue for the past 20 years, chlorambucil has maintained its popularity in both France and North America for the treatment of most connective tissue disease and associated inflammatory eye diseases (Luqmani, Palmer and Bacon, 1990).

Mode of Action

Chlorambucil is a cytotoxic drug (a nitrogen mustard derivative) and belongs to the group of drugs known as alkylating agents. Alkylating agents are chemically very active substances which bind with DNA within the cell nucleus resulting in cell death at the point of cell division.

Pharmacokinetics

Administered orally, chlorambucil is rapidly absorbed and then both chlorambucil and its metabolites are excreted in the urine.

PHENYLBUTAZONE

Introduced in 1949 for the treatment of arthritis and gout, phenylbutazone is said to be one of the oldest and strongest non-steroidal anti-inflammatory drugs and is often prescribed for its suppressive properties. However, because of reported toxic side effects, phenylbutazone is currently only prescribed for ankylosing spondylitis under hospital specialist supervision.

Mode of Action

Phenylbutazone acts to inhibit the biosynthesis of prostaglandins (Moll, 1983).

Pharmacokinetics

Administered orally with food (because of gastric irritation), like other NSAIDs, phenylbutazone is almost entirely absorbed from the gastrointestinal tract (as it is not bound irretrievably by food). Elimination is via the kidneys following conversion by the liver into glucuronides and/or additional metabolites (Hart and Klinenberg, 1985).

DAPSONE

Known principally as an antileprotic drug, it has also proved effective as an anti-malarial drug, and in the treatment of both RA and psoriatic arthritis.

Mode of Action

Related to sulfonamide antibacterials, dapsone produces a depressant effect on the immune system.

Pharmacokinetics

Taken orally, dapsone is absorbed rapidly, with excretion via the kidneys in the urine.

MINOCYCLINE

Minocycline is a broad spectrum antibiotic, prescribed for the treatment of tetracycline-sensitive organisms, certain strains of meningitis, acne and for the treatment of RA.

Mode of Action

The mode of action of minocycline is unclear but it is thought to inhibit pro-inflammatory enzymes.

Pharmacokinetics

Following absorption, minocycline spreads widely throughout the body, including a variable penetration across the meningeal barrier into the cerebrospinal fluid. Excretion of the greater part of the drug is slowly via the kidneys.

MYCOPHENOLATE MOFETIL

Mycophenolate mofetil (MMF) is a pro drug of the active metabolite of mycophenolic acid. It is a suppressor of T and B cell proliferation and adhesion and inhibits monophosphate dehydrogenase that eventually blocks the progression to DNA synthesis and proliferation.

2.4 BIOLOGIC THERAPIES

Susan Oliver

INTRODUCTION

This section will focus on the new therapies (biologic therapies) that have been introduced over the last five years and are usually prescribed when traditional DMARDs have failed to adequately control the disease process in inflammatory joint disease.

DMARDs have been recognized as playing an essential part in controlling inflammatory joint diseases and are the first line treatment for RA and other inflammatory joint diseases (for example, PsA and AS). DMARDs control the disease by suppressing the autoimmune response and reducing the potential for joint erosions and long-term damage. However it is clear that maintaining control of the disease and reducing joint damage remain suboptimal for many patients despite treatment with DMARDs.

There are now a number of new medications that have a specific and more targeted action on the cell-to-cell interactions of the immune response. These include therapies such as anti-interleukin 1 receptor antagonist (IL-1ra), anti-tumour necrosis factor alpha (anti-TNFα) and more recently anti-cluster differentiation 20 (CD 20) B cell depletion (B cell depletion). A general term frequently used to refer to all of these new biologically engineered therapies is 'biologic therapies'.

Biologic therapies follow DMARDs in the treatment pathway and are advocated as appropriate treatment when traditional DMARDs (usually at least two DMARDs) have failed to control the disease (Ledinghan and Deighton, 2005). The initial rationale for placing such therapies at this point in the treatment pathway reflects the need for clinicians to gain a greater insight into using these therapies in routine clinical practice, enabling them to develop a sound knowledge of risks and benefits of such therapies, but also related to the costs of treatment, which can range from approximately £8,000–10,000 per annum per patient. However, more recently there has been an increasing recognition that these therapies are effective in methotrexate naïve patients and early aggressive treatment may improve long-term outcomes (Furst *et al.*, 2005).

Biologic therapies have improved the quality of life for many individuals with moderate to severe RA (Maini *et al.*, 2004). Studies also reveal that not only is progressive joint damage halted, but there is early evidence that repair of joint erosions can be seen; something not experienced with traditional therapies and a factor that adds a very important dimension in treatment for those with RA (Furst *et al.*, 2005). Optimal treatment benefits are achieved when biologic therapies are co-prescribed with methotrexate (Furst *et al.*, 2005).

However, for the practitioners caring for individuals treated with these therapies there are important issues that need to be considered in pre-screening and monitoring of patients receiving biologic therapies (RCN, 2003). This section will outline the key issues that need to be considered.

BIOLOGICALLY ENGINEERED THERAPIES (BIOLOGICS)

The use of biotechnology has enabled scientific knowledge to manipulate and redesign key aspects of the body's own cell-to-cell communications and interactions. A range of new therapies have been, and continue to be, developed for inflammatory joint diseases as a result of this work. A key component of these specifically designed therapies is that of disarming pro-inflammatory cytokines responsible for driving autoimmune responses (Oliver and Mooney, 2002). Cytokines are proteins or glycoproteins that act as important intercellular messengers travelling through blood and the lymphatic systems to communicate important pro- or anti-inflammatory responses.

Therapeutic targets have been identified for the cytokines interleukin 1 (IL−1) and tumour necrosis factor alpha (TNFα) and more recently B cell depletion of CD20 B cells. Further specific cell-to-cell interactions have identified new thera-peutic pathways that are currently being researched and it is likely that some of these will be licensed within the next few years.

The reader should refer to other key documents in the management of patients receiving biologic therapies. These include:

- Guidance on eligibility criteria, screening and management of those being treated with anti-TNFα prepared by the British Society for Rheumatology (BSR, 2002, 2005).
- Guidelines for the patient taking immunosuppressants, steroids and the new biologic therapies. Vaccinations in the immunocompromised person (BSR, 2002; DoH, 1996). Immunizations against infectious disease.
- The British Thoracic Society (BTS, 2005) guidelines for the assessment and treatment of tuberculosis in patients due to start anti-TNF therapy (BTS, 2005)
- The Royal College of Nursing Guidance on assessing, managing and monitoring biologic therapies for inflammatory arthritis (RCN, 2003)
- National Institute of Clinical Excellence (NICE) guidance for etanercept and infliximab for the treatment of RA.
- Background information on the use of rixutimab in the treatment of non-Hodgkin's lymphoma (NICE, 2002). NICE proposes to review rituximab for RA in their appraisal programme this year.

This section will give an overview of how these biologic therapies provide a new and more effective approach to treating conditions that are driven by a faulty immune response (autoimmunity). Autoimmune diseases can result in a range of conditions depending upon the tissues affected. Examples of inflammatory joint conditions include RA, PsA and AS.

CLASSIFICATIONS – BIOLOGIC THERAPIES

All biologic therapies have been developed using technology manipulating immunoglobulins. This technology involves designing immunoglobulins so that they can specifically disarm cytokines or their receptors and, as result, stop their normal mode of action. Biologically engineered immunoglobulins are made up of foreign proteins. These proteins may be made up using technology that incorporates either all human or part human/part animal immunoglobulins demonstrating the different components of three biologic therapies and their constituent parts.

Immunoglobulins (Antibodies)

Immunoglobulins belong to a family of large protein molecules also known as antibodies. Immunoglobulins are produced by B cells in response to a challenge to the immune system. B cells that have had no antigen/antibody reaction are called 'naïve' B cells and therefore produce a good but not highly specific immunoglobulin response (or targeted bullet) on first contact or prior to clonal expansion. Immunoglobulins can become more specific with the ability to recognize an antigen following initial interaction with the antigen resulting in a more rapid and effective response in subsequent challenges to the immune system. When an immunoglobulin develops a specific targeted response it is said to have a 'shared epitope' – that is, a perfect match between the immunoglobulin and the antigen, matching in a similar way to a lock and key, with the lock being the antigen and the key being the immunoglobulin.

MODE OF ACTION – GENERAL

The mechanism of action of traditional DMARDs is not fully understood but it is likely that their effect on immune suppression is suboptimal based upon the limited understanding of their non-specific actions on cytokine production and cell replication. Compared to DMARDs and corticosteroids, biologic therapies have a more specific and targeted effect at cell level. Biologic therapies act by mimicking the normal immune processes, effectively preventing or displacing a cytokine from 'locking' into its defined receptor. This has the consequence of preventing the activation of pro-inflammatory cytokines responsible for ensuring an 'inflammatory cascade'. When activated an inflammatory cascade results in the classic signs of inflammation (heat, redness, swelling, loss of function and pain).

Biologics have a direct cell-to-cell effect on specific targeted cytokines but also have a less clearly mapped action on other closely related or possibly directly linked communicating cytokines that also have an effect on the inflammatory cascade and ultimately the effects that these responses have on other tissues as a consequence of the cytokine activation. (For further reading see Dinarello and Moldawer, 2002, Oliver, 2003, 2004.)

Knowledge of cytokines and their effects continues to be researched with well over 150 cytokines clearly identified. These cytokines are classified into families (for example anti-TNFα or interleukin 1) and are described as either pro- or anti-inflammatory cytokines. Pro-inflammatory cytokines have been identified as playing an important part in driving an inflammatory response (Dinarello and Moldawer, 2002).

Research continues on key cytokines and chemokines (smaller molecules than a cytokines but playing a similar role in the immune response) as well as looking at different stages of the cell-to-cell interactions in the immune pathway as the focus for future therapeutic targets.

Biologic therapies and other key cells-to-cell interactions that might be amenable to therapeutic manipulation are the focus of research for a number of chronic autoimmune conditions. As research continues it is possible that current therapies will be identified as effective treatments for a number of other autoimmune conditions.

ADVERSE REACTIONS TO BIOLOGIC THERAPIES

As with all injected foreign proteins (e.g. blood transfusion) there is the potential for the body to develop antibodies to the protein and/or hypersensitivity reactions. The likelihood of an individual experiencing an anaphylactic reaction to an agent is influenced by age, gender, atopy, route of exposure and prior exposure as well as history of prior anaphylactic reactions (Winbery and Lieberman, 1995).

A detailed discussion on the incidence of infusion reactions and an algorithm to guide practitioners has been described by Cheifetz *et al.* (2003) in the management of Crohn's disease. Table 2.6 provides an overview of management. Adverse responses for immediate and delayed reactions can be categorized as mild, moderate or severe (according to severity and signs of symptoms).

Immediate Reactions (Within the First 24 Hours)

Cheifetz (2003) suggests reactions should be categorized in simple terms such as immediate and delayed, but also considered based upon immune (antibody/antigen reactions) or non-immune mediated reactions (such as dose-dependent drug toxicity, secondary effects of drug or drug—drug interactions).

Severe anaphylaxis type reactions (antibody/antigen reaction) are considered to be driven by IgE-mediated acute hypersensitivity events although Cheifetz *et al.*'s study in the use of infliximab did not support this finding. However anaphylaxis type reactions do appear to occur more frequently in individuals with a history of atopy or previous history of infusion-related reactions. In these cases, retreatment should be commenced at a slower rate (usually slowing the normal rate by half) initially and then gradually increasing in line with normal treatment regimes if all observations are satisfactory (see Tables 2.7 and 2.8).

Delayed Reactions

Delayed reactions can occur after 24 hours and up to 14 days after treatment and often present in the form of arthralgia, myalgia, urticarial rash, fever or malaise.

Table 2.6 Biologic prescribing issues.

Treatment	Screening	Cautions	Contra indications	Withdrawal treatment	Additional comments
1) Anakinra (Kineret)					
• 100 mg daily by subcutaneous injection • Monotherapy • NICE recommendations: Not for the treatment of RA (2003)	• See BSR (2005) BTS (2005) and RCN (2003) guidance for inflammatory arthritis	• History of recurrent infections or with those who have underlying conditions which predispose to infection (see anti-TNFα guidelines for outline of risk factors) • History of asthma (risk of serious infections) • Moderate renal impairment (CL$_{cl}$ 30 to 50 ml/minute)	• Hypersensitivity to *E. Coli* derived proteins • Severe renal impairment (CL$_{cr}$ <30 ml/minute) • Persistent neutropenia (<1.5 x 10^9/l) • Pregnant or breastfeeding women	• Serious allergic reactions to anakinra • Severe renal impairment • If serious infections – do not recommence until infection treated and resolved • Stop treatment if neutropenic (<1.5 x 10^9/l) or persistent neutropenia (<1.5 x 10^9/l) • Pregnancy • Malignancy	• Concurrent administration of anakinra and anti-TNFα is not recommended (associated with increased risk of serious infections) • No data to suggest anakinra rarely associated with increased incidence of tuberculosis (Furst *et al*. 2005). • Blood monitoring for monthly white cells counts (for first six months) and quarterly thereafter • Should not receive live vaccines whilst on treatment

2) Adalimumab (Humira)

• 40 mg every other week can be as a monotherapy or in combination with methotrexate (sometimes prescribed with other DMARDs)
• Treatment of adults with:
  • Moderate to severe RA
  • Active and progressive psoriatic arthritis (monotherapy)
	• See BSR (2005) BTS (2005) for and RCN (2003) guidance for inflammatory arthritis	• History of recurrent infections or with those who have underlying conditions which predispose to infection (See anti-TNFα guidelines for outline of risk factors)
		• History of malignancies or if develop malignancy whilst on treatment
		• In psoriatic arthritis – elevations of ALT were more common than in RA
		• In mild heart failure (NYHA class I/II)
			• Hypersensitivity to the active substances in the treatment
			• Pregnant or breastfeeding women
			• Active tuberculosis or other severe infections (e.g. chronic leg ulcers, persistent or recurrent chest infections, in-dwelling urinary catheter)
			• Sepsis of native joint within last 12 months or sepsis of a prosthetic joint within the last 12 months (indefinitely if joint remains in situ)
			• Moderate to severe heart failure (NYHA class III/IV)
			• Clear history of demylinating disease
				• Drug-related toxicities
				• Serious allergic reactions to treatment
				• If serious infections – do not recommence until infection treated and resolved (see guidance re tuberculosis (BTS))
				• Pregnancy (temporary withdrawal)
				• Malignancy
				• Inefficacy – according to BSR (2005)
				• New symptoms of congestive heart failure or worsening mild heart failure
					• Some patients may receive 40 mg every week if on monotherapy
					• Post-clinical data – anaphylaxis has been reported
					• Should not receive live vaccines whilst on treatment. (Treat with live vaccines four weeks before starting treatment.) Pneumococcal vaccinations may result in lower titres
					• Treatment should be withheld for 2–4 weeks prior to surgery. Restart after surgery if no evidence of infection and good wound healing
					• Auto-antibodies have been identified with all anti-TNFα therapies – the exact significance is not fully understood. However, if lupus-like symptoms develop, treatment should be stopped

Table 2.6 (Continued).

Treatment	Screening	Cautions	Contra indications	Withdrawal treatment	Additional comments
3) Etanercept (Enbrel) 50 mg once a week combination with methotrexate (sometimes prescribed with other DMARDs) • Treatment for adults with: • Moderate to severe RA • Moderate to severe plaque psoriasis (monotherapy) 25 mg twice weekly (50 mg twice weekly can be prescribed for up to 12 weeks) • Psoriasis – indicated where failed to respond or contraindicated to treatment of other systemic therapy including cyclosporine, methotrexate or PUVA	• See BSR (2005) of RA, BTS (2005) and RCN (2003) guidance for inflammatory arthritis	• History of recurrent infections or with those who have underlying conditions which predispose to infection (see anti-TNFα guidelines for outline of risk factors) • Rare cases on pancytopenia and very rare cases of aplastic anaemia: caution in patients who have a previous history of blood dyscrasias • Co-prescribing with sulfasalazine – statistically significant decrease in white blood counts • In psoriatic arthritis – elevations of ALT were more common than in RA	• Hypersensitivity to the active substances in the treatment • Pregnant or breastfeeding women • Active tuberculosis or other severe infections (e.g. chronic leg ulcers, persistent or recurrent chest infections, in-dwelling urinary catheter) • Sepsis of native joint within last 12 months or • Sepsis of a prosthetic joint within the last 12 months (indefinitely if joint remains *in situ*) • Moderate to severe heart failure (NYHA class III/IV) • Clear history of demylinating disease	• Drug-related toxicities • Serious allergic or anaphylactic reactions to treatment • If serious infections – do not recommence until infection treated and resolved • Pregnancy (temporary withdrawal) • Malignancy • Inefficacy – according to BSR (2005)	• Should not receive live vaccines whilst on treatment. (Treat with live vaccines 4 weeks before starting treatment. Can be given 2–3 weeks after last dose of etanercept (see BSR vaccination guidelines (2002) • Pneumococcal vaccinations may result in lower titres • Treatment should be withheld for 2–4 weeks prior to surgery. Restart after surgery if no evidence of infection and good wound healing • Auto-antibodies have been identified with all anti-TNFα therapies – the exact significance is not fully understood. However, if lupus-like symptoms develop, treatment should be stopped

Infliximab (Remicade)

- 3 mg/kg body weight by intravenous infusion 0-,2-,6-, and 8-weekly thereafter
- Co-prescribed with methotrexate (is sometimes prescribed with other DMARDs)
- Treatment of adults with:
- Active RA
- Active and progressive PsA in combination with methotrexate 5 mg/kg body weight 0,2,6 and 8 weekly thereafter
- AS: 5 mg/kg body weight 0-,2-,6- and then every 6–8 weeks thereafter (if responds to treatment in first 6 weeks)
- Also indicated in severe active Crohn's disease

- See BSR (2005), BTS (2005) and RCN (2003) guidance

- History of recurrent infections or with those who have underlying conditions which predispose to infection (see anti-TNFα guidelines for outline of risk factors)
- Very rare cases of jaundice and non-infectious hepatitis. If jaundice and/or raise ALT > 5 times upper limit of normal discontinue treatment and investigate
- Hepatitis B reactive can occur – evaluate chronic carriers

- Hypersensitivity to the active substances in the treatment
- Pregnant or breastfeeding women
- Active tuberculosis or other severe infections (e.g. chronic leg ulcers, persistent or recurrent chest infections, in-dwelling urinary catheter)
- Sepsis of native joint within last 12 months or sepsis of a prosthetic joint within the last 12 months (indefinitely if joint remains *in situ*)
- Moderate to severe heart failure (NYHA class III/IV)
- Clear history of demylinating disease

- Drug-related toxicities
- Serious allergic reactions to treatment
- If serious infections – do not recommence until infection treated and resolved
- Pregnancy (temporary withdrawal)
- Malignancy
- Inefficacy – according to BSR (2005)

- Post-clinical data – anaphylaxis has been reported
- Should not receive live vaccines whilst on treatment (Treat with live vaccines 4 weeks before starting treatment)
- Treatment should be withheld for 2–4 weeks prior to surgery. Restart after surgery if no evidence of infection and good wound healing
- Auto-antibodies have been identified with all anti-TNFα therapies – the exact significance is not fully understood. However, if lupus-like symptoms develop treatment should be stopped

Table 2.6 (Continued).

Treatment	Screening	Cautions	Contra indications	Withdrawal treatment	Additional comments
4) Rituximab (Mabthera) • Currently licensed for NHL • Treatments (unlicensed – new or extension to license expected) for RA in published data include: • Currently being used for RA in patients who have failed treatment with anti-TNFα therapies	• Review bloods prior to treatment; particular focus should be on neutrophils and platelets • Careful screening of signs of reactivation of hepatitis B infections in those with a history of hepatitis B • Practical advice should include checking that those receiving treatment are free of infections (e.g. good skin integrity, no current infection or recent close contact with infections such as varicella)	• Severe cytokine release syndrome (CRS) associated with tumour lysis syndrome (TLS). Both of these syndromes appear to present less commonly with RA-treated patients • Review cardiac status as angina pectoris, myocardial infarction, atrial flutter, etc. have occurred. Monitor closely those with history of cardiac/and or cardiotoxic chemotherapy • Hypotension can occur (consider temporarily withholding anti-hypertensive treatment for 12 hours prior to treatment) • Neutrophils <1.5 x 10^9/l and plate counts < 75 x 10^9/l	• Hypersensitivity to the active substances in the treatment • Pregnant or breastfeeding women	• If serious infusion-related reactions that fail to respond to re-challenge after appropriate prophylactic treatment • Current information remains limited for RA patients	• Treatment information currently published related to clinical trials in RA and the treatment of NHL • Review latest published information in reputable journals and latest data from pharmaceutical company producing rituximab

1) For full details please refer to: Summary of Product Characteristics Amgen (2005), British National Formulary (September, 2004). BSR Guidelines for prescribing TNFα blockers in adults with rheumatoid arthritis (2005), British Thoracic Society (2005), British Society of Rheumatology vaccination guidelines (2002).

2) For full details please refer to: Summary of Product Characteristics Abbott Laboratories Ltd (2005), British National Formulary (September, 2004). BSR Guidelines for prescribing TNFα blockers in adults with rheumatoid arthritis (2005), British Thoracic Society (2005), British Society of Rheumatology vaccination guidelines (2002).

3) For full details please refer to: Summary of Product Characteristics Schering Plough Ltd (2005), British National Formulary (September, 2004). BSR Guidelines for prescribing TNFα blockers in adults with rheumatoid arthritis (2005), British Thoracic Society (2005), British Society of Rheumatology vaccination guidelines (2002).

4) References: Summary of Product Characteristics Rituximab (Roche Products Ltd, 2005), British National Formulary (September 2004).

Table 2.7   Key issues in caring for individuals receiving biologic therapies.

Nurse/practitioner screening prior to starting treatment

Patient has had an opportunity to discuss their treatment options and has made an informed decision about starting therapy. Consent documented for treatment and data collection for BSR Biologics Register data.

Patients need to fulfil the eligibility criteria for treatment (National Institute of Clinical Excellence; NICE 2002) and the British Society for Rheumatology according to disease (RA, ankylosing spondylitis, psoriatic arthritis; BSR, 2005).

Screening for risks of tuberculosis should be undertaken for all patients receiving anti-TNFα therapies according to the BTS guidelines (BTS, 2005). Those who have risk factors should be referred to the prescribing physician for consideration of referral to respiratory or immunology physician.

If co-prescribed with a DMARD that they are continuing on this treatment and monitoring is satisfactory.

Confirmation that women of childbearing age are not pregnant and (both men and women) are aware they must use an effective contraceptive.

Patients should be free of infections or any potential foci of infection (such as chest infections, indwelling catheter or sepsis of prosthetic joint within the last 12 months). Also ensure there is no recent contact with chicken pox or herpes zoster.

Immunizations should be reviewed and if time allows and patient is well enough ensure immunizations are undertaken 4 weeks prior to starting treatment (BSR, 2002).

Ensure no malignancy or pre-malignancy state (excluding basal cell carcinoma or malignancies diagnosed and treated more than 10 years previously).

Exclude any history or new symptoms of heart failure or demyelinating disease.

Treatment issues general

Provide written information and contact details for support about their treatment and ensure they know when they should seek urgent advice.

Question to ensure there are no new symptoms or pending investigations awaited (e.g. for possible malignancy).

Training and competencies have been assessed in storage, administration and monitoring issues related to self-administration of subcutaneous therapy if treated with anakinra, etanercept or adalimumab.

Infusion issues (infliximab or rituximab): Ensure that

Full screening has been undertaken and patient has an opportunity to ask questions.

Assessment and disease activity criteria have been fulfilled for data collection (such as the BSR Biologics Register) and review of treatment benefits.

Pre-infusion monitoring has been carried out and these are with in normal range (vital signs − temperature, pulse, respirations, blood pressure) and urinalysis. Patient has been weighted if appropriate.

Have received appropriate prophylactic drug therapy prior to starting an infusion.

Clinical management plans or protocols for infusion regimes are adhered to and recorded.

All infusion-related reactions are monitored carefully and managed promptly according to local and national guidelines. If severe reactions occur (e.g. dyspnoea, hypotension) treatment should stop and appropriate treatment administered promptly.

Table 2.7   (Continued).

Recommence infusions following a reaction are started slowly and appropriate medical support and full resuscitation equipment readily available.

Post-infusion: Ensure that

Post-infusion observations are satisfactory, the patient is asymptomatic and all details are recorded.

Information and contact numbers have been provided to the patient about follow-up care and what to do if an adverse event occurs.

Table 2.8   Screening and management of infusion-related reactions.

Baseline

General screening

Ensure the patient is free of infection and review any changes in health status (e.g. new investigations for suspected cardiac, neurological or malignancy issues). If of childbearing potential confirm effective contraceptive used.

Check any issues re venous access. The appropriate site for a cannular can sometimes be difficult with consideration required for poor skin integrity, bruising or painful joints.

Practitioners should review blood results before proceeding and check for any documentation of human anti-chimeric antibodies (HACA). The presence of HACA is an additional indicator of potential infusion-related reactions. The co-prescription of a DMARD reduces the risks of HACAs developing.

Check, if prescribed, that the patient is still taking their disease-modifying drugs (usually methotrexate). The risk of infusion-related reactions may be higher if not co-prescribed a DMARD. If stopped DMARD, check the time frame from stopping treatment and refer to prescribing physician.

Enquire on history of atopy or previous infusion-related reactions.

Review baseline blood results (check for any abnormalities and report to prescribing physician or review protocols/guidelines on treatment pathway).

Undertake any data collection and consent that is required (e.g. consent for treatment/or BSR Biologics Register or Disease Activity Assessments).

For individuals on anti-hypertensive agents who are treated with rituximab the prescribing physician may elect to withhold anti-hypertensive medications for 12 hours prior to the infusion.

Pre-administration

If prescribed administer pre-medication prior to starting infusion (e.g. paracetamol and/or antihistamine). If prescribed rituximab review concordance with between infusion oral steroid treatment and ensure 100mg intravenous methylprednisolone pre-treatment is administered.

Patients should have their general well-being (e.g. flushed or chest pain) and observations recorded prior to the infusion and every 30 minutes during the infusion (blood pressure and pulse).

Advise patient to report if they have unexplained/new symptoms such as breathlessness, pruritis, fever, chills or chest pain.

Infusion-related reactions (acute)

Mild to moderate

If patient experiences symptoms stop treatment and treat according to severity of reaction and according to local protocols. Mild or moderate infusion reactions usually occur within two hours of the initial infusion (although they may commence within a few seconds of commencing treatment). They may necessitate temporarily withholding the treatment but usually respond to reduction in the rate of infusion and possibly treatment with paracetamol and diphenhydramine. If observations are satisfactory and symptoms are mild (e.g. headache) and treatment is not required the physician may decide to re-start the infusion at a slower rate and with frequent monitoring. If the infusion then continues without event subsequent infusions can be undertaken with caution.

Moderate to severe

If the patient experiences significant changes in vital signs (e.g. diastolic blood pressure decreases between 15–20 mm Hg) or the patient experiences symptoms that indicate hypersensitivity or in the treatment of rituximab, severe cytokine release syndrome (e.g. severe dyspnoea, bronchospasm, urticaria, fever, hypotension), *stop* infusion. Treat aggressively according to local anaphylaxis protocol (usually would include pain relief, antihistamines, intravenous saline or brochodilators, corticosteroids and/or epinephrine, oxygen). For those treated with rituximab the infusion should not be recommenced until complete resolution of all symptoms and normalization of laboratory values and chest X-ray findings.

The infusion may be resumed (at the discretion of the physician and consent from the patient) but must recommence at no more than one half of the previous rate (Roche, 2005, personal communication). If a severe adverse reaction occurs for a second time the prescribing physician should review the decision to continue subsequent treatments on a case-by-case basis.

Recommencing treatment following an infusion-related reaction

For those patients attending for a subsequent infusion having had a previous serious infusion reaction a physician should be at hand for the next treatment, if the decision to re-treat has been taken.

Commence infusions at slower rate and ensure frequent observations of vital signs until patient stable (e.g. every 15 minutes). Gradually increase rate and maintain observations and observe carefully until patient stable.

If a further severe infusion-related reaction occurs, *stop* infusion and treat aggressively according to local protocols. Review with prescribing physician.

Delayed infusion reactions

Usually present with arthralgia, myalgia, urticarial rash, fever and malaise. These are usually managed by prescribing paracetamol, antihistamines and occasionally steroids if required.

References: Summary of product characteristics for infliximab (Schering Plough, 2005) and rituximab (Roche Products, 2005). For infliximab see also Cheifetz *et al.* (2003).

BIOLOGIC THERAPIES – TREATMENT OPTIONS

Interleukin-1 Receptor Antagonist (IL-1ra)

Anakinra (kineret)

Classification

Anakinra – a biologically engineered monoclonal antibody working as an interleukin-1 receptor antagonist. Anakinra is indicated for the treatment of RA in combination with methotrexate when there is an inadequate response to methotrexate alone.

Mode of Action

In normal joints interleukin-1 receptor antagonist (IL-1Ra) modifies the activity of interleukin 1 (IL-1; a pro-inflammatory cytokine). IL-1Ra binds to interleukin 1 receptors (IL-1R1) and by doing so competitively prevents binding of IL-1 into their receptors reducing the number of receptors available for IL-1 to lock into and cause an inflammatory response. This is the body's normal response to maintain equilibrium and ensure an appropriate level of inflammatory response. The loss of self-tolerance (recognition and acceptance of tissues that belong to self) results in an autoimmunity condition upsetting the usual immunological balance. Anakinra is the only IL-1Ra therapy licensed for RA. Maximum plasma concentrations of anakinra occur three to seven hours following subcutaneous injection. The plasma half life ranges from four to six hours.

Anakinra has been shown to have limited value for the majority of RA patients, based upon current criteria for evaluating effectiveness of treatment using the Disease Activity Score (DAS 28) although research continues into the therapeutic benefits in other conditions (e.g. osteoarthritis). It has been suggested that in RA despite suboptimal DAS scores, there may be benefits in the reduction of long-term joint damage over time although further research will be needed (Strand and Kavanaugh, 2004).

Administration of Anakinra

Anakinra 100 mg daily is administered subcutaneously using a pre-filled syringe preferably at the same time each day, and should be co-prescribed with a once-weekly dose of methotrexate (weekly dose of methotrexate may vary according age, and renal and hepatic function).

Indication for Use

Anakinra should be prescribed for the treatment of RA in combination with methotrexate, where there is an inadequate response to methotrexate alone.

In theoretical terms the combined treatment of anakinra with an anti-TNFα was initially thought to be an ideal therapeutic option. However this has been shown to significantly increase risks of infections and therefore co-prescribing is not recommended (Amgen, 2005).

No dose adjustment is required for the elderly (more than 65 years of age), or those with hepatic or mild renal impairment. Caution is advised for those with moderate renal impairment.

Anakinra is contraindicated in severe renal impairment. Patients with persistent neutropenia (<1.5 x 10^9/l) should be excluded from treatment with anakinra (see Table 2.6 for additional guidance on screening and management).

The risks related to co-prescription of methotrexate need to be considered in the management of patients with hepatic or renal impairment (National Patient Safety Agency, 2005). Individuals who have hypersensitivity to *E. coli* should not be treated with anakinra.

Anakinra was reviewed by the National Institute of Clinical Excellence in 2003 and was not seen to be cost-effective based upon the evidence available at that time.

Side Effects

Allergic Reactions

The most frequently reported side effect ($>10\%$) in all clinical trials has been that of mild to moderate injection site reactions (ISRs). These were usually mild and self-limiting urticarial or maculopapular rashes; however, if severe reactions occur, treatment should be discontinued and appropriate treatment given. Discontinuation due to ISR was seen in only 7% of patients (BSR, 2002). ISRs most frequently occurred within the first four weeks of treatment (see also section on infection and injection site reactions).

Blood disorders

Blood disorders (neutropenia) were seen in $1-10\%$ of patients in clinical trials. It is recommended that pre-screening of white count should be undertaken, if neutropenic (below <1.5 x 10^9/L) treatment should not be initiated. Regular blood monitoring (monthly for the first six months and then quarterly thereafter) are advised. If neutrophils drop below (below <1.5 x 10^9/L) treatment should be stopped (Amgen, 2005; BSR, 2002).

Infections

There is an increased risk of serious infections (particularly upper respiratory tract infections) (1.8% in treated group compared to placebo 0.7%). In clinical trials and post-marketing experience some opportunistic infections have been seen including fungal, mycobacterial and viral pathogens (Amgen, 2005). Infections are commonly bacterial infections; once treated and resolved anakinra can usually be restarted.

Anakinra has not been associated with reactivation of latent tuberculosis (Furst, et al., 2005). The risks of reactivation of TB appear to be greater for anti-TNFα treatments (BTS, 2005). The BTS guidance may be helpful in assessing general risk factors related to TB exposure although it is important to note the management guidelines are related to anti-TNFα therapies and not specifically for anakinra. However, the co-prescribing of methotrexate and the potential for patients who fail on anakinra to progress to anti-TNFα makes this a sensible principle to apply in assessing patients.

Lymphomas and Malignancy

As there is limited data on the impact of treatment on malignancies it is recommended that individuals with pre-existing malignancy should not be treated with anakinra (Amgen, 2005). Patients treated with anakinra have an increased risk of lymphoma compared to the general (non-RA) population; however, the rate for malignancy is comparable to the RA population (two- to threefold increase compared to the general non-RA population) (Amgen, 2005).

Drug Interactions

Drug interactions have not been extensively investigated although in clinical trials non-steroidal anti-inflammatory drugs, corticosteroids and disease-modifying drugs were co-prescribed and no interactions were observed (Amgen, 2005, Tesser et al., 2004). Studies observing toxic interactions related to methotrexate when co-administered with anakinra did not demonstrate any reductions in clearance rates (Amgen, 2002).

Pregnancy and Breastfeeding

As with all new therapies there is insufficient data on the use of anakinra in pregnant or breastfeeding women and therefore treatment should not be prescribed if the patient is at risk of pregnancy, pregnant or breastfeeding. Women of childbearing potential must be advised to use an effective means of contraception when treated with anakinra.

Immunization

There is limited data available on the effects of vaccinations in patients receiving anakinra (Amgen Ltd, 2005).

Live vaccines are contraindicated for both anakinra and methotrexate. Where possible it is helpful to ensure patients have their immune status reviewed for any vaccinations required at least four weeks before starting any biologic therapy. Readers should refer to additional guidance on management of patients who are immunosuppressed and/or are also co-prescribed methotrexate (DoH, 1996 and the BSR, 2002). There is no data on the secondary transmission of infection by live vaccines.

Anti-Tumour Necrosis Factor Alpha (Anti-TNFα)

Anti-TNFα therapies consist of the three currently licensed therapies. These are:

1. Adalimumab (Humira) licensed for:
   (a) RA (severe, active and progressive)
      (i) Dose range 40 mg every other week as a single dose (in combination with methotrexate)
      (ii) Dose may be increased to 40 mg every week (for monotherapy)
   (a) Psoriatic arthritis 40 mg every other week as a single dose.

2. Etanercept (Enbrel) licensed for:
   (a) RA (severe, active and progressive)
      (i) Dose of 50 mg once weekly either as combination therapy with methotrexate or as a monotherapy
   (b) Plaque psoriasis
      (i) 25 mg twice weekly or
      (ii) 50 mg twice weekly for up to 12 weeks reducing to 25 mg twice weekly.

3. Infliximab (Remicade) licensed for:
   (a) RA (severe, active and progressive)
      (i) 3 mg/kg of body weight in combination with methotrexate (0-, 2-, 6- and 8-weekly thereafter)
   (b) AS (severe axial symptoms and elevated serological markers)
      (i) 5 mg/kg body weight 0-, 2- and 6-weekly − if no response after three doses no additional treatment.
   (c) PsA (active progressive)
      (i) 5 mg/kg body weight 0-, 2-, 6- and 8-weekly thereafter.

These three therapies will be discussed individually although the next section will refer to the key issues common to all three anti-TNFα therapies.

GENERAL ISSUES RELATED TO THE MODE OF ACTION – FOR ALL ANTI-TNFα THERAPIES

The release and activation of the cytokine TNFα triggers a cascade of responses from other pro-inflammatory cytokines. Tumour Necrosis Factor alpha (TNFα) is a pivotal cytokine in the inflammatory response. Activating inflammation is achieved when the TNFα cytokine is released and locks into a T Cell Receptor (TCR) for TNFα resulting in a cascade of responses from other pro-inflammatory cytokines.

There are two types of TCR for TNFα that bind with comparable affinity − p55 and p75. TCR for TNFα can be soluble or tissue-bound. Some anti-TNFα therapies can block soluble and tissue-bound receptors.

There are variations in the specific interactions with TNFα tissue and soluble receptors, as well as the structure and composition of each of the anti-TNFα therapies, plasma half lives and routes of administration. The variations between therapies may also explain some differing benefits in specific disease areas although the full significance of the differing therapeutic options is not completely understood and remains an area of close scrutiny and expert discussions. For example it has been suggested that the ability of etanercept to block lymphotoxin α may explain the benefits achieved in JIA as Lymphotoxin α is identified in inflamed joints of JIA patients.

SIDE EFFECTS THAT SHOULD BE CONSIDERED FOR ALL ANTI-TNFα

Table 2.7 provides an overview of the issues to consider for each of the biologic therapies (see also the details related to each therapy individually). The common points that should be considered regularly are:

- The need to consider all possible opportunistic infections.
- Awareness of allergic reactions related to the injected proteins.
- Clinical indications that might be related to tuberculosis or re-emergence of latent tuberculosis.
- Indications of chronic heart failure or exacerbations of previously mild disease.
- Exacerbations or new symptoms suggestive of demyelinating disease.
- Potential withdrawal of treatment if new malignancies or investigations suggestive of malignancies present.
- Blood monitoring for abnormalities.
- The avoidance of pregnancy or breastfeeding whilst being treated with biologic therapies.
- Care with immunization – live vaccines should not be administered and treatment with other vaccines may be suboptima.
- Planned management of patients receiving surgery to ensure adequate withdrawal prior to surgery and recommencement of therapy when wounds are free of infection.

Some side effects seen in patients treated with anti-TNFα are only partially explained in research trials and subsequent clinical practice. These include reports of exacerbations of chronic heart failure and demyelinating diseases.

Allergic Response to Anti-TNFα Therapies (see also Anakinra and Infliximab sections)

As all the anti-TNFα therapies consist of foreign proteins (immunoglobulins) there is a small risk of allergic reactions. Serious allergic reactions have been reported in post-marketing surveillance for all biologic therapies – adalimumab, anakinra, etanercept and infliximab. Treatment should be withheld and appropriate treatment administered.

Infusion or Injection Site Reactions

There is the potential for any foreign injected protein to cause an immune-mediated response. The most common reactions for the therapies administered subcutaneously are injection site reactions (approximately 20%−36% in treated groups compared to 9−14% in control groups). These are usually mild and self-limiting and resolve without treatment. Some patients may benefit from topical hydrocortisone cream if the rash is symptomatic or discomfort persists.

A guidance document and training package for subcutaneous administration of biologic therapies and patient self-administration of anti-TNFα therapies has been developed by the Royal College of Nursing (RCN, 2003) as well as by the specific patient education material prepared by the pharmaceutical companies. In the management of the patient it should be remembered that some patients may also be co-prescribed methotrexate either orally or as a subcutaneous injection (by once-a-week injection) and care needs to be taken in ensuring that injection sites are rotated.

Autoantibodies

Auto-antibodies can develop at any time during an individual's lifetime without receiving biologic therapies; however they can also develop during treatment with biologic therapies. The co-prescribing of a DMARD (particularly methotrexate) may reduce the potential of auto-antibodies developing in individuals treated with an anti-TNFα therapy (Weber, 2004) The presence of auto-antibodies may in rare cases result in the individual developing lupus-like symptoms, which usually resolve on cessation of treatment (Furst et al., 2005). The presence of antibodies increases the risk of infusion/injection sites reactions.

Blood Monitoring

Many patients receiving biologic therapies will also be co-prescribed a DMARD requiring regular blood monitoring (BSR, 2006). However, it is important to note that research evidence from anti-TNFα therapies has occasionally included abnormal haematological findings. These include rare cases of pancytopenia and very rare cases of aplastic anaemia (in very rare cases resulting in fatal outcomes) and abnormal hepatic dysfunction (Furst et al., 2005). The severity and incidence of haematological problems varies between each of the therapies although this can be a complex picture with the patient group, co-morbidities, level of disease activity and previous immunosuppression (or current treatment) with disease-mofying drugs. However, clinical practice should include screening prior to starting treatment and regular monitoring, assessment and review of individuals treated with an anti-TNFα even if treatment is not co-prescribed with a DMARD such as methotrexate.

Cardiac

Clinical examination and history taking should evaluate cardiac status. Treatment with anti-TNFa therapies should not be considered for individuals with a New York

Heart Classification (NYHC) III/IV. Clinical trials and post-marketing surveillance have identified a risk of mortality for individuals with NYHC III/IV (Bozkurt, 2000). For individuals with NYHC I/II treatment should be considered with caution (Abbott Laboratories Ltd, 2005; Schering Plough, 2005; Wyeth Pharmaceuticals, 2005).

Infections Including Tuberculosis

Tuberculosis

All anti-TNFa therapies have the potential to increase the risk of infections, including the re-emergence of latent tuberculosis (TB) (Furst et al., 2005).

All patients should be closely questioned and examined for possible TB infections prior to starting treatment. This should include detailed questioning of those who travel to areas of high prevalence of TB or who have had close contact with relatives who travel to areas with a high prevalence of TB (BTS, 2005). Referral to a respiratory or immunology physician may be required for those who have close contact with TB or relatives with TB or have previously been infected with TB (treated or partially treated), and those who have symptoms suggestive of TB (fever, weight loss). Further assessment and possible prophylactic regimes to treat previously untreated or latent tuberculosis may be required well before the patient can commence anti-TNFα. The British Thoracic Society (BTS) have developed guidelines specifically to address these issues (BTS, 2005).

Reactivation of TB is at its highest in the first 12 months of treatment although for individuals treated with infliximab the majority of cases occurred within 3 cycles of treatment (median range approximately 12 weeks) (BTS, 2005).

Practitioners undertaking assessments and screening of patients prior to starting treatment and during regular monitoring and review should bear in mind the risks of infections including TB, and be vigilant in getting prompt treatment for infections.

Other Infections

A rigorous approach for all patients treated with anti-TNFα should be applied when screening and reviewing patients, particularly in relation to the risk of opportunistic infections. As TNFα is implicated in the regulating of temperature the normal immune response may be compromised and the usual signs of infection may not be present; for example, one of the classical signs of infection such as a raised temperature may be absent. The co-prescribing of additional immunosuppressant therapies (such as steroids or DMARDs) compounds this problem.

Preliminary data from the BSR Biologics Register show that infection rates are broadly similar across all anti-TNFα therapies and broadly similar to the control groups with active disease (treated with DMARDs) but not receiving biologic therapies (Dixon, 2005).

Serious infections (including bacterial, mycobacterium, viral and fungal) have been identified, with some fatalities occurring with all anti-TNFα therapies. A range of infections have been seen including:

- Upper and lower respiratory infections, including rarely pneumonia.
- Tuberculosis (chiefly although not completely related to re-emergence of latent tuberculosis).
- Sepsis/septic arthritis, cellulitis, fungal dermatitis.
- Varicella.
- Reactivation of hepatitis B (in chronic carriers).

For an extensive list and detailed data on the risks related to infections the reader should refer to the summary of product characteristics for each of the therapies (Abbott Laboratories, 2005; Schering Plough, 2005; Wyeth, 2005).

Treatment should not be started in the presence of a serious infection. If serious infections occur, treatment should be discontinued and only recommenced once the infection has been adequately treated and the infection has resolved (BSR, 2005).

There remains uncertainty about the effects of treating individuals who have HIV with anti-TNFα and therefore therapy should not be recommended if HIV is identified until additional evidence is available.

Lymphomas and Malignancy

There is a theoretical risk of malignancy (as yet unproven) as a result of tumour necrosis factor alpha blockade. Observational studies (such as the BSR Biologics Register) will provide important evidence of the long-term risks of patients receiving biologic therapies, and preliminary data published in 2006 do not indicate any major influence on mortality in the early years after first anti-TNFα use (Watson et al., 2002). The RA population who have severe disease have a two- to threefold increase in the risk of malignancy as a result of their condition and traditional (non-biological) medications (Askling et al., 2005a, 2005b).

As there is limited evidence at present, treatment with anti-TNFα should not be commenced where malignancy is suspected until appropriate investigations have been carried out. In addition those with pre-existing malignancies or previous history of malignancy (within the last 10 years) should only be treated with caution and following a review of the potential risks and benefits to the individual (BSR, 2005).

Neurological

Treatment with anti-TNFα therapies has exacerbated demyelinating diseases (such as multiple sclerosis) (Robinson et al., 2001). Treatment for individuals with a strong family history, pre-existing or recent onset central nervous system or demyelinating disorders should be considered with caution (BSR, 2005). If neurological symptoms develop, treatment should be stopped and investigations undertaken.

PREGNANCY AND BREASTFEEDING

As clinical trials on humans have not been carried out to evaluate the potential risks related the pregnancy or the unborn child none of the biologic therapies should be prescribed if attempting to conceive (or father) a child. The co-prescription of a DMARD such as methotrexate should mean that individuals prior to starting treatment with a biologic should already have been using an effective contraception (adequate contraception should be continued for at least six months after stopping biologic therapy). Preliminary observational data shows that there are no major congenital malformations or evidence of maternal harm in patients treated with all biologic therapies (Hyrich *et al.*, 2005).

Immunoglobulins can be excreted in human milk and therefore a biologic should not be administered to mothers who are breastfeeding. In some circumstances the clinician together with the patient may need to make a careful risk—benefit analysis for both mother and child to decide the best option for management (either stop the biologic or advise that the child is bottle-fed).

For individuals who have been prescribed methotrexate it is recommended that at least a six-month period should elapse before attempting conception; the same length of time is recommended for infliximab (which is co-prescribed with methotrexate). Five months free of treatment is recommended on cessation of adalimumab (personal communication, Abbott Laboratories, December 2005). Withdrawal of methotrexate co-prescription must also be considered and manufacturer advice varies on the length of time from withdrawal of methotrexate before attempting to conceive (between three and six months).

IMMUNIZATION

Live vaccines must not be administered to individuals receiving anti-TNFα therapies (with or without methotrexate or another DMARD) (BSR, 2002). It is therefore useful, if patients are well enough, that time should be allowed to review and plan any necessary immunizations at least four weeks before starting treatment. One study suggests that pneumococcal vaccinations may result in a poor response (BSR, 2005) and others have demonstrated anti-TNFα treated patients to have similar response to controls following vaccination with pneumococcal vaccination although methotrexate does seem to reduce immune response.

If immunizations are to be given they should ideally be administered four weeks prior to starting treatment or at least six months after the last infusion of infliximab or two to three weeks after the last dose of etanercept (BSR, 2005). There is no current advice for adalimumab on the time to elapse before it is safe to administer a vaccine. Additional guidance can be sought from the centre for disease control and prevention for those who are immunosuppressed (www.cdc.gov or www.dh.gov.uk).

Specific guidance on immunization for TB is included in a guidance document produced by the BTS (2005).

SPECIFIC INFORMATION ON ANTI-TNFα

Adalimumab (Humira)

Adalimumab is a recombinant human monoclonal antibody and works by binding specifically to TNFα and preventing the normal TNFα function of locking into p55 and p75 cell surface receptors. The bioavailability following a 40 mg subcutaneous dose was 64%. Absorption and distribution is slow with a peak serum concentration reached at approximately 5 days after administration and a half life for adalimumab of approximately 12−14 days (Abbott Laboratories, 2005).

Indication for Use

Adalimumab is indicated for the treatment of adults with moderate to severe RA following inadequate response to DMARDs and for active and progressive psoriatic arthritis (PsA) when previous response to DMARDs has been inadequate.

Administration

Adalimumab is administered by subcutaneously pre-filled syringe in a dose of 40 mg every other week. Adalimumab can be prescribed as monotherapy but for optimal benefit should be prescribed with methotrexate (for RA patients). Those individuals already receiving methotrexate should continue with their treatment when prescribed adalimumab. For individuals with RA on monotherapy an increase in dose to 40 mg every week may be indicated (Abbott Laboratories, 2005).

Specific Additional Comments

For those with renal or hepatic impairment, there is no specific guidance for individuals receiving adalimumab. If co-prescribed with methotrexate guidance from the British Society for Rheumatology monitoring guidance (2006) and advice from the National Patient Safety Agency should be reviewed (National Patient Safety Agency, 2005).

Etanercept (Enbrel)

Etanercept is a human TNFα receptor p75 fusion protein using recombinant deoxyribonucleic acid (DNA) technology. Etanercept is slowly absorbed following subcutaneous injection reaching maximum concentration approximately 48 hours after a single dose. The half life is approximately 70 hours (Wyeth Pharmaceuticals, 2005).

Indication for Use

Etanercept can be prescribed as monotherapy or in combination with methotrexate for the treatment of adults with active RA who have failed to respond adequately to DMARDs and PsA who have failed or are contraindicated/intolerant of DMARDs. It can also be prescribed for adults with RA who have active and progressive disease not previously treated with methotrexate.

Contraindications

See Table 2.6 and for further information refer to Summary of Product Characteristics and BSR Guidelines (2005).

Administration

Etanercept 50 mg is administered by subcutaneous injection once weekly in 1 ml of water. For moderate to severe plaque psoriasis the usual dose is 25 mg twice weekly or if needed etanercept can be administered at a dose of 50 mg twice weekly for up to 12 weeks reducing to 25 mg twice weekly.

Specific Additional Comments

For those with renal or hepatic impairment, there is no specific guidance for individuals receiving adalimumab. If co-prescribed with methotrexate guidance from the National Patient Safety Agency should be reviewed (National Patient Safety Agency, 2005).

Infliximab (Remicade)

Infliximab is a monoclonal antibody that binds with high affinity to both soluble and trans-membrane TNFα inhibiting the normal activity of TNFα (Figure 2.1). Infliximab is administered by intravenous infusion usually over a two-hour period. The median terminal half life at 3, 5 and 10 mg/kg doses ranged from 8–9. 5 days. In most patients infliximab can be detected in the serum for at least 8 weeks after a single dose of 3 mg/kg. It may be that repeated treatments with infliximab might increase this time frame, although the data was studying Crohn's disease with doses of 5 mg/kg with infliximab detected in serum for 12 weeks after administration (Schering Plough, 2005).

Indication for Use

Infliximab is indicated in the treatment of active RA when the response to DMARDs (including methotrexate) has been inadequate and for severe progressive RA not previously treated with DMARDs. For those with RA, infliximab should be prescribed in combination with methotrexate. It is also indicated for the treatment of PsA when the disease is active and progressive and has failed to respond adequately to DMARDs and in the treatment of AS for those who have axial symptoms and have failed to respond adequately to conventional therapy. It is also licensed for the treatment of Crohn's disease.

Contraindications

Evidence of hypersensitivity to mouse or mouse dander. See Table 2.6 and for further information refer to Summary of Product Characteristics and BSR Guidelines (2005).

Administration

Infliximab is administered by intravenous infusion initially, usually over a two-hour period at a dose of 3 mg/kg of body weight for RA and 5 mg/kg body weight for AS and PsA. Infusions are administered following the first infliximab treatment at two and six weeks and then every eight weeks thereafter.

Side Effects that Should Be Considered for All Anti-TNFα Treatments

The long half life of infliximab means that monitoring of side effects or re-emergence of latent TB should be continued for up to six months after cessation of treatment.

Infusion Reactions (see also Reactions)

Infliximab is administered intravenously usually by infusion over a two-hour period. Infusion-related reactions (non-specific symptoms such as fever, chills) are reported as ranging from 5−15% (Cheifetz *et al.*, 2003; Schering Plough, 2005; Shergy *et al.*, 2002). Serious infusion reactions (chest pain, hypertension, hypotension or dyspnea) occur in less than 1% of patients treated with infliximab (personal communication, Schering Plough, 2005).

Sany *et al.* (2005) studied infusion-related reactions and found that pre-medication with betamethasone provided no additional benefit in reducing infusion-related reactions. Infusion-related reactions are more common on the third and fourth infusion and approximately 3% of patients discontinued treatment due to infusion reactions. Individuals receiving a diphenhydramine as a pre-medication had a higher rate of infusion-related reactions (Wasserman *et al.*, 2004).

Although the majority of infusion reactions are mild and do not result in discontinuation of treatment, a small percentage (<1%) can be severe and include anaphylactic reactions that will require emergency treatment including adrenaline, antihistamines and corticosteroids (Schering Plough, 2005). (see Table 2.8).

If patients are re-treated after a prolonged period of time they should be monitored carefully. The episodic treatment (rather than regular maintenance treatment) with infliximab appears to exacerbate the risk of infusion-related reactions (Cheifetz *et al.*, 2003). The risk is reduced if patients continue their DMARDs therapy (Schering Plough, 2005).

It is recommended that infliximab is administered particularly in the first year of treatment, usually over a two-hour period and post-infusion observations continue for one to two hours. There are some differing infusion regimes evolving with developing clinical expertise. Shortened infusion and observation times have been used for those who are established on treatment, and for those who do not have a history of atopy or have experienced a previous infusion reaction. Buch *et al.* (2004)suggests that the risks of infusion-related reactions were high up to and including the fifth infusion and as a result subsequent infusions can be administered at a faster rate.

Delayed hypersensitivity reactions (myalgia, arthralgia fever, rash or facial oedema, dysphagia) are uncommon and appear to be exacerbated by increasing drug free intervals of less than a year (Schering Plough, 2005).

Auto-antibodies (see also general section on auto-antibodies)

When methotrexate is co-prescribed with infliximab the risk of antibodies against the infliximab monoclonal antibody (human anti-chimeric antibodies, HACA) is reduced. Infusion-related reactions are seen more frequently in individuals who have developed antibodies to infliximab.

Rituximab (Mabthera) B Cell CD 20 Depletion

Mode of Action

Rituximab is a genetically engineered anti-CD20 monoclonal antibody that acts by selectively depleting the number of circulating pre B and mature B cells. B cells expressing CD20 antigen develop during a specific phase of the B cells' maturity. This means that the overall integrity of the immune system is not compromised and is designed to sustain remission.

A number of research studies have focused on the role of B cells as a key player in the immunopathogenesis of RA (Shaw *et al.*, 2003). Apart from producing immunoglobulins, B cells may have additional stimulatory effects in inflammatory arthritis and may include:

- Acting as antigen-presenting cells and encouraging co-stimulation of T cells.
- Activating T cells.
- Secreting pro-inflammatory cytokines and chemokines.
- Producing rheumatoid factor (RF). Positive RF is linked to aggressive disease and may be implicated in enhancing stimulus to T cells.

Indication for Use

Rituximab has been used to treat non-Hodgkin's lymphoma (NHL) (Roche, 2005) for a number of years but it is possible that this licence could be extended to include the treatment of RA in patients who have failed anti-TNFα and are RF-positive. Although as yet unlicensed at time of going to press rituximab is being used for patients with severe RA that has failed to respond to anti-TNFα, and therefore it is important for practitioners to be aware of this treatment option.

Treatment with rituximab should always be given with a pre-medication (pain reliever and anti-histamine). Steroids should also be prescribed if rituximab is not administered as a combination with cyclophosphamide, doxorubicin hydrochloride;

oncovin (vincristine) and prednisolone (CHOP) or cyclophosphamide, vincristine and prednisolene (CVP) chemotherapy.

Rituximab has a long half life (up to 152.6 hours) after the first infusion and has been detected for three to six months following treatment (Roche, 2005).

Contraindications

Hypersensitivity to any component of rituximab or murine proteins.

Administration

An intravenous infusion of methylprednisolone (100 mg), paracetamol and antihistamine should be administered before each treatment of an intravenous infusion of rituximab of a fixed dose of 1000 mg rituximab. Treatment usually consists of 2 infusions administered 2 weeks apart (day 1 and day 15). A brief course of oral glucocorticoids should also be prescribed between first and second infusion (British National Formulary (BNF, 2004; Cohen *et al.*, 2006).

Side Effects and Cautions

The research and clinical experience of rituximab is extensive in the field of NHL although clinical experience in the treatment of RA and other inflammatory arthritidies is in its early years to date. Early studies appear to show that there are a reduced number of adverse events compared to those seen in patients with NHL (36% of RA-treated patient compared to 75% of those with NHL) for their first infusion and 10% during the second infusion. It remains to be seen, with greater clinical experience, if the wider aspects of the side effects profile for RA will vary from NHL (Emery *et al.*, 2006).

Cardiovascular

In clinical trials 18.8% of patients' cardiovascular events were reported with the most frequent reports related to hypotension and hypertension. Individuals treated with anti-hypertensives may need to have their treatment withheld for 12 hours prior to infusion. Rixutimab should be used in caution in individuals treated with cardiotoxic chemotherapy or who have cardiovascular disease as exacerbations of angina, arrhythmia and heart failure have been seen (BNF, 2004).

Haematological/Immunoglobulin

Haematological abnormalities (e.g. thrombocytopenia, neutropenia, anaemia) occurred in a minority of patients and were usually mild and reversible. Blood monitoring should be undertaken and if neutrophils are below $1.5 \times 10.^9/l$ or platelet counts are below $75 \times 10.^9/l$ treatment should be withheld until a medical opinion/review is undertaken.

Autoantibodies

There is a theoretical risk that human anti-chimeric antibodies (HACA) may develop from the biologically engineered rituximab, made up of human/mouse chimeric antibody. To date the incidence is low (<1%) and rarely associated with any clinical symptoms (Stahl *et al.*, 2004).

Infections

Bacterial, viral and to a lesser extent fungal infections have been identified in patients receiving rituximab, with severe infections occurring in 3.9% of patients in clinical trials. Some of these infections occurred during the treatment period (1.4%) and others presented during the follow-up period (2.5%) (Roche Products Ltd, 2005).

Very rare cases of hepatitis B reactivation have been reported in individuals who were also receiving cytotoxic chemotherapy whilst being treated with rituximab (Roche Products Ltd).

Infusion-related reactions (see also adverse reactions in general section)

The most common adverse events during or following rituximab treatment are mild to moderate infusion reactions (occurring in approximately 9% of patients) and are related to the rate of the infusion, usually occurring within two hours of the initial infusion (Hainsworth, 2003).

Patients with HACA titres may have allergic or hypersensitivity reactions when treated with other diagnostic or therapeutic monoclonal antibodies. Data in the treatment of NHL state that the incidence of infusion-related reactions are seen in approximately 50% (Roche Products Ltd, 2005). However, this data may not reflect the RA experience as some reactions seen in NHL are related to tumour lysis syndrome (TLS) and cytokine release syndrome (CRS), which may be specific to NHL and the specific tumour burden.

Infusion reactions include fever, chills, rigors and sometimes hypotension and dyspnoea and generally resolve quickly although in post-marking surveillance some fatal outcomes have been reported for those with severe reactions (Roche Products Ltd, 2005). It is therefore essential that full resuscitation support is readily available.

See Table 2.8 for general advice on the management of infusion-related reactions.

Drug Interactions

No data are currently available on drug interactions and the knowledge of agents capable of causing depletion of normal B Cells is as yet not known.

Pregnancy and Breastfeeding

Women (and men) of childbearing potential should use an effective method of contraceptive during treatment and up to 12 months from cessation of treatment as rituximab has a long half life (although proportional to the dose administered).

Women should not breastfeed whilst on rituximab.

Immunization

B cell depletion typically lasts for several months following treatment and it is therefore important to consider the immunization status of individuals prior to commencing treatment with rituximab and to complete all immunizations at least four weeks prior to the first administration of rituximab (Roche products, personal communication, 2005). Live vaccines should not be administered.

BIOLOGIC THERAPIES – PATIENT ISSUES

Patients should have had the opportunity to discuss all aspects of their treatment and be able, where appropriate, to select the treatment that best suits their needs. Risks and benefits should be explained and consent should be documented. All advice and information provided should be supported by written information and clear guidance on when to stop treatment and seek urgent medical advice.

The RCN guidance on training patients in the self-administration of subcutaneous therapies and detailed information on the management of patients prior to infusions will be a useful tool for practitioners (RCN, 2003). Additional guidance on management of rituximab infusions can be seen in Table 2.8.

Individuals treated with anti-TNFα therapies should be easily identified and treated promptly for infections. As a result specific patient alert cards have been developed for the patient to use to inform healthcare professionals and other care workers or dentists to inform them of key issues related to anti-TNFα therapies. These alert cards can be accessed easily (Arthritis and Research Campaign, 2005).

Biologic therapies will play an increasingly important role in the treatment of a range of autoimmune conditions and as such it is imperative that practitioners in all care settings have the expertise to support the patient in the assessment, management and ongoing monitoring of biologic therapies.

2.5 THE USE OF STEROIDS IN THE TREATMENT OF RHEUMATIC DISEASE

Corticosteroid drugs are synthetic derivatives of the body's naturally occurring corticosteroid hormones, which are produced in the cortex of the adrenal glands. The principal corticosteroid of the human adrenal cortex is cortisol (hydrocortisone) derived from the hydroxylation of cortisone. The adrenal gland production of corticosteroids is controlled by the hypothalamus and the pituitary gland via a negative feedback system. Corticosteroids consist of androgenics, mineralocorticoids and glucocorticoids.

GLUCOCORTICOIDS

These are responsible for:

- carbohydrate, protein and fat metabolism;
- the maintenance of blood sugar levels;
- the body's response to both physical and psychological stress;
- the suppression of inflammation and the immune response (Christiansen and Krane, 1993).

Much research has taken place to isolate the glucocorticoid that possesses precise anti-inflammatory and immunosuppressive properties but to date it remains elusive.

Therefore, the role of systemic steroids in the management of rheumatological disorders is complex because, whilst they are very effective anti-inflammatory and immunosuppressive agents, they are also associated with potentially serious side effects even with relatively low doses, which may cause significant morbidity.

Systemic steroids currently prescribed in the treatment of rheumatological disorders include hydrocortisone (cortisol), prednisolone, cortisone and methyl prednisolone.

Mode of Action

Corticosteroids act by binding to specific cytoplasmic receptors which then enter the nucleus where they cause the production of certain mRNAs (ribonucleic acid) coding for various proteins. The beneficial effects of systemic steroids are partly related to increased production of lipocortin and decreased production of the inflammatory response – for example, cytokines, prostaglandins and leukotrienes. The exact effects on the lymphocyte function are still poorly understood. It is not yet possible to separate different corticosteroid effects by using different corticosteroid analogs, indicating that their actions are similar and their relative potencies relate to their structure and plasma half life (Kirwan, 1994) (see Table 2.9).

THE USE OF STEROIDS IN RHEUMATOID ARTHRITIS

In a review of clinical trials of corticosteroids in RA it was concluded that in both short- and long-time studies corticosteroids are effective inflammatory agents, significantly better than placebos and NSAIDs in the relief of pain and stiffness (George and Kirwan, 1990). Work by Kirwan (1995) has demonstrated that patients with early RA who received prednisolone 7.5 mg daily for two years experienced less radiological joint damage (in the hands) than did those individuals receiving placebos. A systematic review from the Cochrane database concluded that prednisolone in doses of less than 15 mg daily may be used intermittantly in patients with RA, especially if the condition could not be controlled by other drugs (Gotzsche and Johansen, 2005). The review highlighted that the lower the dose of steroid the

Table 2.9   Half life of commonly used corticosteroids.

Short-acting: 8−12 hours
   Cortisone
   Cortisol

Intermediate acting: 12−36 hours
   Prednisolone
   Prednisone
   Methylprednisolone
   Triamcinolone

Long acting: 36−72 hours
   Paramethasone
   Dexamethasone
   Betamethasone

less risk of adverse side effects. Bone protection therapy should be commenced at the initiation of treatment with steroids.

However, the problem with using steroids for control of synovitis is that benefits are not sustained unless increasing doses are employed. This increases the risk of steroid side effects and it often becomes very difficult to decrease or stop the steroids.

CORTICOSTEROID SPARING AGENTS

This term is used to describe drugs which are prescribed in order to make it easier to reduce the corticosteroid dose, while at the same time controlling the underlying disease. Azathioprine, cyclophosphamide and methotrexate can all be used for this purpose.

ADVERSE EFFECTS OF CORTICOSTEROIDS (SEE TABLE 2.10)

The Immune System

Corticosteroids are powerful immunosuppressants, which affect both humoral and cell-mediated immune responses. Although corticosteroids can be valuable in the treatment of autoimmune diseases they can also be potentially life-threatening because high levels of corticosteroids will also reduce the formation of antibodies and the white cell count of patients, therefore permitting the invasion of bacteria or viruses and the spread of infection. Patients on long-term corticosteroids may also be predisposed to staphylococcal, gram-negative, tuberculous and listeria infections (Christiansen and Krane, 1993; Kirwan, 1994).

Table 2.10   Adverse effects of corticosteroids.

Metabolic: a) obesity: changes due to fat redistrubution result in cushingoid features such as a moon face; b) glucose protein metabolism: hypergylcemia and insulin resistance occur.

Decreased resistance to infection: due to immunosuppression. Candida and herpes zoster infection can occur along with a variety of bacterial infections.

Musculoskeletal: a) muscule wastage due to protein catabolism; b) tendon rupture occurs with direct injection into a tendon; c) osteoporosis due to a reduction in calcium absorption into the bones and increase in calcium excretion. Vertebral wedge and crush fractures are a frequent complication of treatment; d) corticosteroid withdrawal syndrome occurs with long-term use of steropids and as a result of too rapid a withdrawal. Symptoms include myalgia, fatigue, malaise, anorexia, nausea and weight loss.

Gastrointestinal: a) peptic ulceration due to the inhibition of gastric prostaglandins which maintain the integrity of the gastric mucosa; b) pancreatitis.

Ophthalmic including cataracts and glaucoma

Central nervous system: psychosis, euphoria and depression

Skin including acne, striae, alopecia, bruising and skin atrophy

Growth retardation

Adrenal suppression

Glucose Metabolism

The problem of glucose intolerance with patients receiving corticosteroids was initally highlighted in the late 1940s. The suggested mechanisms of glucose intolerance are as follows:

- decreased insulin secretion;
- increased hepatic glucose production;
- impaired peripheral glucose metabolism.

Methods of Administration

- orally;
- intravenous pulses;
- intra-articular injection;
- intra-muscular injection;
- soft tissue injection.

Pharmacokinetics

Following oral administration of prednisolone, absorption takes place quickly within the gastrointestinal tract and is rapidly metabolized within the liver, with excretion via the urine. Its action on the tissues is of a much longer duration than its presence in the blood (George and Kirwan, 1990).

Treatment Regimen

The factors that dictate the treatment regimen include the actual disease, its severity and the clinical response. Kirwan (1994) divides the treatment regime into three dose-related ranges:

- Low daily doses (up to 15 mg) to treat polymyalgia and symptomatic RA.
- High daily doses 20−60 mg for serious disease − for example, temporal arteritis, dermatomyositis, lupus erythematosus.
- Very high doses (pulsed methylprednisolone) for acute or life-threatening crisis.

THE USE OF CORTICOSTEROIDS IN OTHER RHEUMATOLOGICAL CONDITIONS

The symptoms of PMR and temporal arteritis (TA) often overlap. No controlled trials have been conducted to provide guidance on the best treatment dosage with corticosteroids (Kirwan, 1994). Although practice will differ, PMR is often treated with an initial dose of 15 mg prednisolone daily reducing slowly over 18−24 months governed by blood inflammatory parameters and clinical symptoms. One potential problem is to commence too high a dose of prednisolone accompanied by too rapid a reduction in dosage overtime. This will often result in an exacerbation of original symptoms.

The treatment of TA requires a much higher dose of steroid, usually 60−100 mg daily.

Collagenosis

The use of steroids will be largely determined by the nature of the collagenosis complication rather than by the collagenosis itself − for example, in the case of SLE many individuals with mild disease manifestations may not require steroids.

Inflammatory Muscle Diseases

Dermatomysitis and polymyositis patients are treated with medium to high daily dose steroids initally. This will often be accompanied with a cytotoxic agent such as azathioprine or methotrexate.

Vasculitis

Management of vasculitis involving major organs (e.g. Wegener's granulomatosis, rheumatoid vasculitis, polyarteritis nodosa) will necessitate the use of high dose steroids orally or intravenous pulse therapy.

BONE MINERAL METABOLISM

Studies have revealed that cytoplasmic glucocorticoid receptors are present in bone cells, which appear to influence calcium intake and excretion and the factors that regulate hormones, cytokines and growth factors. Therefore, prolonged steroid therapy possesses multifaceted adverse effects on bone mineral metabolism which precipitate growth retardation in children, osteoporosis, long bone and vertebral fractures. The adverse effects of steroids that affect bone material metabolism include their effects on:

- Osteoblasts: steriod therapy has been shown to reduce circulating osteocalcin levels which affect osteoblast activity thus inhibiting bone formation. Studies have also revealed that bone matrix synthesis is affected within 24 hours of the administration of steroids (Godschalk and Downs, 1988; Reid et al., 1986).
- Osteoclasts: steriod therapy is thought to have a dual accelerating effect of bone reabsorption (1) by directly stimulating osteoclasts or (2) indirectly under the influence of parathyroid hormone (PTH).
- Gastrointestinal absportion of calcium: the consensus of opinion is that steroids suppress the intestinal absorption of calcium although the reason remains unclear.
- Excretion of calcium: a decrease in the reabsorption of calcium within the kidneys has been shown to occur in patients. Although glucocorticoid receptors are present in the kidney their precise mode of action on calcium reabsorption/excretion is unclear (Fuller and Funder, 1976).
- Vitamin D: extensive research regarding the effects of steroids and 25-hydroxyvitamin D levels has revealed conflicting evidence; hence the suggested osteopenic effects of steroids in relation to 25-hydroxyvitamin D levels remains controversial.
- Parathyroid hormone (PTH): PTH-regulated blood phosphorus and calcium levels via its actions on the intestines, bone tissue and kidneys. A normal concentration of calcium (2.2−2/6 mmol/1) is essential for normal physiology. However, numerous studies have demonstrated that steroids stimulate the parathyroid glands and increase PTH levels, which stimulate osteoclasts to accelerate bone resorption (Cosman et al., 1992; Gray et al., 1991).
- Growth retardation: since the early 1950s growth retardation in children has been a recognized side effect of long-term steroid therapy, although the precise mechanisms remain elusive. It is suggested that steroid therapy has a direct effect and an indirect consequence on both the osteoblast and cartilage cells, which consequently suppresses the growth of linear bone and impedes epiphyseal closure (Loeb, 1976). The prevention of growth retardation is helped by prescribing an alternate-day regimen (Clarke and Fitzgerald, 1984; Guest and Broyer, 1991; Polito et al., 1986).

Studies of bone loss in adults treated with cortisteroids do not clearly suggest a threshold dose below which osteoporosis can be avoided (Kirwan, 1994), although there does appear to be a consistent relationship between doses above 7.5 mg daily and the rate of bone loss.

PEPTIC ULCERATION

Evidence from controlled studies of corticosteroid therapy suggests that the increased risk of peptic ulceration is considerably lower than is widely believed (Cooper and Kirwan, 1990). However, corticosteroids may exacerbate the ulcergenic properties of NSAIDs (Piper et al., 1991).

ATHEROSCLEROSIS

Prolonged corticosteroid therapy may accelerate the development of atherosclerosis (Cooper and Kirwan, 1990), with lower limb atherosclerosis occuring in as many as 60% of corticosteroid-treated patients with RA. The evidence linking corticosteroid therapy with atherosclerosis is still considered controversial but, in time, even a small effect could have considerable clinical significance.

REDUCING THE DOSE OF CORTICOSTEROIDS

High doses of corticosteroids are often used for only short periods and can be reduced rapidly with little adverse effect. The exact mode of reduction will depend on the control of the clinical situation. Patients treated with moderate to low doses of corticosteroid over a longer duration of time may develop a corticosteroid withdrawal syndrome when their treatment is reduced. This can include the symptoms of myalgia, fatigue and nausea and has been reported in as many as 70% of patients treated with 30 mg prednisolone daily for longer than three months (Dixon and Christy, 1980).

One approach to try and avoid this is to reduce the corticosteroid treatment very slowly, often by as little as 2.5 mg daily every two months down to 7.5 mg daily, then introduce further graduated reductions of 1.0 mg daily or by 1.0 mg on alternate days.

The administration of exognous steroids may result in the suppression of the body's own (endogenous) steroid production. Therefore, when exogenous steroids are withdrawn, the adrenal gland may fail to produce adequate cortisol, resulting in a steroid crisis with a failure of cortisol production. This in turn results in hypotension, hypoglycaemia and electrolyte imbalance. All patients on steroid treatment should carry a steroid card with them.

The withdrawal of steroids can lead to a marked flair in symptoms of the disease process, which may necessitate the patient being recommended on steroids.

PULSED CORTICOSTEROIDS

Pulse therapy involves the intravenous infusion of a large dose of corticosteroid (usually 500 mg−1 g of methylprednisolone) over 30−60 minutes. There are many different treatment regimens in practice but most include a course of three pulses on alternate days, followed by a resting phase of around six weeks (Kirwan and the Arthritis and Rheumatism Council Low Dose Glucocorticoid Study Group, 1995). It may be used to bridge the time interval between initiation and response to DMARDs or, when a patient has an acute flare of their RA, to induce remission. A review of the use of pulsed methylprednisolone (Weusten, Jacobs and Bijlsma, 1993) shows few or minor side effects. Those who have experienced severe adverse effects of the cardiovascular system, or experienced infection, had existing compromised cardiovascular and immune systems as a result of their disease or due to concomitant drug therapy (Kirwan, 1995).

INTRAMUSCULAR CORTICOSTEROIDS

Intramuscular injections of corticosteroid may be used to reduce the symptoms of a flare in RA, or be administered prior to the initiation of DMARD where it is known that these medications take many months before benefit can be assessed. It is important to give the injection deep into the muscle to prevent muscular atrophy occurring. Choy *et al.* (1993) found that intramuscular methylprednisolone was superior to equivalent oral doses in their study of corticosteroids and gold therapy.

INTRA-ARTICULAR/SOFT TISSUE INJECTIONS OF CORTICOSTEROIDS

Intra-articular and soft tissue injections are interventions used in the management of rheumatology disorders that offer an effective supplement to systemic therapies in the control of inflammatory joint disease. In comparison to oral corticosteroids, they are well tolerated and safe if administered appropriately. The Royal College of Nursing Rheumatology Forum has produced guidelines on the use and administration of intra-articular injections, including contraindications for the administration (see Appendix 2.B).

2.6 DISORDERS OF PURINE METABOLISM: GOUT

Gout is caused by inflammation induced by microcrystalline uric acid in the form of monosodium urate monohydrate in joints and soft tissues. A usual but not essential prerequisite for the condition is a raised plasma level of urate, which is derived from endogenous and dietary nucleoproteins (Snaith and Adebajo, 2004).

HYPERURICAEMIA

Uric acid is the product of purine metabolism and hyperuricaemia can occur either from an overproduction of uric acid (20–25% patients) or when the kidneys fail to excrete uric acid (75% of patients). Excessive hyperuricaemia may then result in the formation of uric acid crystals, which are deposited in various parts of the body, more commonly in the joints of the foot, hand and knee. However, uric acid crystals may also form torphi in soft tissues or as stones in the kidney.

Prevalence

The prevalence of gout is 5−10 per 1000 adults in the United Kindom. It can occur in young men with a family history of gout, middle-aged men with hypertension, obesity and cardiovascualr disease and in older men and women secondary to diuretic use (Snaith and Adebajo, 2004).

Clinical Features

70% of patients present with an acute attack of gout, which is typically characterized by a sudden onset of podagra (an acute, red, painful swelling at the metatarsophalangeal joint of the great toe), although both the knee and hand may also be affected. Patients with acute attacks may also present with a raised erythrocyte sedimentation rate, pyrexia and leucocytosis.

Precipitating Factors

- A sudden raised level of uric acid (greater than 430 umol/1 resulting either from an oversecretion from the liver or impaired kidney excretion).
- Obesity.
- Alcohol.
- Hypertension.
- Severe dietary restriction.
- Diuretics.
- A sudden fall of uric acid levels following the administration of allopurinol or uricosuric drugs.
- Trauma.
- Surgery.
- Severe systemic illness.

If episodes of acute gout reoccur and remain untreated, gout develops into a chronic condition in which erosions of both cartilage and bone may occur along with deposits of trophi. Trophi are composed of sodium biurate and appear as small hard chalky or cheesy deposits which may discharge and ulcerate. Consequently, chronic gout may result in joint deformities and subsequent functional impairment.

Diagnosis

The examination of synovial fluid by polarized light microscopy is used to identify monosodium uric acid crystals. The identification of these crystals provides the clinician with a definite diagnosis of gout, thus excluding either sepsis or pseudogout.

The crystals present in pseudogout are calcium pyrophosphate. The correct diagnosis is paramount to ensure that patients are not prescribed treatment unnecessarily (Currey, 1988).

Diagnosis Features

- Hyperuricaemia (although not all patients with hyperuricaemia have gout).
- X-rays in early acute attacks are unremarkable. However, the appearance of classic 'punched out' erosions (radiolucent urate tophi) appear later with chronic gout.
- Following susbequent episodes of gout, examination of the patient may reveal tophaceous deposits in the helix of the ear, bursae, tendon sheaths and kidney parenchyma.

Treatment

The management of gout is planned in two stages: initially the management of the acute inflammatory joint symptoms, and secondly the long-term management of persistent hyperuricaemia.

First-Stage Treatment

The aim of initial therapy is to suppress the inflammatory process induced by the deposit of uric acid crystals, which may be present in and around joints, tendons and in the kidney parenchyma. Hence, non-steroidal anti-inflammatory drugs are the first line of treatment. The NSAID prescribed will depend on both the patient's tolerance and the clinician's preference. The initial dose required is usually twice the normal maintenance dose for three days, reverting to the maintainance dose until resolution is achieved (Snaith and Adebajo, 2004), usually by 14 days.

In those patients for whom NSAIDs are contraindicated, colchicine is prescribed but is often not tolerared at its full dose. Oral or parental steroids are also effective but septic arthritis must be excluded before their use. If using oral prednisolone it can be prescribed at 30 mg daily tapering to zero over 10 days (Snaith and Adebajo, 2004).

Colchicine

Derived from the autumn crocus *colchicum autumnale*, colchicine is an ancient remedy which has been prescribed since the eighteenth century for the treatment of gout (Emmerson, 1994).

Mode of Action

Colchicine is an alkaloid that halts both the inflammatory response and the deposit of uric acid crystals, although its precise mode of action is complicated and not entirely understood.

Pharmacokinetics

Following administration, colchicine is absorbed through the upper small bowel, metabolized by the liver and then excreted both in the bile and intestinal secretions. As 20% is excreted unchanged in the urine, the dose of colchicine should be adjusted accordingly for those patients who have pre-existing renal disease (Emmerson, 1994).

Treatment Regimen

Initially patients are prescribed 1mg, followed by 0.5 mg every 2 hours which usually has an effect within 24 hours of commencement of therapy. However, because the therapeutic regimen may mirror the toxic dose, dosage continues until either:

- The maximum total dose is attained (10mg).
- The gout subsides.
- Side effects are experienced (diarrhoea and vomiting).

NB: colchicine 0.5 mg 2−3 times daily may also be prescribed concurrently with initial long-term treatment of hypouricaemic drugs to prevent further attack of acute gout. Adverse effects are shown in Table 2.11.

Drug Interactions

Ciclosporin: increased plasma levels − therefore possible risk of both nephroxity and myotoxicity.

Second-Stage Therapy: Long-Term Treatment

The aim of long-term treatment of gout is to prevent the possible consequences of further episodes of acute gout (joint deformity, loss of joint function, and kidney damage).

Table 2.11   Adverse effects of colchicine.

Nausea/vomiting
Abdominal pain
Gastrointestinal haemorrhage
Rashes
Renal and hepatic impairment
Peripheral neuritis
Myopathy
Blood disorders (with prolonged therapy)

The hypouricaemic drug most commonly prescribed is allopurinol, which is a xanthine-oxidase inhibitor which acts to inhibit the production of uric acid. Other hypouricaemic drugs include probenecid and sulfinpyrazone, which are both uricosuric drugs that block the tubular reabsorption of filtered urate in the kidneys and therefore increase the excretion of uric acid via the kidneys. Second-stage therapy, therefore, is prescribed to prevent recurring acute attacks of gout by maintaining uric acid levels that fall within normal blood plasma parameters.

Indications for the prescription of second-stage therapy:

- Hyperuricaemia with recurrent episodes of acute gout.
- Visible tophi and/or erosions revealed by radiological examination.
- Associated renal impairment.

Allopurinol

Allopurinol acts by inhibiting xanthine oxidase, the product that enables the conversion of xanthine and hypoxanthine to uric acid (Edwards and Boucher, 1991). Because of its low incidence of side effects, allopurinol is the most widely used drug for the long-term prophylaxis of gout. Its added advantage is that it can also be prescribed for those patients with renal impairment or those who have kidney stones (which are conditions contraindicated for treatment with uricosuric drugs).

Treatment Regimen

A dose of 100 mg once daily initially for one week (initial dose for both the elderly and patients with renal dysfunction should be reduced to 50 mg to prevent toxicity; Gibson, 1988), increasing over two to three weeks to a maintenance dose (dependent on either blood plasma or urinary uric levels) of 200−600 mg daily in divided doses. Tablets should be taken after food.

Uricosuric Drugs

Probenecid

Treatment Regimen

- Week one: 250 mg twice daily.
- Week two: 500 mg twice daily.
- Maintenance dose up to 2 g daily in divided doses according to uric acid levels. Tablets are to be taken after food.

Sulfinpyrazone

Treatment Regimen

Initially 100 mg−200 mg daily, increasing over two to three weeks to 600 mg daily.

Maintenance dose (when uric acid blood plasma falls within normal levels) may be possible to reduce to 200 mg daily. Tablets to be taken with either food or milk.

Compliance of long-term therapy is dependent on patient education regarding the differing actions of both initial and long-term therapies. To prevent further attacks of gout, patients should receive health promotion regarding the risk factors that can precipitate an acute episode of gout.

Benzbromarone is more potent than probenecid or sulfinpyrazone and it can be used in patients with renal impairment and in conjunction with allopurinol. It does increase the risk of stone formation so a high fluid intake is important (Snaith and Adebajo, 2004).

Diet and Lifestyle

Dietary advice can prevent futher attacks of gout.

- Weight reduction.
- Saturated fats replaced with unsaturated fats.
- Relative increase in protein intake.
- Many beers contain guanosine which is converted into uric acid by gut bacteria.
- Alcohol taken without food is catabolized to lactate and other ketones that compete with urate for excretion via the renal tubule.
- Alcohol also decreases the conversion of allopurinol to the effective metabolite oxipurinol.
- Fortified wines may contain oxalates, which contribute to the formation of stones.
- Coffee and tea are diuretics and can interfere with assays for urate (Snaith and Adebajo, 2004).

For more information on gout contact: www.ukgoutsociety.org

2.7 NURSE PRESCRIBING

The Crown Report on Prescribing, Supply and Administration of Medicines (DoH, 1999) provided the framework for the development of prescribing for nurses. The report describes two types of nurse prescribers.

- Independent prescribers who diagnose patients and then prescribe an appropriate medication.
- Supplementary prescribers who are responsible for the care of the patient once the diagnosis and treatment plan has been determined by an independent prescriber. For example, a patient with inflammatory symptoms will be reviewed by the rheumatologist. Once a diagnosis of RA has been established and the need for DMARDs established the rheumatologist could refer the patient to a rheumatology nurse for the instigation of a DMARD and the necessary ongoing surveillance.

The recommendations of the Crown Report were implemented in three stages.

- Patient group directions (PGDs) for the supply and administrations of medicines (DoH, 2000a). (Appendix 2.C contains an example of a PGD that enables nurses to administer intramuscular Depomedrone to patients with rheumatoid arthritis.)
- Independent prescribing for nurses (DoH, 2000b).
- Supplementary prescribing for pharmacists and nurses (DoH, 2002).

WHO SHOULD PRESCRIBE?

The National Prescribing Centre (NCP) (2005) have suggested the following criteria that may help to identify nurses who would benefit from becoming prescribers. These include nurses who:

- Run their own clinics or services, which would include most rheumatology clinical nurse specialists.
- Work in isolation from other prescribers (although to a lesser extent with supplementary prescribers who need to work in partnership with an independent prescriber).
- Could complete episodes of care if they were able to prescribe.
- Are likely to be able to prescribe for more than one medical condition.
- Hold additional qualifications whereby their professional expertise would facilitate prescribing for specified medical conditions.

INDEPENDENT PRESCRIBING

The first extended nurse prescribers qualified in 2002. The main goal was to have competent nurse prescribers who could treat patients in four specific areas:

- minor illness;
- minor injuries;
- health promotion;
- palliative care.

These areas were chosen as they represent the commonest reasons for patients requiring input from their GPs and the introduction of the extended nurse prescribers (ENPs) formulary was to enable nurses to prescribe in these four domains, in a safe, quick and effective manner to benefit the patients and free up GP time. Consequently the initial nurse prescribing courses were aimed at nurses working in walk-in centres or running minor injury clinics. The ENPs formulary is a list that contains over 70 symptoms and specific conditions for which the nurse prescriber can prescribe (see www.nurse-prescriber.co.uk).

Acute musculoskeletal conditions for which an ENP can prescribe include:

- acute chronic back pain (uncomplicated);
- neck pain (uncomplicated);

- soft tissue injury;
- sprains;
- low back pain;
- knee pain;
- osteoarthritis;
- rheumatoid arthritis.

Independent prescribing is appropriate in the following circumstance:

- The nurse works remotely from a doctor, seeing patients independently for those conditions listed in the nurse prescriber extended formulary (NPEF).
- The doctor could see and treat other patients while the nurse sees some patients.
- The nurse is competent to assess, diagnose and make treatment decisions for the patient.

It is not suitable for prescribing for complex medical conditions or for patients with several co-morbidities (Department of Health Medicines and Healthcare Products Regulatory Agency, 2005a).

From spring 2006, qualified extended formulary nurse prescribers and pharmacists who are independent prescribers will be able to prescribe any licensed medicine (except controlled drugs) for any medical condition. Extended formulary nurse prescribers will be known as nurse independent prescribers (NIPs) and supplementary prescribers as nurse supplementary prescribers (NSPs).

SUPPLEMENTARY PRESCRIBING

The Department of Health define supplementary prescribing as a voluntary prescribing partnership between an independent prescriber and a supplementary prescriber to implement an agreed, patient-specific, clinical management plan with the patient's agreement (Hennell, 2004).

Once the patient has been diagnosed by the independent prescriber (who in this situation has to be a doctor) a clinical management plan (CMP) is required that has to involve both the independent and supplementary prescriber (in this case a rheumatology nurse).

The Department of Health (2002) state that the CMP should:

- Be patient-specific.
- Be agreed by both the independent and supplementary prescribers before supplementary prescribing begins and supported by the intended recipient.
- Specify the range and circumstances within which the supplementary prescriber can vary the dose, frequency and formulation of the medicines identified.
- Specify when to refer from supplemntary prescriber to independent prescriber.
- Contain relevant warnings about known sensitivities of the patient to particular medicines, and include arrangements for notification of adverse drug reactions.
- Contain the date of commencement of the arrangment and a date for review (not normally longer than one year for patients with chronic conditions).

Supplementary prescribers can prescribe all medications currently prescribed by doctors with the exception of unlicensed medicines (except in specific circumstances) – see Department of Health web site: www.doh.gov.uk/ supplementaryprescribing/plan.htm.

Supplementary prescribing is appropriate in the following circumstances:

- Patients with long-term conditions, who can be managed by a nurse or pharmacist and some allied health professionals (AHPs) between reviews by the doctor.
- Nurses or pharmacists (and some AHPs) who are competent to manage the patient's condition.
- There is a close working partnership between the independent prescriber (doctor) and the supplementary prescriber, who have access to the same patient record.

Supplementary prescribing is not suited to an urgent prescribing situation because an agreed CMP is required before prescribing can begin (DoH, 2005a).

EDUCATIONAL PREPARATION

Potential nurse prescribers must undertake a Nurse and Midwifery Council (NMC) approved course at level three (first degree level) consisting of at least 26 taught days plus 12 days learning and assessment in practice working with a designated medical practitioner.

PROFESSIONAL RESPONSIBILITIES

As with all areas of practice, nurse prescribers must act within their own level and area of competence acknowledging the scope and limitations of their role. In order to promote safe and effective practice there must be clearly defined policies, support mechanisms and audit systems (Cully, 2005). The National Prescribing Centre (2002) have produced a useful resource reminding nurses of their legal and professional accountability and duty of care.

EVALUATION OF PRESCRIBING

National research evaluating the first two years of extended formulary prescribing demonstrated that it was well received by nurses, patients and doctors and had a positive impact on patient care because of improved access (Latter, 2005). Nurse prescribers felt that:

- they were confident in their prescribing practice;
- extended prescribing had a positive impact on patient care and enabled nurses to make better use of their skills;
- the limited nursing formulary imposed unhelpful limitations on their practice;
- they had received support from their medical practitioner (Latter, 2005).

An audit of the prescribing practice of rheumatology nurses in one rheumatology department over a 10-month period demonstrated that the majority of patients requiring a prescription were patients with RA (81%) and the commonest drug prescribed was methotrexate (35%) (Hennell, 2005). All patients were satisfied with specialist nurses issuing a prescription. The specialist nurses have a greater sense of job satisfaction and are autonomously able to complete episodes of care. It also provides medical staff with more time to manage patients with complex medical needs (Hennell, 2004).

Clinical Management Plan
  Name of patient: Mrs B. Davenpot
  Patient identification e.g. ID number, date of birth: 04/04/1944
  Patient medication sensitivities/allergies: penicillamine
  Current medication: diclofenac 75mg BD; co-codamol.
  Medical history: Hypertension
  Independent prescriber: Dr H.
  Contact details: tel./e-mail/address
  Supplementary prescriber: Nurse X.
  Contact details: tel./e-mail/address
  Condition(s) to be treated: active rheumatoid arthritis
  Aim of treatment: to suppress disease activity
  Treatment plan:

- Commence methotrexate 7.5 mg weekly for eight weeks.
- After eight weeks increase methotrexate by increments of 2.5 mg every fortnight until a dose of 15 mg in reached.
- Commence folic acid 5 mg daily.
- Observe full blood count (FBC), AST and ALT weekly for the first month and then monthly.
- Observe for dry cough or breathlessness.

Indication: methotrexate
Preparation: oral
Dose schedule: as above
When and who to refer to: Dr H. if change, no improvement (after four months) or if adverse event occurs.
  Guidelines supporting treatment plan:

- Inhouse protocols (January 2006).
- Current BNF (September 2005).
- Oxford Handbook of Rheumatology (Hakim and Clunie, 2002).

Review and monitoring requirements: weekly for the first month and then monthly.
  Process for reporting adverse drug reactions (ADRs): yellow card.
  Documentation and record keeping: hospital case notes and patient's computerized record.

Name and agreement of independent prescriber/supplementary prescriber, date, date agreed with patient.

There are various useful websites for nurse prescribers including:

- Department of Health: www.dh.gov.uk
- NHS Modernisation Agency: www.modern.nhs.uk/cwp
- Medicines and Healthcare Products Regulatory Agency: www.mhra.gov.uk
- National Prescribing Centre: www.npc.co.uk
- Prescribing News: www.nurse-prescriber.co.uk
- Prodigy: www.prodigy.nhs
- Royal Pharmaceutical Society of Great Britain: www.rpsgb.org.uk.

2.8   SELF-MEDICATION

If the treatment of RA is to be effective, patients must have the ability to adjust drug administration according to the changing activity of their disease (Hill *et al.*, 1991). It is vital in patients with chronic inflammatory conditions who take medications for a long period of time as there is a clear need to assess both the safety and efficacy of the drug regime (Hopkins, 1990), especially as it is the patient who will be responsible for administering prescribed medications at home. Healthcare professionals can no longer assume that people are passive recipients of care, and patients will require information to administer medicines safely and effectively (Kennedy, 1981).

Beardsley, Anderson Johnson and Kabat (1983) define drug self-administration procedures as specific education strategies that contain the necessary knowledge and behavioural components to effect better compliancy. (The whole area of adherence is discussed in further depth in Chapter 4.)

THE CASE FOR SELF-MEDICATION

The conventional system of drug administration from a ward trolley often neglects to address the need for individual education nor does it seek to prepare patients to administer drugs within their own home environment following discharge. All the nurse has to do is to administer and sign that the prescribed drug has been given. This is despite the fact that health education has become a major part of the nurse's role (Bird, 1990). This traditional system frequently provides dosages at incorrect times and unfortunately is not error-free (Johnson and Giles, 1993). It should no longer be acceptable to the profession and we should aim to provide patients with a personal pharmacy (Corrigan, 1989). Webb (1990) states that the traditional approach of batch processing suits staff convenience rather than being governed by patient need; whereas a holistic humanitarian approach to nursing care necessitates considering people as individuals and providing care in partnership with them.

An important but often neglected area of discharge planning is whether a patient is being discharged home without adequate knowledge of their tablets or with containers that they cannot open. The NMC has recommended that self-administration projects be established during a hospital stay to provide patients with the necessary knowledge and confidence to continue with a high degree of compliancy on discharge (Sutherland, Morgan and Sample, 1991).

Many patients, particularly those in the older age group, are taking medications when they are admitted to hospital. Quilligan (1990) offers a framework for ensuring that older patients are given enough support in learning about their tablets. It follows the structure of the nursing process:

Patient Assessment

- Does the patient understand their condition and the purpose of their medications?
- Does the patient want to learn more about their medications and are they able to do so?
- Can the family be involved in the process?

Planning and Implementation

- Use realistic joint goals on agreed topics and if possible conduct the sessions when the family can be present.
- Limit the teaching to 3 topics in a 15-minute-maximum session.
- Discuss the patient's worries and check previous knowledge.

Evaluation

- Ongoing assessment of managing tablets and the teaching programme is required.

ADVANTAGES OF SELF-MEDICATION

Patients have the chance to familiarize themselves with their medications and the opening of the containers/packaging. They would be able to discuss any needs or concerns whilst the nurse would have the opportunity to assess patient knowledge, evaluate previous teaching and identify those patients who will need ongoing support from the community services.

A programme of self-medication may help to reduce the number of drug errors as it would incorporate extensive patient education and provide the opportunity for supervised practice of drug administration. Nurses reported that those patients who had self-medicated in hospital had a better understanding of all aspects of their drug regime (Bird, 1990). Work by Scrivin and Bryan (1987) found that patients were very appreciative of a self-medication programme and medication errors reduced from 17.9% to 6.9% after the programme had been introduced. Also, if patients experience accidental overdoses it is safer for this to occur in the hospital rather than the home environment.

Self-medication returns control to the patient, promoting comfort and demonstrating trust (Bird, 1990). A self-medicating patient will not be woken at 6 a.m. or stay awake until after midnight for sedation, or seek out a nurse for analgesia. Corrigan (1989) found that patients would question if the tablets looked different and were likely to refuse steroids until after breakfast. Webb (1990) found that most patients took in the process of self-medication very quickly, feeling unrushed over administration and enjoyed having something positive to do.

STAGES IN THE IMPLEMENTATION OF SELF-MEDICATION

- Planning — this is often considered the most important stage and cannot be rushed. It is vital to the overall success of the programme to gain the cooperation and support of all those involved including the ward staff, doctors and (crucially) the pharmacist.
- Assessment — in some units this will be a dual process involving both the pharmacist and the nursing staff. The patient will be assessed on their understanding as to the purpose of their medications, their safety in administration (i.e. timing and dosage), potential side effects to report and their psychomotor skills in the handling and reading of their medications. It is at this stage that the nurse will enter into a therapeutic partnership with the patient, offering support and education on an individualized basis to both the patient and their family as required. Table 2.12 lists the information that patients will require to know about their medications. An assessment document is often used to highlight any perceived problems and to determine the level of supervision required.
- Accountability can be a major concern to nurses when they consider implementing a self-medication programme. It can generate concerns of losing control

Table 2.12   What patients need to know about their medication (Quilligan, 1990).

The name of the drug
How it is taken
Its intended action
What dosage to take
The side effects
The time of day it is to be taken
How many tablets to take and how often
Whether to take it with food
What to do if a dose is omitted
Check the expiry date
Not to stop essential medicines without first contacting the doctor
Whether any special storage is required
Can you drive?
Not to take any non-prescription drugs without first consulting the doctor

over drug administration whilst still holding the same degree of responsibility. In fact, the nurse is not losing any element of control but is able to utilize the skills of educator, guide and supporter in a more constructive manner to ensure that patients are safely and knowledgeably administering their tablets. It could be argued that there are more concerns about accountability in the traditional system of drug administration as nurses could be engaging in the provision of medicines without ascertaining the patient's knowledge and understanding of the therapy. Bird (1990) states that the anticipated problems that nurses fear of patients forgetting to take their tablets, taking too many tablets or gaining access to other people's drugs seldom occurs in practice.

- Implementation – in some units a staging process is used. The assessment process will determine the level the patients enter the programme and what degree ofsupervision is required – for example:

  - Level One – the nurse administers the medicines providing full explanation.
  - Level Two – the patient administers the medicines with nurse supervision.
  - Level Three – the patient administers the medicines without supervision (Sutherland, Morgan and Sample, 1991).

Some areas have introduced memory aids in the form of calendar cards, which have been shown to lead to fewer errors when compared with written or verbal instructions (Wandless and Davie, 1997).

- Evaluation –various degrees of supervision have been used, generally including at least daily discussions and observations of the patient's progress. Evaluation should include the obtainment of both the patient's and the nurse's views on progress.

2.9   COMPLEMENTARY MEDICINE

Alternative and complementary medicine is the aggregate of diagnostic and therapeutic practices and systems that are separate from, and in contrast to, conventional scientific medicines (Champion, 1994). Table 2.13 demonstrates the different types of complementary medicines available today.

A third to almost 100% of patients with RA admit to using some form of complementary therapies (Ernst, 1998). Reasons for using complementary therapies include dissatisfaction with conventional medicines and the need for psychological support (Moore, 2000; Jacobs, Kraaimaat and Bijlsma, 2001). Many nurse practitioners actively recommend complementary treatments to patients (Sohn and Cook, 2002).

Table 2.13   Complementary therapies.

Acupuncture
Aromatherapy
Chinese medicine
Diet
Herbalism
Holistic medicine
Homeopathy
Massage
Naturopathy
Osteopathy
Reflexology
Spiritualism
Yoga

DIET

The extensive research into dietary treatments of RA has been reviewed by
Buchanan *et al.* (1991) and the results remain inconclusive. Individual dietary
manipulation may be beneficial to selected patients (Darlington *et al.*, 1986; Panush
et al., 1983) but it is difficult to generalize from these findings and further study
with sound methodological design is required.

Patients are extremely interested in this area and invest both time and money,
striving to obtain relief from their symptoms. Dozens of publications vie with each
other to suggest yet another method of ridding sufferers of pain and inflammation —
often contradicting each other. Trials have shown that the green-lipped mussel
extract (Seatone) does not work but its sales continue (Champion, 1994).

Surveys have found that many patients with RA consume diets that are marginally
inadequate in several essential nutrients (Kowsari *et al.*, 1983; see Table 2.14).
There is no sound evidence that the pharmacologic doses of vitamins used to treat
arthritis have definite therapeutic efficacy. However, there is work to suggest that
vitamin C, and perhaps vitamin E as an oxidant, could slow the progression of
osteoarthritis (Champion, 1994).

RA is associated with moderate hypochromic normocytic anaemia, which is
caused by a reduction in endogenous iron metabolism rather than dietary deficiency
(Smith, Driscoll and Coniff, 1985). Abnormalities in iron metabolism tend to be
corrected as disease activity is suppressed.

Diets rich in fish oil containing N-3 fatty acids, along with a reduction of N-6
fatty acid intakes, have been associated with improvements in pain and stiffness.
Some authors claim that fish oils will help inflammation by reducing arachidonic
acid and leukotrienes production (Chaitow, 1997). Dietary fish oils may prove to

be more effective when used in combination with specific anti-inflammatory agents (Champion, 1994).

Dietary Advice for Patients

For patients with OA:

- Reduce carbohydrates and fats.
- Keep weight down.
- Exercise regularly.

For patients with RA:

- Eat a well-balanced diet that contains minerals and vitamins.
- Eat more fruit and vegetables.
- If weight loss is experienced, increase carbohydrate intake.
- Seek advice regarding drug therapy.

For patients with gout:

- Advice on weight management.
- Reduction of high purine foods.
- Reduction in alcohol intake.

For patients with osteoporosis, see Chapter 3.

MASSAGE

Body massage is a method of manually manipulating the tissues of the body by either stroking, percussion or applying pressure. These actions increase the circulation of blood and lymph, and induce relaxation by soothing sensory nerve endings in the skin (Goldberg, 1991). There have been verbal reports from patients with RA and fibromyalgia that this form of intervention reduces pain and enhances sleep but evaluation from a critical perspective remains limited.

Table 2.14 Nutrients that can be lacking in the diet of patients with RA.

Calcium
Carbohydrates
Folacin
Magnesium
Pantothenic acid
Vitamin B6

AROMATHERAPY

Aromatherapy is the use of essential oils to promote healing in both a physical and a psychological manner. Methods of application include massage, bathing, compresses and steam inhalations. Aromatherapy professes to provide pain relief, reduce inflammation and to maintain joint mobility in patients with RA (Worwood, 1993). Advice must be sought from a qualified aromatherapist before treatment can be instigated.

REFLEXOLOGY

Reflexology is a form of massage applied to the reflex areas present in both the feet and hands. It is suggested that these reflex areas correspond with a specific area of the body and can stimulate the natural healing powers of the body (Dougans and Ellis, 1992).

Reflex areas suggested to ease the symptoms of RA include:

- The diaphram to reduce muscle tension.
- The shoulder and arm to enhance circulation and nerve conduction.
- The hip and leg to aid healing.
- The spine to improve flexibility and to balance the nervous system.
- The solar plexus to promote deep breathing and relaxation.
- The parathyroid glands to maintain homeostasis with both calcium and potassium levels.
- The liver to remove toxins from the body.
- The adrenals to stimulate cortisone production, maintain mineral balance and enhance muscle tone (Norman, 1992).

ACUPUNCTURE

Acupuncture is believed to change the vital energy which flows in the body and connects the internal organs with the superficial parts of the body (Beinfield and Korngold, 1992). It is currently used for musculoskeletal conditions by orthodox, complementary and alternative practitioners (Champion, 1994).

HERBAL MEDICINE

Herbal derivatives are widely used in orthodox rheumatology (Champion, 1994) – for example:

- Salicylates (willow bark).
- Colchicine (Autumn crocus).
- Opiates (opium poppy).
- Quinine (cinchana bark).

Controlled trials of other herbal treatments have proved inconclusive. Herbal preparations may be taken as tablets, infusions — such as tea — tinctures or added to baths. Popular herbs for rheumatism include aloe vera, comfrey, devil's claw, feverfew and evening primrose oil.

NATUROPATHY

This is a mixture of traditional folk wisdom, empiricism and selections of biomedical science. The basic principles (Champion, 1994) are:

- the healing power of nature is fundamental;
- treat the cause rather than the effect;
- ill health results from a lowering of resistance due to diet, stress etc.

HOLISM

Treatment involves a combination of counselling, nutritional advice, herbal medicine and homeopathy remedies.

2.10 GLUCOSAMINE

Biological compounds such as hyaluronans, chrondroitin sulfate and glucosamine are now used routinely in the treatment of osteoarthritis. Although not yet proven these compounds may be potentially chondroprotective, in that they may favourably modify the natural progression and course of OA (Towheed et al., 2005). Glucosamine is a natural substance and a building block of the glycosaminogly-cans (CAG) and glycoproteins in the ground substance of the articular cartilage (Towheed et al., 2005). Glucosamine is usually taken in a daily dose of 1500 mg.

Adverse effects are likely to be mild and predominantly affect the GI tract and are reversible on discontinuation of glucosamine. Concerns about glucosamine affecting glucose homeostasis, increasing insulin resistance and/or impairing insulin secretion (Monauni et al., 2000) appear not to be founded. Research by Scroggie, Albright and Harris (2003) and Tannis et al. (2004) found that normal doses of glucosamine supplemetation did not cause glucose intolerance in healthy adults.

Randomized trials comparing glucosamine to NSAIDs suggest that glucosamine produces similar symptomatic benefits as NSAIDs but with fewer adverse effects (Towheed et al., 2005). A meta-analysis (Richy et al., 2003) comparing the structural and symptomatic efficacy of glucosamine in relation to placebo found an improvement in symptoms as well as in joint space narrowing. Two randomized controlled studies (Pavelka et al., 2002; Reginster et al., 2001) have demonstrated that patients prescribed glucosamine had no significant progression of cartilage loss, suggesting that glucosamine may indeed modify the natural radiological progression of OA of the knee.

PATIENT INFORMATION LEAFLET: GLUCOSAMINE

(This is a modified version of the information sheet used in the rheumatology clinic at the Haywood Hospital, Stoke on Trent).

Glucosamine is a dietary supplement that may be effective in the treatment of osteoarthritis.

WHAT HAPPENS IN OSTEOARTHRITIS?

Healthy cartilage covers the ends of your bones within your joints and helps with smooth and pain-free movement. Osteoarthritis occurs when the healthy cartilage starts to wear out causing the bones to rub together. The joint lining may become inflamed, leading to swelling. Cartilage is made up mainly of water, cells called chondrocytes and other substances such as collagen and proteoglycans. These substances give the cartilage its elastic properties and the ability to absorb shock, especially in hips and knees. As we grow older we produce less of these substances and the cartilage wears down.

WHAT DOES GLUCOSAMINE DO?

Glucosamine is a natural substance that helps to provide the building blocks within cartilage. It helps to produce and maintain healthy cartilage. Exactly how it benefits the cartilage in osteoarthrits is unknown.

WHAT ABOUT THE RESEARCH?

Studies have looked at the effect of glucosamine in the treatment of osteoarthritis. It has been found to reduce pain and improve function in some people. There is also some evidence that it may slow the progression of the condition.

DOES IT WORK WITH EVERYONE?

As with other forms of medication and supplements, everyone can respond differently, and there is no guarantee that it will help. There is no proven evidence that glucosamine helps in other types of arthritis.

ARE THERE ANY SIDE EFFECTS?

Glucosamine is generally well tolerated. Common side effects include nausea, diarrhoea and stomach upset which resolve on stopping glucosamine. There is very little information available about whether there are any increased side effects taking it long term. Always read the information provided with glucosamine.

WHAT DOSE DO I NEED?

The current recommended dose is 1500 mg (1.5 g) of glucosamine sulfate per day.

DOES MY DOCTOR NEED TO PRESCRIBE IT?

Some doctors will prescribe it. It is also available over the counter in pharmacists and health food shops.

WHEN WILL I NOTICE A DIFFERENCE?

Benefit can be variable and it is worth taking for at least six months before assessing whether it has been helpful.

2.11   CAPSAICIN

Capsaicin (trans-8-methyl-N-vanillyl-6-nonenamide) is the alkaloid which makes chillies hot. Interest has centered on the use of capsaicin as a topical analgesia for a variety of conditions characterized by pain that are not responsive to analgesia or NSAIDs (Zhang and Wan Po, 1994). Local application of capsaicin to the peripheral sensory endings in the skin results in depletion of substance P from the neurone, both peripherally and centrally (Fitzgerald, 1983). One randomized placebo-controlled trial in osteoarthritis has reported an improvement in pain levels (Deal *et al.*, 1991).

CONCLUSION

Drug therapy plays an important role in the management of inflammatory arthritis. It is hoped that this chapter has provided information on the wide-ranging aspects of medications, enabling the nurse to share this knowledge with the patient so that a mutual understanding of care management can evolve.

APPENDIX 2.A   WHAT HAPPENS NEXT?

For each scenario, state what, if any, drug intervention you would recommend:

- 45-year-old man with chronic ankylosing spondylitis. Previous bleeding duodenal ulcer. Found to be *H. pylori*-positive. NSAID stopped and treated with triple therapy. Ulcer healed on gastrocopy. Attends for review appointment. Stiff as a board. Can't do his exercises. Current treatment: co-codamol only.
- A 74-year-old woman. Chronic generalized osteoarthritis. Now presents with a several-month history of a superimposed inflammatory arthritis which is clinically very active and is causing significant disturbance to her quality of life. PMH: Peptic ulcer 1970; vagotomy and pyloroplasty 1973. Hypertension. Current treatment: atenolol, ramipril, bendrofluazide, hydralazine, co-codamol. ESR 40, C-reactive protein (CRP) 15, X-rays soft tissue swelling ++, no erosions.

- 77-year-old woman with RA for 12 years. Established erosive disease. Joints troublesome — hands, wrists, shoulders. Clinically low grade synovitis in these areas. PMH: chronic obstructive pulmonary disease (COPD) with recurrent infections. Smoker. Treatment: co-codamol, Slo-Phyllin, frusemide, zoton. Salbutamol, seretide and combivent inhalers.
- 81-year-old man with RA and ?mycetoma left lung cavity. Meloxicam was recently changed by GP to celecoxib. PMH: No ischaemic heart disease/cardiovascular disease (IHD/CVD). Previous thoracotomy. Treatment prednisolone 2mg, sulfasalazine 2g, zoton, celecoxib, weekly fosamax.
- 65-year-old man with chronic ankylosing spondylitis. PMH: Gout, asthma, renal stones, bleeding peptic ulcer detected because of anaemia after 15 years on voltarol suppositories. Now asymptomatic from gastrointestinal aspect and haemoglobin (Hb) stable. Treatment: co-codamol and losec. Spine and peripheral joints getting worse.
- 25-year-old male driver. Presents with an eight-month history of a sero-negative inflammatory oligoarthritis affecting knee, forefoot (dactylitis), and sacroiliac joints. Quite symptomatic despite diclofenac slow release 75mg twice daily (bd). PMH : Nil of note. On examination (O/E) synovitis in affected areas. ESR 3 CRP 4. X-rays: suspicion of erosion third and fourth MTPs.
- 35-year-old woman with a 3-month history of inflammatory joint symptoms involving hands, wrists, shoulders and feet. PMH: Nil of note. Non-smoker. Rx: Over-the-counter (OTC) ibuprofen or paracetemol. O/E Synovitis in MCPs, wrists and MTPs. Stiff shoulders. ESR 40, CRP 20, RF-positive. X-rays non-erosive.

Case scenarios kindly provided by Dr A. B. Hassell, Consultant Rheumatologist, Haywood Hospital, Stoke on Trent.

APPENDIX 2.B GUIDELINES FOR NURSES ON THE USE AND ADMINISTRATION OF INTRA-ARTICULAR INJECTIONS

1. What is an expanded role?
   Role extension refers to nurses carrying out tasks not included in their normal training for registration. Most of these tasks relate to medical technical interventions usually carried out by doctors (Wright, 1995).
2. Accountability:
   The scope of professional practice (UKCC, 1992) acknowledges that nurses are involved in negotiating the boundaries of practice and should be responsive to the needs of patients and clients. The onus is on individual nurses to recognize their own levels of competence and decline any duties or responsibilities unless they are able to perform them in a safe and skilled manner. Nurses are also individually accountable for maintaining and improving their knowledge and should be familiar with the contents of the following documents:

   (a) UKCC Exercising Accountability 1989;

   (b) UKCC Scope of Professional Practice 1992;

   (c) UKCC Code of Professional Practice 1992;

   (d) UKCC Standards for the Administration of Medicine 1992.

3. What are intra-articular injections?

   These are injections into the synovial joints. Long-acting steroids are generally used for joint injections (and hydrocortisone is used for soft tissue injections).

4. Indications for joint injections:

   (a) Relief of pain from localized inflammation of the joint (e.g. Rheumatoid Arthritis);

   (b) Relief of pain from soft tissue discomfort;

   (c) To aid mobilization;

   (d) To assist with rehabilitation (e.g. physiotherapy);

   (e) To improve function.

5. Contraindications of joint injections:

   (a) Local infection;

   (b) Intra-articular fracture;

   (c) Anticoagulant therapy;

   (d) Bleeding disorders.

6. Preparation the nurse must undertake prior to the administration of intra-articular injections:

   The nurse must be able to demonstrate evidence of competency in the administration of intra-articular injections in accordance with the Scope of Professional Practice (UKCC, 1992).

   (a) Evidence of competency should indicate that the nurse has knowledge of:

      (i) Anatomy and physiology of the joints and soft tissues;

      (ii) Drugs used and their effects and side effects;

      (iii) Indications and contraindications for intra-articular injections;

      (iv) Potential complications;

      (v) Aspiration and injection technique.

   (b) Evidence of assessment of competency should be available.

   (c) The employer must have precise knowledge of the employee's activities, and agree to them being undertaken by the employee; in accordance with vicarious liability.

7. The nurse's responsibility when giving intra-articular injections:

   (a) Obtain written instructions from the prescribing doctor detailing the drug, dosage and site of administration.

   (b) Ensure the patient has given informed consent.

   (c) Use an aseptic or no touch technique.

   (d) Aspirate the joint if swollen.

   (e) Send a sample of synovial fluid for culture if it is very opaque, green or foul-smelling.

(f) If no obvious signs of infection or contraindications are present, administer the prescribed drug into the site stated.

(g) Document the drug, dosage and site of administration in the care records.

(h) Provide the patient with after care advice.

8. After care advice:

The nurse must advise patients that:

(a) The joint may be painful for 24 hours after the injection. Take analgesia if necessary.

(b) It may take several days before benefit is felt.

(c) The injected joint should be rested as much as possible 24−48 hours after the injection.

(d) Short-term facial flushing may be experienced.

(e) Localized skin atrophy may occasionally occur.

(f) They should contact the rheumatology department if they have any concerns.

9. Potential complications following the administration of intra-articular injections:

(a) Infections;

(b) Damage to the articular cartilage;

(c) Tendon rupture;

(d) Skin atrophy.

REFERENCES

Wright S. (1995) The Role of the Nurse: Extended or Expanded? *Nursing Standard*, May 10, **9** (33), 25−9.

APPENDIX 2.C: PATIENT GROUP DIRECTION FOR THE ADMINISTRATION OF METHYLPREDNISOLONE INJECTION 40 mg/ml BY INTRAMUSCULAR INJECTION

Reproduced by kind permission of Dr AB Hassell, Consultant Rheumatologist, Haywood Hospital, Stoke on Trent.

1. Reference number:

2. Medicine:

(a) Methylprednisolone (Depomedrone) injection 40 mg/ml.

3. Dose, route and duration:

(a) 120mg methylprednisolone (Depomedrone) intramuscularly, no more frequently than once every four months.

(b) The injection should be administered deeply into the gluteal muscle and aspirate to avoid intravascular administration.

4. Legal status of the medicine:

   (a) Prescription only medicine.

5. Date PGD comes into force:
6. Date PGD expires:
7. Health professionals who may supply or administer this medicine:

   (a) Registered nurses who will have completed the training programme including the Assessment Exercise.

8. Clinical condition/situation to which the PGD applies:

   (a) Active rheumatoid arthritis.

9. Criteria for confirmation of the clinical condition/situation:

   (a) Flare of rheumatoid arthritis.
   (b) Two out of the following three criteria must be present:
      (i) Increased early morning stiffness (over one hour).
      (ii) Polyarticular pain with soft tissue swelling.
      (iii) Raised serum inflammatory markers − for example, ESR over 30, CRP over 30.

10. Description of the circumstances in which further advice should be sought from a doctor (or dentist) and the arrangement for referral:

    (a) Patient is an insulin-dependent diabetic.
    (b) Patient has severe osteoporosis.
    (c) If the patient is taking ciclosporin or warfarin. Ciclosporin can interact with methylprednisolone causing convulsions and methylprednisolone may increase the anticoagulant effects of warfarin.
    (d) Pregnancy.

11. Description of these patients excluded from treatment under the PGD:

    (a) Patients with an infection.
    (b) Patients who have received more than three intramuscular injections of methylpresdnisolone in the past year.
    (c) Patients with a known allergy to methylprednisolone.

12. Details of actions to be taken for patients who do not wish to receive or do not adhere to care under the PGD:
    Patients who do not wish to receive intramuscular methylprednisolone will be referred to the rheumatologist's clinic for a review of their clinical management.

13. Potential adverse reactions:

    (a) Facial flushing. This is a transient reaction and will settle within one to two days.
    (b) Suppresses reaction to skin tests − for example, Heaf test.
    (c) Subcutaneous and cutaneous atrophy.
    (d) Anaphylactic and allergic reactions. Refer to the medical guidelines for management of anaphylactic reactions

14. Patient information/advice to be given:
    (a) Provide the patient with an information sheet.
    (b) Facial flushing may occur 24–48 hours following administration.
    (c) Provide the patient with a blue steroid card to monitor accumulative dosages.

PATIENT INFORMATION SHEET ON INTRAMUSCULAR DEPOMEDRONE

Steroids can be given in many different ways. They can be injected into a muscle, vein or joint or given as tablets. Steroid injections are usually given only occasionally to treat a flare of arthritis. This information sheet deals only with injections in to the muscle.

1. Why am I having a steroid injection?
   If your arthritis has recently become more active you may have noticed more joint pain and swelling and an increase in the stiffness of the joints, particularly in the morning. The steroid injection should help to reduce these problems.
2. How long will the injection take to work?
   The injection works quickly and you should notice a benefit within a few days.
3. What are the possible side effects?
   All drugs including injections can cause side effects. The after effects of the injection can lead to:

   (a) facial flushing;
   (b) an upset of diabetes.

   The side effects listed below are a feature of long-term treatment with steroids and should not occur with occasional injections:

   (a) weight gain;
   (b) thinning of the bones;
   (c) easy bruising;
   (d) stomach pain;
   (e) thinning of the skin;
   (f) muscle weakness;
   (g) mood changes;
   (h) cataracts.

If you suffer from epilepsy then it is possible that steroids can make this worse. Steroids can reduce reactions to skin tests – for example, Heaf tests.

Warning

If you have not had chicken pox but come in to contact with someone who has chicken pox or herpes zoster or you develop either of these yourself, you should contact your doctor immediately.

What do I do if I experience any problems?

- If you experience any side effects following the injection, contact the Arthritis Helpline. If you develop a fever, contact your own doctor.
- If you have any operations or other illnesses over the next two to three months it is important that you inform the doctor and show your blue card.

ASSESSMENT EXERCISE REGARDING THE ADMINISTRATION OF METHYLPREDNISOLONE INJECTION 40 mg/ml BY INTRAMUSCULAR INJECTION

When you have completed the exercise below you need to have it assessed by the nurse consultant.

1. Which of the following clinical conditions does this PGD apply to?

   (a) Psoriatic arthritis.
   (b) Ankylosing spondylitis.
   (c) Rheumatoid arthritis.
   (d) Lupus.

2. Which of the following clinical criteria must be present for a patient to be eligible for a methylprednisolone intramuscular injection?

   (a) Widespread pain.
   (b) Increased early morning stiffness lasting over one hour.
   (c) Increased stiffness after inactivity lasting over one hour.
   (d) A hot, painful, swollen joint.
   (e) Polyarticular pain with soft tissue swelling.
   (f) Raised inflammatory markers.

3. Which of the following conditions/situations would prevent the administration of methylprednisolone?

   (a) Hypertension.
   (b) Insulin-dependent diabetic.
   (c) Renal impairment.
   (d) Infection.
   (e) Severe osteoporosis.
   (f) Osteoarthritis.
   (g) Known allergy to methylprednisolone.

4. Name two medications that interact with methylprednisolone.
5. Which of the following are potential adverse reactions to methylprednisolone?

   (a) Increased pain.
   (b) Facial flushing.
   (c) Epistaxsis.
   (d) Suppressed reaction to skin tests − for example, Heaf test.
   (e) Anaphylactic and allergic reactions.

(f) Mouth ulcers.

(g) Subcutaneous and cutaneous atrophy.

6. What advice would you give to a patient who rings the day after an injection experiencing facial flushing?

7. What action would you take in the event of an anaphylactic reaction following the administration of methylprednisolone?

8. What is the dose and route of administration of methylprednisolone in this PGD?

9. What is the maximum number of injections over a 12-month period of time?

CASE SCENARIOS

WHAT WOULD YOU DO IN THE FOLLOWING SITUATIONS?

- Mrs T. has RA. She is very weepy with a history of widespread pain and stiffness. Her inflammatory markers are stable. She had an intramuscular injection of methylprednisolone six months ago and is requesting another one.
- Mr A. has recently commenced phenylbutazone for his SA. He has back pain and peripheral arthritis with objective swelling. He asks whether anything can be given to help him with his pain and stiffness in the short term as he has been informed that the phenylbutazone will take many months to work.
- Mrs J. has RA with objective evidence of polyarticular pain with soft tissue swelling and raised ESR and CRP. She has developed a cough over the last week. She enquires whether she can have an injection of methylprednisolone.
- Mr W. has RA. Over the last month his early morning stiffness has increased to four hours and his ESR has risen to 60. He also has hypertension and is a long-standing insulin-dependent diabetic. He enquires whether he can have an injection of methylprednisolone.
- Mrs B. has RA with increased early morning stiffness and polyarticular pain and stiffness. She enquires whether she can have an injection of Methylprednisolone.

REFERENCES

Abbott Laboratories Ltd (2005) *Adalimumab. Summary of Product Characteristics.* Abbott Laboratories, Berkshire.

Amgen (2002) *Internet Product Monograph,* Amgen Ltd, Cambridge.

Amgen (2005) *Summary of Product Characteristics: Anakinra,* Amgen Ltd, Cambridge.

ARMA (Arthritis and Musculoskeletal Alliance). (2005) www.arma.uk.net

Arthritis and Research Campaign. (2005) www.arc.org.uk

Askling, J., Fored, C.M., Baecklind, E. (2005a) Haematopoietic malignancies in rheumatoid arthritis, lymphoma risk and characteristics after exposure to tumour necrosis factor antagonists. *Arthritis and Rheumatism,* **64**, 1414–20.

Askling, J., Fored, C.M., Brandt, L. *et al.* (2005b) Risk of solid cancers in patients with rheumatoid arthritis and after treatment with tumour necrosis factor antagonists. *Annals of Rheumatic Diseases*, **64**, 1421−6.

Austin, H.A., Klippel, J.H., Barlow, J.E. *et al.* (1986) Therapy of lupus nephritis: controlled trial of prednisolone and cytotoxic drugs. *New England Journal of Medicine*, **314**, 614−9.

Australian Acute Musculoskeletal Pain Guidelines Group. (2004) Evidence based management of acute musculoskeletal pain − a guide for clinicians. *Brisbane Academic Press*, www.nhmrc.gov.au

Bagley, C.M.J., Bostick, F.W. and De Vita, V.T. (1973) Clinical Pharmacology of Cyclophosphamide. *Cancer Research*, **33**, 226−33.

Beardsley, R., Anderson Johnson, C. and Kabat, H. (1983) A drug self administration programme. A behavioural appproach to patient education. *Contempary Pharmacy Practice*, **5** (3), 156−60.

Beinfield, H. and Korngold, E. (1992) *Between Heaven and Earth: A Guide to Chinese Medicine*, Ballentine, New York.

Bersani-Amado, C.A., Das Duarte, A.J., Tanji, M.M. *et al.* (1990) Comparative study of adjuvant induced arthritis in susceptible and resistant strains of rats. Analysis of lymphocyte sub populations. *Journal of Rheumatology*, **17**, 153−8.

Bird, C. (1990) *Patient Self Medication*, The Medicine Group UK Ltd, London, pp. 22−6.

Bird, H. (2004) Drug treatment for fibromyalgia. *Musculoskeletal Care*, **2** (2), 90−100.

Blocka, K., Frust, D.E., Landaw, E. *et al.* (1982) Single dose pharmacokinetics of auranofin in rheumatoid arthritis. *Journal of Rheumatology*, **9** (Suppl. 8), 110−9.

Bombardier, C., Laine, L., Reicin, A. *et al.* (2000) Comparison of upper gastrointestinal toxicity of rofecoxib and naproxen in patients with rheumatoid arthritis. *New England Journal of Medicine*, **343**, 1520−8.

Borel, J.F., Fever, C., Gubler Hu and Stahelin, H. (1976) Biologic effects of ciclosporin A: a new antilymphocyte agent. *Agents and Actions*, **6**, 468−75.

Bozkurt, B. (2000) Activation of cytokines as a mechanism of disease progression in heart failure. *Annals of Rheumatic Disease*, **59** (1), 90−3.

Brant K. (2004) Non-surgical treatment of Osteoarthritis; a half century of advances. *Annals of Rheumatic Diseases*, **63** (2), 117−22.

Bresalier, R.S., Sandler, R.S., Quan, H. *et al.* (2005) The adenomatous polyp prevention on vioxx trial investigations. Cardiovascular events associated with rofecoxib in a colorectal adenoma chemoprevention trial. *New England Journal of Medicine*, **352**, 1092−102.

Brook, A. and Corbett, M. (1977) Radiographic changes in early rheumatoid arthritis. *Annals of the Rheumatic Diseases*, **36**, 71−3.

Brooks, P.M. (1990) *Slow Acting Anti-Rheumatic Drugs and Imminosuppressives. Bailliere's Clinical Rheumatology*, Balliere Tindall, London.

Brooks, P.M. (1994) Non steroidal anti-inflammatory drugs, in *Rheumatology*, (eds J. Klippel and P. Dieppe), Mosby Year Book, Europe Limited, pp. 51−6.

Brown, R.S. and Bottomley, W.K. (1990) The utilisation and mechanism of action of antidepressants in the treatment of chronic facial pain − a review of the literature. *Anaesthetic Programme*, **37**, 223−9.

BSR (British Society for Rheumatology) (2002) *British Society of Rheumatology Vaccination Guidelines*, BSR, London.

BSR (British Society for Rheumatology) (2005) *Guidelines for Prescribing TNFα Blockers in Adults with RA*. BSR, London.

BSR (British Society for Rheumatology) (2006) *BSR and BHPR Guideline for Disease Modifying Anti-rheumatic Drug (DMARD) Therapy.* www.rheumatology.org.uk

BTS (British Thoracic Society Standards of Care Committee) (2005) Recommendations for assessing risk and managing Mycobacterium Tuberculosis infection and disease in patients due to start anti TNFalpha treatment. *Thorax*, **60**, 800−5.

Buchanan, H.M., Preston, S.J., Brooks, P.M. and Buchanan, W.W. (1991) Is diet important in rheumatoid arthritis? *British Journal of Rheumatology*, **30**, 125−34.

Carrette, J., Bell, M.J.K., Reynolds, W.J. *et al.* (1994) Comparison of amitriptyline, cyclobenzaprine and placebo in the treatment of fibromyalgia. A randomised, double-blind clinical trial. *Arthritis and Rheumatism*, **37**, 32−40.

Caruso, I., Sarzi Puttini, P.C. and Bocassini, L. (1987) Double blind study of dothiepin versus placebo in the treatment of primary fibromyalgia syndrome. *Journal of International Medical Research*, **15**, 154−9.

Chaitow, A.L. (1997) Diet for arthritis and rheumatism. *International Journal of Alternative and Complementary Medicine*, **15** (4), 29−32.

Champion, G.D. (1994) Unproven remedies, alternative and complimentary medicine, in *Rheumatology* (eds J. Klippel and P. Dieppe), Mosby Year Book, Europe Limited, Section 3, 13.1−12.

Champion, G.D., Graham, G.C. and Ziegler, J.B. (1990) The gold complexes, in *Slow Acting Anti-Rheumatic Drugs and Immunosuppressives Bailliere's Clinical Rheumatology* (ed. P.M. Brooks), Bailliere Tindall, London, pp. 491−534.

Cheifetz, A., Smedley, M. and Martin, S. (2003) The incidence and management of infusion reactions to Infliximab. A large centre experience. *American Journal of Gastroenterology*, **98**, 1315−24.

Christiansen, C. and Krane, S. (1993) *Advances in Corticosteroids: A Seminar in Print*, Adis International Inc, USA.

Choy, E.H.S., Kingsley, G., Corkhill, M.M. and Panayi, G.S. (1993) Intramuscular methylprednisolone is superior to pulse oral methylprednisolone during the induction phase of Chrysotherapy. *British Journal of Rheumatology*, **32**, 734−9.

Clarke, J.H. and Fitzgerald, J.F. (1984) Effects of exogenous corticosteroid therapy on growth in children with HBs Agnegative chronic aggressive hepatitis. *Journal of Pediatric Gastroenterology and Nutrition*, **3**, 72−6.

Cohen, M.L. (1994) Principles of pain and pain management, in *Rheumatology* (eds J. Klippel and P. Dieppe), Mosby Year Book, Europe Limited, Section 3, 41−6.

Cohen, S., Emery, P., Greenwald, M. *et al.* (2006) Rituximab for RA refractory to anti-tumor necrosis factor therapy. *Arthritis and Rheumatism*, **54** (a), 2793−806.

Cooper, C. and Kirwan, J.R. (1990) The risk of local and systemic corticosteroid administration. *Bailliere's Clinical Rheumatology*, **4**, 305−32.

Corrigan, M.S. (1989) Primary pharmacy. A patient self help service. *The Pharmaceutical Journal*, October, 458−600.

Cosman, F., Nieves, J., Gordon, S. *et al.* (1992) High dose IV steroids acutely depress serum phosphorous and elevate 1, 25 (OH2) prior to an increase in PTH. *Journal of Bone and Mineral Research*, **7**, S168.

Cronstein, B.N. (1996) Molecular therapeutics. Methotrexate and its mechanism of action. *Arthritis and Rheumatism*, **39**, 1951−60.

Cully, F. (2005) Understanding developments in non-medical prescribing. *Nursing Times*, **101** (34), 30−3.

Currey, H.L.F. (1988) *Acute Monoarthritis Differential Diagnosis and Management: Collected Reports on the Rheumatic Diseases*, Arthritis Research Campaign, Chesterfield.

Darlington L.G., Ramsey, N.W. and Mansfield, J.R. (1986) Placebo – controlled blind study of dietary manipulation therapy in rheumatoid arthritis. *Lancet*, **1** (8475), 236–8.

Davis, B. (2000) *Caring for People in Pain*, Routledge, London.

Day, R. (1994) Pharmacologic approaches SAARD, in *Rheumatology* (eds J. Klippel and P. Dieppe), Mosby Year Book, Europe Ltd, Section 3, 8.1–10.

Deal, C.L., Schnitzer, T.J., Lipstein, E. *et al.* (1991) Treatment of arthritis with topical capsaicin: a double blind trial. *Clinical Therapeutics*, **13**, 383–93.

Del Pozo, E., Graeber, M., Elford, P. and Payne, T. (1990) Regression of bone and cartilage loss in adjuvant arthritis rats after treatment with ciclosporin A. *Arthritis and Rheumatism*, **33**, 247–52.

Department of Health. (2000a) *Patient Group Directions (England Only) Health Service Circular 2000/026*, DoH, London.

Department of Health. (2000b) *Consultations on Proposals to Extend Nurse Prescribing*, DoH, London.

Department of Health. (2002) www.doh.gov.uk/supplementaryprescribing

Department of Health Medicines and Healthcare Products Regulatory Agency. (2005a) *Consultation on Options for the Future of Independent Nurse Prescribing by Extended Formulary Nurse Prescribers*, MHRA, London.

Deodhar, A.A., Brabyn, J., Jones, P.W. *et al.* (1995) Longitudinal study of hard bone densitometry in rheumatoid arthritis. *Arthritis and Rheumatology*, (Suppl. 41), D183.

Dinarello, C.A. and Moldawer, L.L. (2002) *Proinflammatory and Anti-inflammatory Cytokines in Rheumatoid Arthritis: A Primer for Clinicians*, 3rd edn, Amgen, Thousand Oaks, CA.

Dixon, R. and Christy, N. (1980) On the various forms of corticosteroid withdrawal syndrome. *American Journal of Medicine*, **68**, 224–300.

Dixon, W. (2005) The incidence of serious infections is not increased in patients with rheumatoid arthritis treated with anti-TNF drugs compared to those treated with traditional DMARDs. Results from a prospective study. *Arthritis and Rheumatism*, **54** (8), 2368–76.

DoH (Department of Health) (1996) *Immunisation Against Infectious Diseases*, DoH, London.

DoH (Department of Health) (1999) *Review of Prescribing, Supply and Administration of Medicines* (Crown Report), DoH, London.

Donnelly, S., Scott, D.L. and Emery, P. (1992) The long term outcome and justification for early treatment, in *Management of Early Inflammatory Arthritis. Bailliere's Clinical Rheumatology* (ed. P. Emery), Bailliere Tindall, London, pp. 251–60.

Dougans, I. and Ellis, S. (1992) *The Art of Reflexology*, Bath Press Limited, Great Britain.

Dwight, M.M., Arnold, L.M., O'Brien, H. *et al.* (1998) An open clinical trial of venlafaxine treatment of fobromyalgia. *Psychosomatics*, **39**, 14–7.

Easterbrook, M. (1988) Occular effects and safety of anti-malarial agents. *American Journal of Medicine*, **85** (Suppl. 4A), 23–9.

Edwards, C. and Boucher, I. (1991) *Davidson's Principles and Practice of Medicines*, Churchill Livingstone, Great Britain.

Elliot, M.J., Maini, R.M., Feldmann, M. *et al.* (1994) Randomised double-blind comparison of chimeric menoclonal antibody to tumour necrosis factoid (cA2) versus placebo in rheumatoid arthritis. *Lancet*, **344**, 1104–10.

Emery, P., Fleischman, R., Filipowiiz-Sosnouska, A. *et al.* (2006) The efficacy and safety of rituximab in patients with active RA despite methotrexate treatment. *Arthritis and Rheumatism*, **54** (5), 1390–1400.

Emmerson, B.T. (1994) Antihyperuricemics, in *Rheumatology* (eds J. Klippel and P. Dieppe), Mosby Year Book, Europe Ltd, Section 8, 9.1–12.

Eraker, S.A., Kirscht, J.P. and Becher, M.H. (1984) Understanding and improving patient compliance. *Annals of Internal Medicine*, **100**, 258–68.

Ernst, E. (1998) Usage of complementary therapies in rheumatology: a systematic review. *Clinical Rheumatology*, **17**, 301–95.

Evans, I. and Spelman, M. (1983) The problem of non-compliancy with drug therapy. *Drugs*, **25**, 163–76.

Farkouh, M.E., Kirshner, H., Harrington, R.A. *et al.* (2004) Comparison of lumiracoxib with naproxen and ibuprofen in the therapeutic arthritis research and gastrointestinal event trial, cardiovascular outcomes, randomised controlled trial. *Lancet*, **364**, 675–84.

Flendrie, M., Creemers, C.W., Welsing, P.M. and van Riel, P.L.C.M. (2005) The influence of previous and concomitant leflunomide on the efficay and safety of infliximab therapy in patients with rheumatoid arthritis; a longitudinal observational study. *Rheumatology*, **44**, 472–8.

Ferrante, F.M. (1983) Opiods, in *Post Operative Pain Management* (eds F.M. Ferrante and T.R. Vade Boncoeur), New York, Churchill Livingstone.

Fitzgerald, M. (1983) Capsaicin and sensory neurons – a review. *Pain*, **15**, 109–30.

Flowers, R. (1996) The role of Cox1 and Cox2: implications for NSAID development. *Current Opinions in Rheumatology*, **9** (1), 15–19.

Fordham, M. (1986) Psychophysiological pain theories. *Nursing*, **10** (3), 360–4.

Fuller, P.L. and Funder J.W. (1976) Mineralocorticoid and glucocorticoid receptors in human kidney. *Kidney International*, **10**, 154–7.

Furst, D.E., Breedveld, F.C., Kalden, J.R. *et al.* (2005) Updated consensus statement on biological agents, specifically tumor necrosis factor alpha (TNFA) blocking aens and interleukin1 receptor antagonists (IL-1ra) for the treatment of rheumatic diseases. *Annals of Rheumatic Diseases*, **64** (iv), 2–4.

Furst, P.E. and Clements, P.J. (1994) Pharmacologic approaches SAARD 11, in *Rheumatology* (eds J. Klippel and P. Dieppe), Mosby Year Book, Europe Ltd, Section 3, 9.1–10.

George, E. and Kirwan, J.R. (1990) Corticosteroid therapy in RA. *Bailliere's Clinical Rheumatology*, **4**, 621–47.

Gibson, H. (1994) *Psychology of Pain and Anaesthesia*, Chapman and Hall, London.

Gibson, T. (1988) *The Treatment of Gout – a Personal View. Collected Reports on the Rheumatic Diseases*, Arthritis Research Campaign, Chesterfield.

Godschalk, M.F. and Downs, R.W. (1988) Effect of short term glucocorticoids on serum osteocalcin in healthy young men. *Journal of Bone and Mineral Research*, **3**, 113–5.

Goldberg, A.G. (1991) *Body Massage*, 2nd edn, Redwood Press Limited, Great Britain.

Goodwin, J.S. and Regan, M. (1982) Cognitive dysfunction associated with naproxen and ibuprofen in the elderly. *Arthritis and Rheumatism*, **25**, 1013–5.

Gotzsche, P.C. and Johansen, H.K. (2005) Short term low dose corticosteroids versus placebo and non-steroidal anti-inflammatory drugs in rheumatoid arthritis. *The Cochrane Database of Systemic Reviews*, No CD000189.

Gough, A.K., Lilley, J., Eyre, S. *et al.* (1994) Generalised bone loss in patients with early rheumatoid arthritis occurs early and relates to disease activity. *Lancet*, **344**, 23–7.

Gray, R.E.S., Doherty, S.M., Galloway, J. *et al.* (1991) A double blind study of deflazacort and prednisolone in patients with chronic inflammatory disorders. *Arthritis and Rheumatism*, **34**, 287–95.

Guest, G. and Broyer, M. (1991) Alternate day corticosteroid therapy and growth in renal transplant patients. *Annales de Pediatrie*, **38**, 401–4.

Guyton, A.C. (1991) *Medical Physiology*, WB Saunders, London.

Haagsma, C., van de Putte, L. and van Riel, R. (1995) Sulfasalazine, methotrexate and the combination in early RA, a double blinded randomised study. *Arthritis and Rehumatism*, **36**, 1501–9.

Hainsworth, J.D. (2003) Safety of rituximab in the treatment of B cell malignancies. Implications for RA. *Arthritis Research and Therapy*, **5** (4), 512–16.

Hakim, A. and Clunie, G. (2002) *Oxford Handbook of Rheumatology*, Oxford University Press, Oxford.

Hart, D. and Klinenberg, J. (1985) *Choosing NSAID Therapy*, Adis Press Ltd, Great Britain.

Hennell, S. (2004) Nurse prescribing in rheumatology: a case study. *Musculoskeletal Care*, **2** (1), 65–71.

Hennell, S. (2005) Presentation of nurse prescribing, delivered to the Staffordshire Rheumatology Centre at Primary Care Science, Keele University, December.

Hill, J., Bird, H.A., Hopkins, R. *et al.* (1991) The development and use of a patient knowledge questionnaire in RA. *British Journal of Rheumatology*, **30**, 45–9.

Hippisley-Cox, J. and Coupland, C. (2005) Risk of myocardial infarction in patients taking cyclo-oxygenase-2 inhibitors or conventional non-steroidal anti-inflammatory drugs: population based nested case control analysis. *BMJ*, **330**, 1366–73.

Hopkins, R. (1990) Sans awareness. *Nursing Times*, **86** (30), 50–1.

Huskisson, E.C., Woolf, P.C., Bourne, H.W. *et al.* (1974) Four anti-inflammatory drugs – responses and variations. *British Medical Journal*, **1**, 1084–9.

Hyrich, K.L., Watson, K.D. and Dixon, W.G. (2005) Pregnancy experiences in women with rheumatic diseases exposed to biologic agents: results from the BSR Biologics Register. *Arthritis and Rheumatism* **54** (8), 2701–2.

Ischemia Research Group and the Ischemia Research and Education Foundation Investigators. Efficacy and safety of the cyclogenase 2 inhibitors parecoxib and valdecoxib in patients undergoing coronary artery bypass surgery. *Journal of Thoracic Cardiovascular Surgery*, **125**, 1481–92.

Jackson, A. (1995) Acute pain: its physionogy and the pharmacology of analgesia. *Nursing Times*, **91** (16), 27–8.

Jacobs, J., Kraaimaat, F. and Bijlsma, J. (2001) Why do patients with rheumatoid arthritis use alternative treatments? *Clinical Rheumatology*, **20**, 192–6.

Jamison, R.M. (1996) Comprehensive pre-treatment and outcome assessment for chronic opioid therapy. *Journal of Pain Symptom Management*, **11**, 231–4.

Johnson, L. and Giles, R. (1993) Prescription for change. *Nursing Times*, **89**, 42–5.

Jones, A. (1997) *Pain and Its Perception. Topical Review series 3 No 10*, Arthritis Research Campaign, Chesterfield.

Jordan, S. (1992) Drugs update: drugs for severe pain. *Nursing Times*, **88** (2), 24–7.

Joyce, D.A. (1990) D – Penicillamine, in *Slow Acting Anti-Rheumatic Drugs and Immunosuppressives. Bailliere's Clinical Rheumatology* (ed. P.M. Brookes), Bailliere Tindall, London, pp. 553–74.

Juni, P., Nartey, L., Reichenback, S. *et al.* (2004) Risk of cardiovascualr events and rofecoxib: cumulative meta-analysisi. *Lancet*, **364**, 2021–9.

Kennedy, B. (1981) Self medication. *Canadian Nurse*, **77**, 366–7.

Kirwan, J.R. (1994) Systemic corticosteroids in rheumatology, in *Rheumatology* (eds J.H. Klippel and P. Dieppe), Mosby Year Book, Europe Ltd.

Kirwan, J.R. and the Arthritis and Rheumatism Council Low Dose Glucocorticoid Study Group. (1995) The effects of glucocorticoid steroid on joint destruction in RA. *New England Journal of Medicine*, **333**, 142–6.

Koes, B.W., Van Tulder, M. and Osteso, R. (2001) Clinical guidelines for the management of low back pain in primary care-an international comparison. *Spine*, **26**, 2504–13.

Kowal, A., Carstens, A.J.H.Jr and Schinitzer, T.J. (1990) Cyclosporin in RA, in *Immunomodulators in the Rheumatic Diseases* (eds D.E. Furst and M.E. Wenblatt), Marcel Dekker, New York.

Ledinghan, J. and Deighton, C. (2005) Update of the BSR guidelines for prescribing TNFα blockers in adults with RA. *Rheumatology*, **44** (2), 157–63.

Loeb, J. (1976) Corticosteroids and growth. *New England Journal of Medicine*, **295**, 547–2.

Lubkin, I.M. (1990) *Chronic Illness Impact and Interactions*, Jones and Bartlett Publishers Incorporated, USA.

Luqmani, R.A., Palmer, R.G. and Bacon, P.A. (1990) Azathioprine, cyclophosphamide and chlorambucil, in *Slow Acting Anti-Rheumatic Drugs and Immunosuppressives Bailliere's Clinical Rheumatology* (ed. P.M. Brookes), Balliere Tindall, London, pp. 595–620.

Maddison, P., Kiely, P., Kirkham, B. *et al.* (2005) Leflunomide in rheumatoid arthritis: recommendations through a process of consensus. *Rheumatology*, **44**, 280–6.

Maini, R.N., Breedveld, F.C. Kalden, J.R. *et al.* (2004) Sustained improvement over 2 years in physical function, structural damage and signs and symptoms among patients with RA treated with Infliximab and methotrexate. *Arthritis and Rheumatism*, **50** (4), 1051–65.

Mease, P., Russel, I.J., Young, L.J. Jr *et al.* (2003) Pregabalin improves pain, sleep and fatigue associated with fibromyalgia syndrome (FMS) in a multi-centred, randomised, placebo controlled monotherapy trial. *Annals of Rheumatic Diseases Supplement: Abstract OP0041*, **62**, 77.

Melzack, R. and Wall, P.D. (1982) *The Challenge of Pain*, Basic Books, New York.

Miller, T.E. and North, D.K. (1981) Clinical injections, antibiotics and imunosuppression – a puzzling relationship (editorial). *American Journal of Medicine*, **71**, 334–6.

Moll, J.M. (1983) *Management of Rheumatic Disorders*, Chapter Hall, London.

Monauni T, Zenti, T.M.G., Cretti, A. *et al.* (2000) Effects of glucosamine infusion on insulin secretion and insulin action on humans. *Diabetes*, **49** (6), 926–35.

Moore, D. (2000) The use of alternative medical therapies in patients with systematic lupus erythematosus. *Arthritis and Rheumatology*, **43**, 1410–8.

Moore, A. (2003) *Bandolier's Little book of Pain*. Oxford University Press, Oxford.

Mouridsen, H.T. and Jacobsen, E. (1975) Pharmacokinetics of cyclophosphamide in renal failure. *Acta Pharmacologica et Toxicologica*, **36**, 409–14.

National Patient Safety Agency (2005) *Methotrexate*, National Patient Safety Agency, London.

National Prescribing Centre (2002) *Signposts for Good Prescribing: A Resource to Help Prepare Nurses, Midwives and Health Visitors for Prescribing Responsibilities* (CD ROM), NPC, London.

National Prescribing Centre (2004) *Monitoring Competency in Prescribing: An Outline Framework to Help Allied Health Professional Supplementary Prescribers*, NPC, Liverpool.

Newman, S., Fitzpatrick, R., Revensen, T. *et al.* (1996) *Understanding RA*, Routledge, London.

NICE (National Institute of Clinical Excellence) (2002) *Guidance on the Use of Etanercept and Infliximab in the Treatment of RA*. Technology Appraisal 36, NICE, London.

Norman, L. (1992) *The Reflexology Handbook*, Bath Press, Great Britain.

Nusslein, H.G., Herbst, M. Manager, B.J. *et al*. (1985) Total lymphoid irradiation in patients with refractory RA. *Arthritis and Rheumatism*, **28**, 1205–10.

Nussmeier, N.A., Whelton, A.A., Brown, M.T. *et al*. (2005) Complications of the COX-2 inhibitors parecoxib and valdecoxib in patients undergoing cardiac surgery. *New England Journal of Medicine*, **352**, 1081–91.

Oliver, S. (2003) The immune system and new therapies for inflammatory joint disease. *Musculoskeletal Care*, **1** (1), 44–57.

Oliver, S. (2004) *Chronic Disease Nursing: A Rheumatology Example*, Whurr Publishers, London.

Oliver, S. and Mooney, J. (2002) Targeted therapies for patients with rheumatoid arthritis. *Professional Nurse*, **17** (12), 716–80.

Ott, E., Nussmeier, N.A., Duke, P.C. *et al*. (2005) the Multicenter Study of Perioperative Pain Society. www.britishpainsociety.org

Pain Society (2005) www.britishpainsociety.org

Panush, R.S., Carter, R.L., Katz, P. *et al*. (1983) Diet therapy for RA. *Arthritis and Rheumatism*, **26** (4), 462–71.

Pavelka, K., Gatterova, J., Olejarova, M. *et al*. (2002) Glucosamine sulfate use and delay of progression of knee osteoarthritis. *Archives of Internal Medicine*, **162**, 2113–23.

Parkin, D.M., Henney, C.R., Quirk, J. and Crooks, J. (1976) Deviation from prescribed drug treatment after discharge from hospital. *British Medical Journal*, **1**, 359–69.

Paulus, H.E., Machlide, H.I., Levine, S. *et al*. (1977) Lymophocyte involvement in RA – studies during thoratic duct drainage. *Arthritis and Rheumatism*, **24**, 867–73.

Pearce, S. and Wardle, J. (1989) *The Practice of Behavioural Medicine*, Oxford University Press, England.

Piper, J.M., Ray, W.A., Doughery, J.R. and Griffin, M.R. (1991) Corticosteroid use and peptic ulcer role of NSAIDs. *Annals of Internal medicine*, **114**, 735–40.

Polito, C., Oporto, M.R., Totino, S.F. *et al*. (1986) Normal growth of nephrotic children during long term alternate day Prednisolone therapy. *Acta Paediatrica Scandinavica*, **75**, 245–50.

Porter, D.R. and Capell, H.A. (1990) The use of Sulfasalazine as a disease modifying anti-rheumatic drug, in *Slow Acting Anti-Rheumatic Drugs and Immunosuppressives. Bailliere's Clinical Rheumatology* (ed. P.M. Brooks), Balliere Tindall, London, pp. 535–52.

Quilligan, S. (1990) When should you take your tablets? *Professional Nurse*, **September**, 639–40.

Ray, W., Stein, M., Hall, K. *et al*. (2002) Non-steroidal anti-inflammatory drugs and the risk of serious coronary heart disease: observational cohort study. *Lancet*, **359**, 118–23.

RCN (Royal College of Nursing) (2003) *Assessing, Managing and Monitoring Biologic Therapies for Inflammatory Arthritis*, Royal College of Nursing, London.

Reginster, J.Y., Deroisy, R., Rovati, L.C. *et al*. (2001) Long term effects of glucosamine sulphate on osteoarthrits progression: a randomised placebo-controlled clinical trial. *Lancet*, **357**, 251–6.

Reid, I.R., Chapman, G.E., Fraser, T.R.C. *et al*. (1986) Low serum osteocalcin levels in glucocorticosteroid-treated asthmatics. *Journal of Clinical and Endocrinological Metabolism*, **62**, 379–83.

Richy, F., Bruyere, O., Ethgen, O. *et al*. (2003) Structural and symptomatic efficacy of glucosamine and chrondroitin in knee osteoarthritis. A comprehensive meta-analysis. *Archieves of Internal Medicine*, **163**, 1514–22.

Rowbotham, D. (1993) Post operative pain. *Prescribers Journal*, **33** (6), 237–43.

Robinson, W.H., Genovese, M.C. and Moreland, L.W. (2001) Demyelinatry and neurologic events reported in association with tumour necrosis factor alpha anatagonism. *Arthritis and Rheumatism*, **44** (9), 1977–83.

Roche (2005) *Rituximab: Summary of Product Characteristics*, Roche Products Ltd, Herts.

Sany, J., Kaiser, M.J., Jorgensen, C. and Trape, G. (2005) Study of the tolerance of infliximab infusions with or without betamethasone premedication in patients with active RA. *Annals of Rheumatic Diseases*, **64**, 1647–9.

Schering Plough (2005) *Infliximab and Occurence of Infusion-related Reactions*, Schering Plough, Berkshire.

Schlegal, S. (1987) General characteristics of NSAIDs, in *Drugs for Rheumatic Diseases*, (eds H. Paulus, D. Furst and S. Dromgoole), Churchill Livingstone, New York.

Scroggie, D.A., Albright, A. and Harris, M.D. (2003) The effects of glucosamine chondroitin supplementation on glycosylated heamoglobin levels in patients with type 2 diabetes mellitus: a placebo controlled trial. *Archives of Internal Medicine*, **163** (13), 1587–90.

Scriven, L. and Bryan, L. (1987) Self medication on a surgical ward. *New Zealand Nurse Journal*, **81**, 25–6.

Shaw, T., Quan, J. and Totoritis, M.C. (2003) B cell therapy for RA, the rituximab (anti-CD20) experience. *Annals of Rheumatic Diseases*, **62** (11), 1155–9.

Shergy, W.J., Isern, R.A., Cooley, D.A. *et al.* (2002) The Prompt Study: open study to assess infliximab safety and timing of onset of clinical benefit among patients with RA. *Journal of Rheumatology.* **29**, 667–77.

Smolen, J.S., Kalden, J.R., Scott, D.L. *et al.* (1999) Efficacy and safety of leflunomide compared with placebo and Sulphasalazine in active rheumatoid arthritis; a double blind randomised, multicentre trial. European leflunomide study group. *Lancet*, **353**, 259–66.

Smith, J., Driscoll, P. and Coniff, R. (1985) *Rheumatology Nursing – A Problem Orientated Approach*, John Wiley & Sons, Ltd, Chichester.

Snaith, M.L. and Adebajo, A.O. (2004) *ABC of Rheumatology*, 3rd edn, BMJ Books, London.

Sohn, P. and Cook, C. (2002) Nurse practitioner knowledge for complementary alternative health care; foundation for practice. *Journal of Advanced Nursing*, **39** (1), 9–16.

Solomon, D.H. (2005) Selective cyclooxygenase 2 inhibitors and cardiovascualr events. *Arthritis and Rheumatism*, **52** (7), 1968–78.

Songsiridej, N. and Furst, D.E. (1990) Methotrexate – the rapidly acting drugs, in *Slow Acting Anti-Rheumatic Drugs and Immunosuppressives Ballieres Clinical Rheumatology* (ed. P.M. Brookes), Bailliere Tindall, London, pp. 574–94.

Speight, T.M. (1987) *Avery's Drug Treatment*, Edinburgh: Churchill Livingstone.

Stahl, H.D., Szecsepassli, L., Szechiaski, J. *et al.* (2003) Rituximab in RA: efficacy and safety from a randomised controlled trial. *Annals Rheumatic Diseases*, Supp.1, 65.

Stein, C. (1991) Peripheral analgesic effects of opioids. *Pain System Management*, **6**, 119–24.

Strand, V. and Kavanaugh, A.F. (2004) The role of interleukin-1 in bone resorption in RA, *Rheumatology*, **43**, Supplement 3, 10–16.

Sutherland, K., Morgan, J. and Sample, S. (1991) Self administering drugs: an introduction. *Nursing Times*, **23**, 19–33.

Tannis, A.J., Barban, J. and Conquer, J.A. (2004) Effects of glucosamine supplementation on fasting and non fasting plasma glucose and serum insulin concentration in healthy individuals. *Osteoarthritis and Cartilage*, **12** (6), 506–11.

Tesser, J., Fleischmann, R., Dore, R. *et al.* (2004) Concomitant medication use in a large international multi-centre, placebo controlled trial of anakinra; a recombinant interleukin 1 receptor antagonist in patients with RA. *The Journal of Rheumatology*, **31.4**, 649–54.

Thompson, P. and Dunne, C. (1995) *NSAIDs Use and Abuse. Collected Reports on Rheumatic Diseases*, Arthritis and Rheumatism Council, Chesterfield.

Topol, E. and Falk, G. (2004) A coxib a day won't keep the doctor away. *Lancet*, **364**, 640−1.

Towheed, T.E., Maxwell, L., Anastassiades, T.P. *et al.* (2005) Glucosamine therapy for treating osteoarthritis (review). *The Cochrane Library* Issue 3.

Trouce, J. and Gould, D. (1990) *Clinical Pharmacology for Nurses*, Churchill Livingstone, London.

Turk, D.C., Dworkin, R.H. and Allan, R.R. (2003) Core outcome domains for chronic pain trials. *Pain*, **106**, 337−45.

Turk, D.C. and Melzack, R. (1992) *Handbook of Pain Assessment*, Guildford, New York.

Turk, J.L. and Parker, D. (1979) The effect of cyclophosphamide on the immune response. *Journal of Immunopharmacy*, **1**, 127−37.

UKCC (1992) *The Scope of Professional Practice*, UKCC, London.

Van de Heij de, D.M.F.M., Van't H of M.A., Van Riel, P.L.C.M. *et al.* (1992) Validity of single variables and composite indicies for measuring disease activity in rheumatoid arthritis. *Annals of Rheumatic Diseases*, **51**, 177−81.

Walker, G. (1994) *ABPI Data Sheet Compendium*, Datapharm Publications Ltd, Great Britain.

Wandless, I. and Davie, J.W. (1997) Can drug compliance in the elderly be improved? *British Medical Journal*, **1**: 359−61.

Watson, C.P.N. (1994) Anti-depressant drugs as adjuvant analgesia. *Journal of Pain Symptom Management*, **9**, 392−401.

Watson, D.J., Rhodes, T., Cai, B. and Guess, H.A. (2002) Lower risk of thromboembolic events with naproxen amongst people with rheumatoid arthritis. *Archives Internal Medicine*, **162**, 1105−10.

Wasserman, M.J., Weber, D.A., Guthrie, J.A. *et al.* (2004) Infusion related reactions to infliximab in patients with RA in a clinical practice setting; relationship to dose, antihistamine pre treatment and infusion number. *Journal of Rheumatology*, **31**, 1912−17.

Webb, C. (1990) Self medication for elderly patients. *Nursing Times*, **86** (16), 46−9.

Weber, R.W. (2004) Adverse reactions to biological modifiers. *Current Opinion, Allergy Clinical Immunology*, **4** (4), 277−83.

Weusten, B.L.A.M., Jacobs, J.W.G. and Bijlsma, J.W.J. (1993) Corticosteroid pulse therapy in active RA. *Seminars Arthritis and Rheumatism*, **23**, 183−92.

Winbury, S.L. and Lieberman, P.L. (1995) Anaphylaxis. *Immunology Allergy Clinician, North America*, **15**, 447.

Woolf, C.J. (1994) The dorsal horn state. Dependent sensory processing and the generation of pain, in *Textbook of Pain* (eds P.D. Wall and R. Melzack), Churchill Livingstone, Edinburgh.

Worwood, V.A. (1993) *The Fragrant Pharmacy*, Bantam Books, London.

Wyeth Pharmaceuticals (2005) Enbrel 50 mg. Wyeth Pharmaceutical, Berkshire.

Yocum, D.E., Allen, J.B., Wahl, S.M. *et al.* (1986) Inhibition by ciclosporin A of streptococcal cell wall induced arthritis and hepatic granulomas in rats. *Arthritis and Rheumatism*, **29**, 262−74.

Zhang, A. and Wan P.O. (1994) The effectiveness of topically applied capsaicin. *European Journal of Clinical Pharmacology*, **46**, 517−22.

3 The Role of the Nurse in Drug Therapy

SARAH RYAN AND MARGARET ANN VOYCE

Learning Objectives

After reading this chapter you should be able to:

- Describe the philosophy that underpins rheumatology nursing.
- Explain the role of the nurse in preparing the patient to commence a DMARD.
- Demonstrate an understanding of the safety monitoring required in the surveillance of DMARDs.
- Discuss the role of community provision for patients with musculoskeletal conditions.
- Explain the drug management of a person with osteoporosis.

Patients with inflammatory arthritis such as RA can experience a range of physical, psychological, social and/or sexual problems. The role of the nurse is to support, guide, educate and empower the patient and their family so that problems can be identified and care that has meaning and relevance for the patient implemented. This has to be a shared process between the patient and the nurse, as conditions such as RA are not curable and the patient must be committed to a long-term treatment plan. Patients with active disease activity (determined by haematological and biochemical markers, X-ray results and clinical findings) will require a combination of drug therapy to reduce symptoms such as pain and stiffness and also to suppress disease activity, minimizing the potential harm that prolonged inflammation can cause. Analgesia and non-steroidal anti-inflammatory drugs can provide symptoms relief and the DMARDs (see Table 3.1) can suppress disease activity. The nurse requires in-depth knowledge regarding the condition and treatment options and will need to employ the skills of educator to provide the patient with sufficient information to contribute to shared decision making prior to the commencement of drug therapy.

3.1 WHAT IS RHEUMATOLOGY NURSING?

Therapeutic nursing has been defined by Powell (1991) as that practice where the nurse has made a difference to the patient's or client's health state and where

Drug Therapy in Rheumatology Nursing: Second Edition. Edited by Sarah Ryan.
© 2007 John Wiley & Sons, Ltd.

Table 3.1 Disease-modifying anti-rheumatic drugs.

- Hydroxychloroquine/chloroquine
- Dapsone
- Sulfasalazine
- Gold injections
- Auranofin
- D-penicillamine
- Ciclosporin
- Minocyline
- Azathioprine
- Methotrexate
- Cyclophosphamide
- Phenylbutazone
- Leflunomide
- Mycophenolate

he or she is aware of how and why this positive difference has occurred. Levine (1973) distinguishes between nursing which is supportive in nature and seeks to prevent further deterioration and that which is therapeutic, promoting adaptation and contributing to the restoration of well-being. The introduction of drug therapy in conjunction with other treatment interventions – for example, exercise – can be seen as fulfilling both a supportive and a therapeutic role, preventing deterioration and leading to an improvement in symptoms, enabling the patient to participate more fully in meaningful life activities.

Caring is the most important value of rheumatology nursing. Although often referred to as a basic requirement there is nothing basic about high quality nursing care, which requires a combination of knowledge, understanding and expertise. Caring involves both an action element in identifying and meeting the needs of the patient and an emotional element, which involves having regard for people as individuals and being concerned about what happens to them (Malin and Teasdale, 1991). It would appear that in many situations the action element remains the dominant feature of nursing practice with interactions with patients governed by their physical care needs, resulting in the neglect of the emotional needs of the patient (Henderson, 1994). Yet we know that from the patient's perspective it is how the individual nurse relates to the patient, the emotional style, that determines whether a patient perceives a care episode as satisfactory or not (Smith, 1992). For care to be effective and holistic in nature the nurse must incorporate both the action and emotional element into care delivery. The adoption of this approach is as important in the instigation of drug therapy as in all treatment interventions, as the patient will have to be satisfied on an emotional level as to the value of drug therapy for compliance to occur.

THE NURSE–PATIENT RELATIONSHIP

The most important element in rheumatology nursing is the relationship that exists between the patient and the nurse. Such a relationship requires both time and knowledge for the nurse to begin to empower the patient so that an informed decision regarding care management can be reached. The relationship needs to be founded on participation. There is the assumption that by involving the patient in their own care they will ultimately obtain the status of participant but it may well be that the patient is participating from the nurse's frame of reference, rather than from their own view point. Asking the patients to write down their expectations regarding drug therapy may provide the starting point from which the partnership can commence.

The factors needed for a therapeutic relationship include:

- Genuine participation.

  It is important to encourage the patient to participate in as many treatment decisions as possible. When a patient chooses a course of action such as commencing sulfasalazine they are more likely to adhere even if the beneficial effects take some time to emerge, which in the case of this particular drug could be anything from two to four months. Informing the patient about different drug options and enabling the patient to choose from them should heighten his or her sense of control.

- The exploration of lay beliefs.

  Until the nurse has spent time exploring the patient's own beliefs about the purpose and outcome of drug therapy it will not be possible to arrive at shared treatment objectives.

- The establishment of realistic goals.

  Trying to reach unrealistic goals will only demoralize and adversely affect self-esteem. If the patient is not informed that DMARDs take many months before benefit can be assessed they could become disillusioned with the treatment if symptoms did not improve after the first few weeks and discontinue the regime.

- The provision of information specific to the individual's situation.

  It is not helpful to be given generalized information and told what percentage of patients respond well to a given treatment. The individual requires information that is relevant to their own particular situation.

- The involvement of significant others.

  It is important that family members are included and assist in care planning so that care options decided can be endorsed and implemented within the patient-supportive framework and within their own social setting.

- Maintaining contact.

  It is important that the patient has access to a knowledgeable practitioner who is familiar with their care, at any time when there is a perceived change in disease activity or self-management. This can be maintained through a telephone helpline system, which provides the patient with a designated point of contact and helps to reduce anxiety and provide support.

3.2   TELEPHONE ADVICE LINES

Telephone advice lines have become an integral part of rheumatology care and are traditionally run by clinical nurse specialists or other heath professionals in extended roles (Thwaites, 2004). This service provides patients with the means of contacting professionals directly involved in their care management, for advice regarding symptoms management and concerns relating to drug therapy. The telephone advice line also provides direct access for other members of the team involved in the patient's medical and nursing care to seek advice. For example, a general practitioner may ring to question whether gold injections should be discontinued due to the slight presence of haematuria on a urinalysis dipstick test. The immediate advice by the nurse to continue will prevent treatment being stopped unnecessarily. It will also enable a consistency to care management to develop between members of primary and secondary healthcare. This will reinforce communication links and promote a greater appreciation of the different roles of these two groups.

3.3   THE PHILOSOPHY OF RHEUMATOLOGY NURSING

A philosophy of practice is required to enable nurses within rheumatology to work as a united team with identified shared goals for patient management. A philosophy consists of a system of beliefs from which core practice evolves. The establishment of a philosophy has to include debate and discussion from all members of the nursing team. It is a statement of purpose and will require commitment from all concerned for it to be integrated into practice. If a shared approach to care is not adopted then disunity and fragmentation of care will occur. A rheumatology nursing philosophy of care can be divided into four main areas which are interlinked and complementary to each other. These include:

- Health.
- Beliefs relating to the environment.
- Beliefs relating to the individual patient.
- Beliefs relating to nursing.

Health

Health is achieved when the patient is able to function on a physical, psychological and social level. This is not a reinstatement of complete well-being in all these spheres of life; rather that the patient perceives that they are able to make a useful contribution to all areas of activity. Health requires adaptations and the development of coping strategies to minimize the symptoms of arthritis. Health does not mean the removal of all symptoms; this would be an unrealistic outcome and an unfair burden to place on patients. Health and illness are not static entries and vary depending on:

- disease activity;
- coping strategies;
- available resources;
- support.

RA is characterized by flares and remissions of disease activity and the patients may find themselves alternating between health and illness or functioning well on a physical level but not on a psychological level. The patient will need to know how to access a knowledgeable nurse when they experience a stage in their condition that presents different or recurring problems, so that the situation can be reassessed collectively and necessary modifications to the treatment programme made.

Beliefs Relating to the Environment

A patient needs to be involved in the planning of all aspects of care to feel committed and able to implement the agreed treatment programme based on the individual's perceived needs (Tones, 1991) and this applies equally to drug therapy. Neglect of individual concerns can lead to non-adherence with treatment. Nurses need to identify any existing internal and external barriers. A patient may not be able to open their medication container due to reduced manual dexterity or be afraid to continue with treatment due to adverse peer pressure. If the orientation of the consultation between the nurse and the patient does not encourage shared discussion, the patient may not feel part of the treatment regime and discontinue their medications if they are not immediately effective.

Beliefs Relating to the Individual Patient

The individual's lay beliefs must be explored before any treatment plan is decided so that the care programme that emerges has both relevance and meaning of the individual concerned. Lay beliefs are usually consistent over time and pertinent to the individual concerned (Donovan, 1991). If a patient has in their lay belief system the thought that drug treatment such as gold has only the potential for damaging side effects to occur and not the potential for improvement they may reject this as a treatment option. The patient will require explanation on the disease process before they can understand the role of drug therapy. If they do not understand that their pain, stiffness and fatigue is related to disease activity they may not perceive drug treatment as a useful adjunct to other therapy.

The individual has a right to be an active not a passive recipient of care so informed decisions can be made and the management of the condition viewed as a shared commitment between the patient and the health professional. Patients may not feel equipped to adapt to this role at first but as the nurse begins to share knowledge with the patient and a therapeutic relationship develops the patient may feel more able to contribute to care decisions.

Beliefs Relating to Nursing

The nurse will be a knowledgeable practitioner using evidence-based practice to underpin holistic care management.

3.4   THE ROLE OF THE NURSE IN DRUG THERAPY

EMPOWERMENT

Once the clinical decision has been made to commence a patient on DMARD therapy, the patient will require to spend time with a knowledgeable practitioner so that the following aspects can be discussed:

* The purpose of the medication.
* The dosage and time of administration.
* Potential side effects.
* Monitoring regime.
* The patient's expectations of treatment.
* The course to take if a problem arises.

Tones (1991) defines empowerment as the process whereby an individual or community of individuals acquire power − that is, the capacity to control other people and resources. By explaining about the particular drug therapy and the rationale for its introduction the patient will begin to determine its acceptability from their particular view point.

Klein (1974) describes five categories of patient involvement:

* Information. This is the process whereby the health professional gives the information to the patient and the patient passively receives it. This will not be useful for commencing patients on drug therapy as the patient will be the individual responsible for the administration of the medication and to adhere with the proposed regime must be committed to the type of treatment being advocated. Patient–physician communication may be the single most important variable affecting adherence (Bradley, 1989). For communication to be successful the nurse must present information clearly whilst the patient needs to seek clarification and ensure that their concerns are addressed (Newman et al., 1996).

Factors that influence effective practitioner–patient communication include: (Newman et al., 1996)

1) The nature of the explanation concerning the diagnosis, and the course and purpose of treatment. When rheumatologists were recorded as having made a clear statement about the purpose of the drug treatment 79% of patients adhered with their therapy compared to only 33% of patients when the explanation offered was not clear (Daltroy, 1993).

2) An overuse of medical jargon, which excludes the patient from shared discussion.

3) A shared agreement of the goals for treatment are essential. Arluke (1980) found that some patients with RA stopped their medication at the first sign of improvement as they held the belief that drug efficacy would reduce over time.

4) The need to obtain the patient's concerns regarding drug treatment. Several studies have shown that practitioners misperceive patients' needs regarding the amount, content and preferred method for providing information (e.g. drug information sheets) on arthritis and its treatments (Potts, Mazzuca and Brandt, 1986).

- Consultation. The health professional may consult the patient and may use the information gained. This will not lead to a shared approach towards treatment management as the practitioner may not have obtained the patient's beliefs, values and expectations, which are all potent factors affecting adherence, not only because of their direct relationship to health behaviour but also because they are subject to misinterpretation unless clarification is sought and will ultimately influence how satisfied the patient is with the consultation.

- Negotiation. Here equality exists and both parties contribute to the decision making and negotiate the treatment. The nurse would begin by ascertaining the patient's concerns regarding treatment and identify potential compliance difficulties and jointly plan how to overcome them (Daltroy, 1993).

- Participation. A patient's values are taken into account and underpin the decision process. A patient may prefer not to commence methotrexate if they drink alcohol regularly and will be more likely to comply with an alternative drug where they do not have to abstain from alcohol.

- Veto-participation. The patient holds the right not to comply with treatment. Liang (1989) describes non-compliance as the ultimate experience of independence. If this occurs it should do so only after full negotiation has occurred and not as a result of ignorance or non-disclosure. The nurse would seek to ascertain the reason why the patient was declining drug therapy. It may be due to a lack of knowledge or apprehensions that have not been discussed. If patients decline therapy they must be given the opportunity to reaccess the service at any time to reassess their condition and other treatment options.

3.5 THE COMMENCEMENT OF DMARDs

PATIENT PREPARATION

The mode of action of DMARDs has been discussed in depth in Chapter 2. Patients often commence DMARDs at a time when their arthritis is in an illness phase with evidence of increased disease activity. This will often cause the patient to experience an increase in symptomatology inducing pain, stiffness, fatigue, low mood and systemic manifestations such as anaemia. The majority of DMARDs take many months before their ability to affect the disease process can be assessed. Patients respond at different times but will require education, support and guidance at the commencement of treatment and on an ongoing basis. The nurse will need, in conjunction with the patient, to plan interventions to enable the patient to cope with increased symptomatology. This may include a combination of exercise, relaxation, pacing activities, review of analgesia or an inpatient stay.

The objective of ongoing education and care provision are to enable the patients to participate effectively in their own management, develop coping skills, make informed choices about their treatment and weigh up the consequences of their action or inaction.

In a comprehensive review of patient education studies, Lorig et al. (1987) demonstrated positive improvement in patient knowledge, self-care beliefs, medication adjustment and compliance; as well as psychosocial characteristics such as anxiety, depression, self-esteem, locus of control and health status.

After the patient has received a full explanation regarding the drug treatment proposed and been given the opportunity to discuss concerns and expressed a commitment to the therapy there may be safety preparation that needs to occur prior to commencement of the named drug – for example, if a patient is to commence methotrexate a chest X-ray will need to be obtained.

MONITORING CLINICS

Patients receiving DMARDs require regular safety monitoring of therapy and assessment of disease activity. This is usually carried out within the holistic framework of a nurse led follow up clinic. The full functions of such a clinic can be seen in Table 3.2.

Running drug monitor clinics is a major component of the nurse specialist role (Phelan et al., 1992; Ryan and Hill, 2004) Nurse-led clinics allow partnership, intimacy and reciprocity to evolve between the nurse and the patient and provide the medium for an ongoing therapeutic partnership to develop in which the nurse will be assessing all care needs and identifying problems that may require a referral

Table 3.2 Functions of a nurse-led clinic (Hill, 1992).

- Assessing the progress of the disease
- Monitoring the progress of the disease
- Monitoring drug response
- Initiating and interpreting clinical and laboratory data
- Acting as educator
- Expert source of referral to other members of the multidisciplinary team
- Research

Table 3.3 Key nursing functions (Wilson Barnett, 1984).

- Understanding illness and treatment from the patient's viewpoint
- Providing continuous psychological care during illness and critical events
- Helping people cope with illness or potential health problems
- Providing comfort
- Coordinating treatment and other events affecting the patient

---

to other members of the healthcare team such as the chiropodist. The clinic will also provide the forum for education and the development of coping strategies. The nurse's role evolves from supportive to therapeutic, instead of concentrating exclusively on preventing deteriorating. The nurse will incorporate essential nursing functions (see Table 3.3) to promote adaptation to the condition for the patient and their families.

For care to be meaningful within an individual context nurses must understand the impact of illness from the patient's view point (Ryan, 1996). The nurse must work actively with the patient to establish realistic achievable goals which incorporate the patient's lay beliefs.

The Operational Workings of a Drug Monitoring Clinic

Patients receiving DMARDs and cytotoxic agents require regular blood tests and in certain cases urinalysis and blood pressure monitoring. The British Society of Rheumatology and the British Health Professionals in Rheumatology have produced guidelines for clinicians and these are available from either society. Kay and Puller (1992) found marked variations amongst respondents in monitoring schedules and in the interpretation of results.

At each visit the patient is seen by the same rheumatology nurse to allow the continuation of the therapeutic relationship. The nurse will:

- Assess safety in administration − for example, ensuring that methotrexate is taken on a weekly basis.
- Monitor and observe for any drug reactions that have occurred − for example, gastrointestinal, skin, urinary abnormalities and chest manifestations.
- Take blood to ascertain any bone marrow suppression leading to a reduction in red blood cells, white blood cells and platelet count; elevation in liver function tests, creatinine levels and urea and electrolytes where indicated. Hill's (1994) research demonstrated that the nurse practitioner is able to identify and instigate appropriate action from blood results.
- Provide the patient with time to discuss any perceived problems or concerns − for example, is it safe to have vaccinations? Is it normal to experience increased stiffness after the administration of intramuscular gold?
- Assess for evidence of increased disease activity − for example, synovitis. This may necessitate a different treatment intervention − for example, the

administration of intra-articular injections. About 12% of nurse specialists within rheumatology are engaged in the provision of intra-articular injections (Phelan *et al.*, 1992) and this number is rapidly increasing as nurses seek to develop their practice around patient need and provide a more comprehensive programme of care expansion and is in accordance with principles established in the scope of professional practice (UKCC, 1992). This framework encourages and supports nurses to develop practice which has been shown to directly benefit patient care, as long as it does not fragment existing care or involve inappropriate delegation of duties. It would be inappropriate, indeed unsafe practice, to develop one's role without first obtaining the necessary theoretical knowledge and practical expertise necessary to ensure understanding and safe practice. Benner (1984) states that an expert nurse requires a combination of academic achievement, recognized clinical expertise and practical experience.

- Access other care needs within a holistic framework (see Figure 3.1) and refer where appropriate to other members of the multidisciplinary team.
- Provide the patient with the telephone helpline − providing a designated point of contact with a knowledgeable practitioner should any problems or concerns arise before the next appointment.

DOCUMENTATION

The Staffordshire Rheumatology Centre uses a computerized drug monitor program. Kay (1989) states that more use could be made of computer technology in drug monitoring. All relevant information about the patient is recorded. This includes demographic data, blood and urine results, medications taken and reasons for discontinuation where appropriate. The computer is programmed to alert the operator to any results that fall outside the normal parameters such as three consecutive falls in platelets. It is also an invaluable communication tool as any member of the nursing and medical team can place a message on the patient's computerized record that will be acknowledged by the nurse conducting the clinic. This may include requests for additional investigations to be made while the patient is in clinic so that they do not have the inconvenience of being recalled. Other units use a metrology graph which includes a visual analogue pain scale, early morning stiffness, articular index, grip strength and the recording of drug regimes. A list of past medication and the reasons for discontinuation is kept on the reverse of the graph. Joint injections, intramuscular steroid injections, infusions, admissions, trauma and even domestic stress are recorded on the chart because they all have a bearing on disease activity. This method of documentation enables the course of the disease to be followed easily (Thompson, Morgan and Fletcher, 1992).

THE USE OF PROTOCOLS

The establishment of protocols to guide decision making, ensure continuity of care and safety in practice requires collaboration and commitment from all health

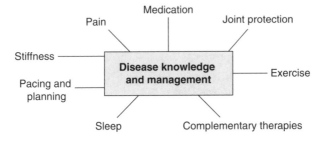

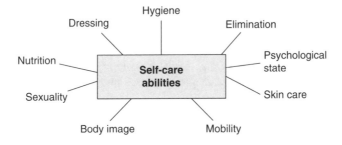

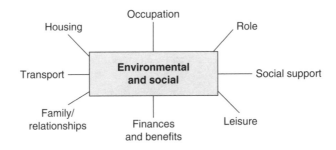

Figure 3.1 The rheumatology nurse forum problem model.

professionals involved in the monitoring and assessment of drug therapy. They provide an educational tool for nurses by ensuring that practice is research-based, and act as a dynamic structure updated when new evidence becomes available. The protocols may cover:

- Urinary abnormalities.
- Gastrointestinal side effects.
- Skin manifestations.
- Chest symptoms.
- Alteration of drug dosages.

Included below are the protocols used for the daily drug monitor clinic at the Staffordshire Rheumatology Centre. This provides an example of the framework we have adopted enabling these protocols to be a fluid and dynamic tool supporting nurses in the decision making process.

DRUG MONITOR CLINIC PROTOCOLS

Reactions can occur in many sites. The nurse needs to:

- Be aware of what to look for.
- Know how to respond.

   1. Skin manifestations. Changes in skin integrity can be related to:

     (a) The disease process − that is, vasculitis and leg ulcers.
     (b) The drugs used for therapy − that is, gold injections.
     (c) Difficulties faced in maintenance of skin integrity.

       (i) Rash

A rash

        − May occur with any medication but is most commonly seen in those patients having gold therapy.
        − Can vary from minor eczematous lesions to severe widespread problem.

If a patient presents with a rash:

        − Ask if they have recently changed their detergent. Consider sun burn, insect bites.

If the rash is isolated to an odd patch, advise E45 cream. Review in a month's time.

   If it is a severe, persistent or generalized rash, this may require a dermatology opinion − arrange referral.

       (ii) Itching

If the itching is:

        − troublesome − continue with treatment. Advise use of E45 cream or antihistamines.. If the scalp is itchy, scaly or dry, advise a coal tar-based solution − for example, Baltar.
        − unbearable − that is, cannot sleep with it − stop the medication and refer to the doctor's clinic.

   2. Urinary manifestations

Urinary abnormalities may be due to:

     (a) The disease itself − amyloid.
     (b) Gold or D-penicillamine and are less likely with sulfasalazine and methotrexate.
     (c) Asymptomatic urinary tract infections, which are common in RA patients.

(d) The ultra-sensitivity of lab stick testing.

   (i) Proteinuria

      – A trace or one + in isolation ignore.

      – ++ repeat dipstick testing, if ++ still present then send midstream specimen of urine (MSSU) (patient and GP will be contacted if infection is present).

      – If patient is symptomatic send MSSU.

      – If MSSU reveals no infection but ++ persists arrange 24-hour urine collection.

      – When sending off an MSSU please record on the form whether or not the patient is taking antibiotics.

      – If +++ protein stop treatment and collect 24-hour urine, unless the patient is known to have proteinuria.

   (ii) Haematuria

      – Confirm that the patient is not menstruating.

      – A trace or one + in isolation ignore.

      – If ++ or +++ MSSU – continue treatment.

      – If the patient has observed blood loss, inform doctor.

   (iii) Nitrate

      – If nitrate positive with protein or blood, send MSSU.

      – Nitrate in isolation ignore.

   (iv) Glycosuria

      – If known diabetic, advise, refer back to diabetic monitoring.

      – If not known to be diabetic arrange random blood sugar (if over 11 mmol = diagnostic of diabetes, and will require fasting blood sugar. Fasting blood sugar of over 8 = diagnostic of diabetes.

3. Mouth

If the patient presents with a sore mouth:

(a) If dentures are worn ensure these are fitted correctly.

(b) For minor ulcers (i.e. one or two in isolation) continue treatment and suggest: Bonjela, Bioral Gel (apply after meals and bedtime), Bioplex mouth rinse.

(c) For major mouth ulcers – that is, acute severe crop, more than two ulcers: The patient may require Difflan mouth wash and Corlan lozenges or Adcortyl in Orabase. Inform GP.

4. Gastrointestinal tract

(a) Anorexia, dyspepsia and nausea can occur with any drug.

(b) Sulfasalazine - if nausea and/or vomiting occurs. Reduce back to the dose that was not causing this problem and increase as per protocol on fortnightly not weekly basis. If a rash occurs desensitization may be appropriate for early onset (first 14 days/rash - require 2/52 monitor and increase as per protocol).

(c) Leflunomide − if loose stools are experienced patients should be encouraged to remain on the medication and treat the bowel problem.

(d) Penicillamine − taste alteration can occur for up to 12−16 weeks. Support and reassure the patient. May require advice on nutritional supplementation.

(e) Methotrexate − if nausea/vomiting occurs split the dosage over the day, or two days. If nausea/vomiting continues to persist, patient will require domperidone (10 mg three times a day).

(f) Remember gastrointestinal intolerance could be due to NSAIDs − advise over-the-counter antacids and, if it persists, to see doctor.

5. Headaches

(a) Common with sulfasalazine, can occur with leflunomide.

(b) If severe stop drug. Reintroduce after one month at two-weekly intervals.

6. Active joint involvement

(a) Joint stiffness - may follow administration of gold.

7. Chest symptoms

Breathlessness with or without a cough in a patient on gold, leflunomide or methotrexate. Inform doctor.

8. Alopecia

Can occur whilst taking cytotoxic drugs − that is, cyclophosphamide or methotrexate. If troublesome or severe inform doctor.

9. Muscle

If the patient notices weakness, double vision, swelling or speech difficulties this raises the possibility of drug-induced myositis (inflammation of muscle) or myasthenia gravis (disorder of the neuromuscular junction) − inform doctor.

Non-Drug-Related Problems

- Septic joint − if patient has a pyrexia and a hot red joint think of sepsis and inform doctor.
- Neck instability − sudden onset of weakness in hands and legs. Recent onset of bladder and/or bowel incontinence − inform doctor.
- Early herpes zoster − if patient on immunosuppressants they may need anti-viral therapy. Stop cytotoxic medication temporarily until herpes zoster has cleared.

Patients who require blood pressure recording.

1. Patients receiving ciclosporin or leflunomide or present with significant protein-urea or haematuria − if the diastolic is greater than 95 Hg discuss with the doctor

Having such a framework enables the nurse to take immediate action when faced with side effects. Ryan (1997) states that during the first year of using such protocols over 800 patients were reviewed in the clinic with only 2% requiring medical referral. Before the instigation of the protocols 16% of patients were referred annually for a medical consultation primarily as a result of limitations being placed on nurse decision making skills.

The protocols can also ensure continuity of care when the patient moves back in to the community setting.

3.6 INVESTIGATIONS

HAEMATOLOGICAL INVESTIGATIONS

The most frequently requested laboratory test is the full blood count (Higgins, 1996). This test examines three groups of cells with different functions: platelets, red cells (erythrocytes) and white cells (leucocytes). Around 2–2.5 mls of venous blood is required in a tube containing an anticoagulant.

Red Blood Cells

RBCs are biconcave disks. Their main function is to transport haemoglobin around the body and supply oxygen to the tissues. The average number of RBCs per cubic millimetre of blood is about 5 million. The number of RBCs available in the circulation is regulated so that there is an adequate source to provide oxygenation of the tissues without stopping blood flow. The RBC has a very flexible structure which allows it to alter shape as it passes through the capillaries without damage. Altitude and the degree of exercise undertaken can affect the number of circulating RBCs.

RBCs derive from a cell known as the haemocytoblast and are produced in the bone marrow.

Vitamin B12 (Cyanocobalamin)

Vitamin B12 is a nutrient that is required for all cells of the body. An absence or reduced supply of vitamin B12 will severely hinder the rate of RBC production, the problem often being the failure to absorb vitamin B12 from the gastrointestinal tract, as occurs in pernicious anaemia. Gastric secretion contains a substance called the intrinsic factor which combines with vitamin B12 in food, so preparing it for absorption by the gut; but in pernicious anaemia the gastric muscosa does not secrete the intrinsic factor and therefore absorption cannot occur.

In the normal process vitamin B12 is stored in large quantities in the liver after being absorbed from the gastric system. The total amount of vitamin B12 required every day to assist in RBC production is less than 1 microgram and the store in the liver is a thousand times that amount.

Folic Acid

Folic acid is part of the vitamin B complex and deficiency can also hinder the production of RBCs.

Anaemia

The typical anaemia of RA is a normocytic normochromic anaemia; the haemoglobin being around 10–12 g/dl. There appears to be a correlation between disease activity and the severity of anaemia. Some disease modifying anti-rheumatic drugs (e.g. gold) may induce anaemia by attacking erythyroid progenitor cells but in other situations studies show that these therapies may normalize erythropiesis (Pincus et al., 1990).

The cause of anaemia in RA is multifactorial. Iron utilization is impaired as indicted by reduced serum iron and transferritin concentration. As with other forms of chronic inflammation there is an increased synthesis of ferritin and haemosiderin, abnormal retention of iron from FBCs by the reticulo-endothelial system and an increase of lactoferritin, which contributes to the binding and lowering of serum iron (Matteson, Cohen and Conn, 1994).

Anaemia means a deficiency of RBCs with haematocritis sometimes as low as 10%. The anaemia of RA can be complicated by:

- blood loss – NSAIDs can cause intestinal blood loss;
- poor nutrition;
- intercurrent infections;
- autoimmune haemolytic anaemia;
- bone marrow suppression secondary to drug treatment – for example, gold.

A macrocytic macrochromic anaemia may be due to vitamin B12 or folate deficiency, alcohol intake or the mechanisms of sulfasalazine or methotrexate (Hernadez et al., 1975).

Leucocytes

When stained and viewed under the microscope it is possible to identify five types of leucocyte. A full blood count measures both their total number and counts the number of each of the five types. This is the differential count. The normal range of values and differential results can be seen in Table 3.4.

The white blood cells (WBCs) are the mobile units of the body's protective system. They are formed in the bone marrow and the lymph nodes prior to being transported in the blood to the different parts of the body where they are used. All WBCs have a limited life span and adequate numbers are maintained through marrow production.

WBCs play a central role in the process of inflammation. The purpose of the inflammatory response is a complex integration of cellular function and although each type of leucocyte has a different and well-defined function they operate in

Table 3.4 White blood cells.

total white blood cell count	$4-11 \times 10^9$ per L
neutrophils (40−75% to total white cells)	$2.5-7.5 \times 10^9$ per L
lymphocytes (20−40% of total white cells)	$1.5-4.0 \times 10^9$ per L
monocytes (2−10% of total white cells)	$0.2-0.8 \times 10^9$ per L
eosinophils (1−6% of total white cells)	$0.04-0.4 \times 10^9$ per L
basophils (less than 1% of total white cells)	$0.01-0.1 \times 10^9$ per L

conjunction communicating via a range of chemical messengers called cytokines (Higgins, 1996). This concept is explained in greater detail in Chapter 1.

Leucocytosis (a raised WBC count) occasionally occurs in RA but it is not a typical feature. If marked it should raise suspicions of a superseded infection (either systemic or a septic arthritis), a post-infected arthritis or one of the varieties of polyarteritis.

Leucopaenia (a reduced WBC count) can occur in systemic lupus erythematosus and in Felty's syndrome but the commonest cause is in the use of DMARDs.

Neutrophils

From 40−75% of circulating WBCs are neutrophils, the first line of defence against bacterial invasions. They are present in large numbers at the place of invasion where they ingest and kill bacteria by a process of phagocytosis.

Monocytes

These are mobile WBCs that filter out of the blood and into the tissues, where they are referred to as macrophages. The key role is probably as an antigen-presenting cell. Lymphocytes cannot respond to naked antigen and it must first be processed by and presented on the surface of an antigen-presenting cell. Macrophages become attached to tissues and remain attached for months, even years. They are involved in the primary clearance of highly resistant bacteria such as mycobacteria.

Monocytes manufacture a range of cytokines that attract or activate other cells involved in the inflammatory response − for example, macrophages produce interleukin 1 which activates a type of lymphocytes to kill viruses (Oppenheim, Koacs and Matsushima, 1986).

Basophils

These are seen only rarely in peripheral blood. They mature in the tissues, becoming mast cells. These cells liberate heparin into the blood to prevent blood coagulation and to assist in tissue repair. The mast cells also release histamine and small quantities of bradykinin and serotonin during inflammation.

Eosinophils

These cells are natural phagocytes. They collect at the site of antigen antibody reaction in the tissues and 'digest' the combined antigen antibody complex after the immune process has performed its function. Eosinophils are involved in the pathogenesis of hypersensitivity (allergic) reactions. Their number is greatly increased in the circulating blood during allergic reactions.

Eosinophils accompanying RA is sometimes associated with extra-articular manifestations (Parrish, Franco and Schur, 1971). Although the pathogenesis is not known, immune complexes may be chemotaxis for eosinophils (e.g. attracted towards the source of the chemical).

Eosinophilia has also been associated with high titre of rheumatoid factor, elevation of serum gammaglobulins and diminished serum complement levels (Matteson, Cohen and Conn, 1994). Pulmonary complications may be associated with eosinophili (Crisp et al., 1982) or it may be associated with drug therapy such as gold.

Lymphocytes

From 20–40% of circulating WBCs are lymphocytes, which are the cells of the acquired immune system although a routine blood count cannot differentiate between them. There are two types – B lymphocytes and T lymphocytes. B lymphocytes produce antibodies and T lymphocytes are responsible for the elimination of viruses and other micro-organisms that infect the cell of the host and are not 'visible' for antibody attack (Higgins, 1996). Both types of lymphocyte function are independent and a normal immune response requires adequate numbers of both B and T lymphocytes.

Causes of Low White Cell Count

A low WBC count is significant because it reduces the body's protection against infection. If the neutrophil count falls below 0.5×10^9 per litre patients are likely to become susceptible to frequently recurring bacterial infections. If levels drop further life is threatened by the risk of overwhelming infection.

Causes of leucopaenia include:

- Felty's syndrome.
- Aplastic anaemia, which is a pancytopenia where reduced production of bone marrow stem cells results in reduced numbers of red cells, white cells and platelets. Aplastic anaemia can be inherited as can pancytopenia although most causes of the latter arise as side effects of cytotoxic drugs.
- Systemic lupus erythematosus.
- Side effect of DMARDs.
- Leukaemia is associated with reduced neutrophil count as bone marrow production of large numbers of abnormal immature white cells continues at the expense of normal white cell production.

- Acquired immune deficiency syndrome (AIDS).
- Hodgkin's disease.

Agranulocytosis

The bone marrow stops producing WBCs, leaving the body unprotected against bacteria and other agents that might invade the tissues. Within two days of production ceasing, ulcers appear in the mouth and colon and severe respiratory infection develops. Bacteria then rapidly invade the surrounding tissues and the blood; without treatment death usually occurs within a week.

Platelets

The number of platelets in each cubic millimetre of blood is normally around 300 000. An increased amount of platelets (thrombocytosis) is a frequent finding in active RA and may well correlate with the number of joints involved, the amount of active synovitis and the presence of extra-articular features. The mechanism of thrombocytosis is uncertain; an increase in the intravascular coagulation with a compensatory increase in platelet production has been suggested (Matteson, Cohen and Conn, 1994). The thrombocytosis does not predispose to an increase in thrombotic events and is not correlated with bone marrow neoplastic changes. A reduced platelet count (thrombocytopenia) is rare in RA except when related to drug treatment or Felty's syndrome.

BIOCHEMICAL INVESTIGATIONS

Hepatic Function

Liver function abnormalities may reflect the anaemia, thrombocytosis and increased erythrocyte sedimentation rate of active inflammatory disease such as RA. Examination of liver histology at this time reveals only minimal non-specific change and some perioportal mononuclear cell infiltration (Matteson, Cohen and Conn, 1994).

Active RA may be associated with an increase in liver enzymes, especially serum glutamic oxaloacetic transaminase (SGOT) and alkaline phosphatase (Fernandes et al., 1979).

Total protein, total albumin and total globulin estimates are also taken. These reflect hepatic function (particularly albumin which is made in the liver) as well as absorption and inflammation. Apart from in lupoid hepatitis, which can mimic RA, bilirubin and SGOT are likely to be normal.

NSAIDs may induce liver enzyme abnormalities and it may be difficult to differentiate between drug effects and disease activity without discontinuation of NSAID therapy. NSAIDs seldom cause serious liver deterioration. Liver involvement may be present in up to 65% of patients with Felty's syndrome (Thorne et al., 1982).

Bone Metabolism

Calcium, phosphate and alkaline phosphatase are all measured. Calcium is bound to protein and this may need a correction factor if protein levels are abnormal as can occur in RA. A slightly raised calcium and raised alkaline phophatase level if of bony origin should alert the clinician to the possibility of osteomalacia. In Paget's disease there is a markedly raised alkaline phosphatase of bony origin. X-ray confirmation of Paget's disease should be sought since secondary cancer in bone can also cause a raised alkaline phosphatase.

Renal Function

Kidney involvement is usually sparse in RA although a low grade nephropathy, glomerulitis vasculitis and secondary amyloidosis have all been described (Matteson, Cohen and Conn, 1994). More commonly renal abnormalities result from agents used in the treatment of RA, notably gold, D-penicillamine, ciclosporin and the NSAIDs (Samuels *et al.*, 1977). The renal involvement caused by nephrotoxic drugs is more likely to be seen first on routine urine testing.

Electrolytes (sodium, potassium, chloride and bicarbonate) together with urea and creatinine are usually measured. The chronic renal failure of connective tissue disorders may produce a raised potassium and a low bicarbonate level. The renal function in a normal population will deteriorate throughout adult life. Urea may be raised because of dehydration but creatinine is less likely to do so under those circumstances. Creatinine is the most sensitive simple estimation of renal damage and a raised level may indicate amyloidosis or chronic renal failure.

Amyloidosis

This may develop in patients with RA as a result of long-standing active inflammation and cause proteinuria. It is not specific to the kidneys and may affect other organs including the heart, liver, spleen, intestines and skin. The diagnosis of amyloidosis is confirmed by biopsy of the involved tissue. Unfortunately the presence of secondary amyloidosis in patients with RA heralds a poor outcome.

ASSESSMENT OF RHEUMATIC DISEASE ACTIVITY

Rheumatoid Factor

This is a commonly requested immunological investigation. Rheumatoid factor (RF) is found in the blood of 75% of patients with RA of more than 12 months duration but in only 40−50% of those with early disease. Therefore the absence of RF does not preclude a diagnosis of RA; indeed the diagnosis of RA is not made on the presence of RF alone but includes a host of other factors. If the RF is absent and the patient has RA the arthritis is said to be sero-negative.

The RF, an IgM/IgG complex of two immunoglobulins, can also be found in other conditions including liver disease, sarcoidosis, subacute bacterial endocarditis and in 4% of healthy adults.

The RF is detected by one or more of the following tests:

- sheep cell agglutination (Rose Waaler) test;
- latex agglutination test.

The Rose Waaler test is given as a titre; below 1:32 is not significant, 1:64 is positive and values above 1:500 usually indicate severe rheumatoid disease.

The Anti-Nuclear Antibody

The ANA is regarded as an initial screening test for systemic lupus erythematosus but is not specific for this condition and if positive the clinician will proceed to request DNA binding from the same patient before confirming a diagnosis of lupus. ANA can occur in other connective tissue disorders such as systemic sclerosis and occasionally in low titre in RA. The ANA titre is important and titres of 1:200 or more in the presence of anti-DNA antibodies are likely to confirm the diagnosis of lupus.

Extractable Nuclear Antigen

The ENA is helpful for the diagnosis of mixed connective tissue disorder (Golding, 1981).

Immunoglobulins

These can provide useful information when the ESR is raised for no obvious reason. In sero-positive RA serum IgM is usually though not always raised representing RF in the blood. Equally there may be a polycolonal increase of all immunoglobulins such as IgA, IgG and IgM.

IgA synthesized in mucous membranes may be raised in Sjögren's syndrome.

Plasma Proteins and Electrophoresis

The alpha 2 globulin is an acute phase reactant which when elevated indicates tissue destruction in the early phases of rheumatic disease. In the later stages a raised gammaglobulin may indicate antibody formation and very high levels can occur in connective tissue diseases, sarcoidosis and myelomatosis (Golding, 1981).

Erythrocyte Sedimentation Rate

The erythrocyte sedimentation rate (ESR) is used as the standard test in many hospitals for evaluating disease activity in rheumatic disease. If inflammation is present in the body the ESR increases. This is due to the changes in the patient's blood. A quantity (2 mls) of anticoagulated blood is sucked into a capillary tube and the speed with which red and white cells settle over a period of one hour is observed. Normal values vary with age and sex. ESR is of value in distinguishing inflammatory polyarthritis from the degenerative conditions.

ESR is elevated in RA, AS, acute gout, PMR, systemic connective tissue disorders, reactive and infective arthritis. A persistently raised ESR should alert the clinician to the possibility of myeloma (a malignant condition of the plasma cells). If suspected, urine should be collected to test for Bence Jones protein, a characteristic protein produced by the cell.

The ESR is not normally elevated in degenerative metabolic joint disease or in soft tissue rheumatism. The Westergren method of establishing the ESR is now universally used. ESRs of up to 20 mm/hr in males and 25 mm/hr in females are accepted as being within normal limits in rheumatological practice (Golding, 1981).

Plasma Viscosity

The plasma viscosity (PV) test mimics ESR evaluation but studies the movement of the plasma in the horizontal rather than the vertical plane. PV eliminates the variation caused by the anaemia of RA which can influence the ESR. High values are found in active RA.

C-Reactive Protein

C-reactive protein (CRP) is an acute inflammatory protein produced by the liver in response to infections, inflammation or acute injury. It rises in active RA falling back to normal levels once the disease has come under control. Changes in the CRP occur faster than in other biochemical assessments. Levels remain normal in systemic lupus erythematosus.

Other Acute Phase Reactants

Fibrinogen, hepatoglobin and caeruloplasmin all behave as acute phase reactants with high levels found in active disease and low values apparent as the conduction comes under control (Golding, 1981).

3.7 URINE TESTING

Urinalysis, the examination of urine, is a valuable tool for the diagnosis of and screening for several conditions. It also plays an important role in the surveillance of drug therapy especially in terms of toxicity. This will be discussed in further depth later on in the chapter. A patient who is asked to supply a specimen of urine for testing requires the following:

- An explanation of the reason for testing.
- Instruction in the method of collecting the specimen.
- The provision of suitable equipment, including a container for the specimen and washing facilities.
- An appropriate environment including wherever possible visual and auditory privacy and adequate time (Cook, 1996).

APPEARANCE

The appearance of the urine should be noted for colour and clarity. Colour changes may be due to endogenous pigments such as haemoglobin (red/brown colour), bilirubin (yellow) or intact red cells (smoky red). Exogenous pigments such as contamination with menstrual blood may also cause colour changes. The administration of sulfasalazine can cause orange discoloration.

Cloudiness is caused by suspended particles which will settle on standing to leave a deposit. Normal urine may contain some renal tubular cells and a few white and red blood cells; these will be prevalent in certain diseases contributing to a cloudy appearance (Cook, 1996).

ODOUR

Normal, freshly voided urine has very little odour but will develop an ammoniacal smell if left for any length of time. Infected urine has a characteristic fishy smell. The urine of patients with anorexia, or a ketoacidosis diabetic person will have a sweet smell. The administration of sulfasalazine and/or D-penicillamine can also cause a characteristic odour.

MEASUREMENT OF SPECIFIC GRAVITY

This can be measured using either reagent strips or a specially calibrated hydrometer. Specific gravity of the urine measures the ability of the kidneys to concentrate or dilute urine. A low specific gravity can occur if a patient has a high intake of fluid or it may indicate renal abnormalities or the presence of diabetes insipidious. A raised specific gravity may indicate dehydration.

Routine testing of urine may detect:

- Glucose. This is not usually found in urine. Its presence may be due to raised blood glucose levels or to reduced renal absorption. It can be associated with conditions such as diabetes mellitus, stress, Cushing's syndrome and acute pancreatitis. Glycosuria occurring in the urine of a patient with rheumatic disease alerts the clinician to the possibility of corticosteroid-induced diabetes mellitus.
- Bilirubin in the urine may be indicative of hepatic or biliary disease. It may also be present if the patient has been prescribed phenothiazides or chlorpromazine leading to a false positive result occurring.

- Ketones. These are not normal constituents of urine; they are the produces of the breakdown of fatty acids. Their presence may indicate starvation, excessive dieting or uncontrolled diabetes (Cook, 1996).
- Blood. Often found to be of no significance but should be investigated if persistent. It may be due to trauma, infection, tumour or stones. Haematuria is an early sign of polyarteritis and 50% of patients with lupus will have small amounts of blood and protein in their urine.
- Protein can indicate a range of conditions including renal disease, urinary tract infection, hypertension, pre-eclampsia or congestive heart failure. Transient positive tests are not always significant, and normal urine contains small amounts of albumin and globulin although not usually at a level that would be detected positively on a reagent strip. When testing for urinary protein a morning specimen of urine is recommended to ensure sufficient concentration (Cook, 1996). Proteinuria may be the first sign of a collagen disease such as polyarteritis. In rheumatoid disease it may indicate urinary infections, nephropathy due to gold or D-penicillamine or be secondary to amyloid diseases. If proteinuria persists a 24-hour urine specimen should be requested; more than 0.15 g protein/24 hours is abnormal. Over 1 g/24 hours is found when there is renal tubular damage and in nephrosis well over 5 g protein/24 hours can occur (Golding, 1981). The presence of albuminuria on routine testing often indicates a simple infection that will require treatment to prevent aggravation of a flare of RA but it may also indicate glomerular dysfunction in conditions such as lupus.
- Urobilinogen. This is normally found in urine but increased levels may indicate liver abnormalities or excessive destruction of red blood cells such as in haemolytic anaemia (Cook, 1996).
- Nitrate. This is not normally present in urine. It is produced when gram-negative bacteria such as *Escherichia coli* convert dietary nitrates (e.g. from the preservative in meat products and cheese and in smoked foods) to nitrites. As *E. coli* is responsible for 80% of urine infections (Talaro and Talaro, 1993), the presence of nitrites is strongly suggestive of urinary tract infection. The specimen for testing should have been in the bladder for at least four hours before voiding to allow sufficient time for the nitrate/nitrite conversion.
- Leucocytes. The presence of leucocytes in the urine is an indication of bladder or renal infection but follow-up testing such as urine culture is required. White blood cells should be sought in the urine when infections such as Reiter's disease are suspected. Early morning specimens are more likely to contain tubercule bacilli than those taken later in the day if the condition is suspected.

RECORD KEEPING

The results of the urinalysis should be recorded in the patient's records as soon as possible after testing. It is worth noting that a negative result on a particular date may acquire significance in retrospect so all results should be recorded in patient's records at the time of testing (Cook, 1996).

3.8 DRUGS THAT REQUIRE SURVEILLANCE

GOLD (MYOCRISIN) THERAPY

Treatment Regime

Gold is used as long-term treatment for inflammatory joint disease (most commonly RA). Initially most patients are given a test dose of 10 mg intramuscularly (IM) and if no adverse effects are experienced progress to 50 mg IM weekly reducing to 50 mg fortnightly as the patient responds, normally around six months. With adequate control, frequency is reduced to monthly (around 12 months) and continued indefinitely until side effects occur. It may take three to six months for patients to respond to treatment with gold. There are vast variations in the implementation of gold therapy. Kay and Puller (1992) found that out of a survey of 100 rheumatologists 89% used a test dose of intramuscular gold but of those who gave a test dose 64% gave a single 10 mg dose, 9% gave 10 mg followed by 20 mg, 4.5% gave 5 mg followed by 10 mg and the remaining rheumatologists gave various slowly increasing incremental doses. Toxicity with injectable gold is common occurring in 30–40% of patients (Day, 1994).

Caution

Elderly, renal or hepatic impairment, urticaria, eczema or inflammatory bowel disease.

Contraindications

- Severe renal or hepatic impairment
- Blood disorders
- Systemic lupus erythematosus
- Significant pulmonary fibrosis
- Porphyria
- Pregnancy and lactation.

Nephrotoxicity. It is the responsibility of the nurse administering the intramuscular injection of gold to test the urine prior to giving the injection. Minor transient proteinuria is common whilst on this therapy. A meta-analysis of clinical trials showed significant proteinuria in patients receiving gold (Day, 1994). A trace of proteinuria can be ignored but increasing proteinuria is an indication to stop gold. Treatment should be discontinued if 24-hour protein urinalysis exceeds over 1 g. Recovery is usual when gold is stopped.

Minor renal effects in the absence of proteinuria has been noted with the elevation of enzymes and tubular cell secretion, but this increased turnover of tubular cells has not been related to decreased tubular function later in life (Ganley, Paget and Reidenberg, 1989). Isolated microscopic haematuria is not usually attributed to gold (Leonard et al., 1987).

Skin Reactions

Dermatitis and oral reactions account for 60–80% of all reactions to injectable gold complexes (Champion, Graham and Zeigler, 1990). Oral mucosal lesions occur less often than rashes. Minor ulcers can be treated symptomatically. Check that ill-fitting dentures are not causing friction. Most rashes are usually erythematous and macular but rarely can exfoliate; 85% of rashes are severely pruritic.

Raised eosinophils may be the forerunner to a rash, and the rash may be associated with a metallic taste and organ toxicity such as proteinuria (Champion, Graham and Zeigler, 1990).

Minor rashes and/or pruritis can be treated symptomatically with aqueous cream or 0.5% hydrocortisone cream.

The nurse will also want to establish that the cause of the rash is related to drug therapy so that the treatment is not discontinued unnecessarily. The nurse will check that the patient has not recently changed their soap, washing powder or commenced new drug therapy. In some units close cooperation with the dermatologist can establish the cause of the rash and/or irritation and thus may provide valuable information in planning long-term care.

Gold should be withheld if there is a widespread pruritis, severe or rapidly progressive rash and/or mouths ulcers/stomatitis as these can be associated with exfoliative dermatitis.

Once moderate rashes and/or pruritis has settled it may be possible to reintroduce gold at a smaller dose.

Haematological Disorders

Neutropenia

It is important to consider whether a decrease in WBCs is due to the disease or related condition (e.g. Felty's syndrome) or to the gold treatment. Careful attention needs to be paid to a rapid and/or progressive downward trend in neutrophils accompanied by a fall in platelets as this is often caused by bone marrow suppression as a direct result of gold treatment. (You can also get neutropenia related to gold without an accompanying fall of other blood cells). Increasing neutropenia will require increased surveillance, possible dosage reduction or cessation of gold.

Eosinophilia

This will occur in up to 50% of patients receiving gold at some stage of their treatment and although it does not generally correlate highly with toxicity it should not be dismissed as in some cases it may herald a toxic reaction to treatment (Elderman, Davis and Owen, 1983).

Thrombocytopenia

This occurs in 1–3% of patients receiving intramuscular gold. It is usually minor but can be serious (Day, 1994). It usually responds well to corticosteroids.

Aplastic Anaemia

This is rare but has a high mortality rate, although the rate for survival is improving (Yan and Davies, 1990).

Inflammation Lung Reactions

Hypersensitivity pneumoconitis, distinguishable from rheumatoid lung by its acute or subacute onset, can occur and will necessitate cessation of gold. Obliterative bronchiolitis has been reported in patients with RA (Penny *et al.*, 1982) but it remains unclear whether this is a result of gold therapy or the condition itself.

Pulmonary Involvement in Patients with RA

Pulmonary involvement in patients with RA is fairly common although the clinical features may be subtle (Matteson, Cohen and Conn, 1994). Pleurisy and pleural effusions may improve spontaneously or require treatment. The occurrence of persistent pleural effusions will lead to fibrosis.

Sero-positive RA patients may develop parenchymal pulmonary nodules which, although usually asymptomatic can cause pleural effusions.

Caplan's syndrome (pneumoconiosis) is characterized by large multiple pulmonary nodules and is seen in individuals who have experienced prolonged exposure to coal dust.

Isolated pulmonary arteritis is a rare complication of RA and is frequently associated with interstitial fibrosis and nodulosis (Gardener *et al.*, 1957).

Neurotoxicity due to Gold

Neurotoxic reactions are uncommon but the following diverse reactions have been noted, including peripheral neuropathy, Guillan Barré syndrome, cranial nerve palsies and encephalopathy.

Vasomotor Reactions

These are often referred to as 'nitroid' reactions and may occur within minutes of administration of the gold injection and necessitate that the patient remains in clinic for a period of time following the injection. Reactions are characterized by weakness, dizziness, nausea, sweating, facial flushing, erythema and hypotension.

Post-Injection Reactions

Apart from the possibility of vasomotor reactions the patient may also experience transient polyarthralgia, myalgia, joint swelling, fatigue and malaise. It can be difficult at times to distinguish these effects from the symptoms of active inflammatory disease.

Incidence Rate of Side Effects

A meta-analysis of clinical trials (Clarke *et al.*, 1989) found that 11% of all patients had to discontinue gold due to side effects experienced. The majority of side effects occur within the first 12 months of treatment and are not related to cumulative dose (Sambrook *et al.*, 1982). Lockie and Smith (1988) published their experience with gold therapy in 1019 patients; the main reasons for discontinuation of gold was skin reactions (36%) and buccal irritation in 13% of patients.

Gold should be stopped if:

- Total white cell count is $<3.5 \times 10^9$ L or neutrophils $<2 \times 10^9$ L
- Platelets $<150 \times 10^9$ L
- Eosinophilia $>0.5 \times 10/L$
- Proteinuria > 1 g/24 hours
- There is a severe or progressive rash.

The majority of adverse reactions to gold resolve spontaneously within weeks to months following cessation of treatment.

AURANOFIN (RIDULA) THERAPY IN RA

Treatment Regime

Auranofin is used in the long-term treatment of RA. The usual dose is 3 mg twice daily. The absorption of gold from auranofin following a single dose is about 20–25% and there is less retention of gold in tissues than occurs with injectable gold. Nevertheless regular blood monitoring is required.

Caution

Elderly, renal or hepatic impairment (moderate) history of urticaria, eczema or inflammatory bowel disease.

Contraindications

- Severe renal or hepatic impairment.
- History of blood disorders.
- Significant pulmonary fibrosis and porphyria.
- Systemic lupus erthematosus.
- Pregnancy and lactation.

Adverse Effects

- Skin
  Rashes. Minor rashes can be treated symptomatically (aqueous cream, 0.5% hydrocortisone cream).
- Mouth ulcers
  Minor ulcers can be treated with Bonjela, Difflam mouth wash or Adcortyl in orabase.
- Gastrointestinal
  Diarrhoea is often the commonest side effect and may respond to the introduction of bulking agents such as bran or to a temporary reduction in dosage. Some patients experience nausea and vomiting and it is recommended that this therapy is taken with food.
- Renal
  Proteinuria
- Haematological
  The nurse must observe for any reductions in neutrophils and platelets.
- Miscellaneous
  Rarely colitis, peripheral neuritis, pulmonary fibrosis, hepatotoxicity with cholestatic jaundice and alopecia have all been reported.

  Auranofin should be stopped if:

- Total white cell count is $<3.5 \times 10^9$ L
- Platelets $<150 \times 10^9$ L
- Proteinuria >1 g/24 hours
- Severe rashes or severe mouth ulcers occur.

D-PENICILLAMINE (DISTAMINE)

Treatment Regime

D-penicillamine is used in the long-term treatment of rheumatoid arthritis and in scleroderma. Treatment is commenced at 125 mg or at 250 mg daily, increasing at four-week intervals by increments of 125 mg daily to 500 mg or 750 mg. The tablets are best taken as a single daily dose an hour before breakfast and not with iron tablets or milk as they interfere with drug absorption. Toxicity is common with this treatment with about 50% of patients with RA experiencing an adverse effect within the first six months of treatment at 600 mg daily resulting in 25% of patient discontinuing with this treatment. The incidence of toxicity increases as the dose increases (Kay, 1986).

Caution

Renal impairment, concomitant nephrotoxic dugs including gold treatment.

Contraindications

- Systemic lupus erythematosus
- Renal impairment
- Pregnancy and lactation.

Drug Interactions

- Antacids and iron: do not take within two hours as this reduces the absorption of D-penicillamine.
- Antipsychotic drugs: may increase agranulocytosis.
- Digoxin: Levels of digoxin can be reduced by concurrent use of D-penicillamine.
- Zinc supplements may reduce the absorption of D-penicillamine.

Skin Reactions

Urticarial, pruritic, macular and papular eruptions of apparent allergic origin account for the majority of skin reactions (Kay, 1986). Minor rashes can be treated symptomatically but severe rashes may necessitate stopping D-penicillamine and this will normally resolve the rash. Autoimmune bilious skin eruptions, typical of the pemphigus group, are the most worrying. Patients who have a penicillin allergy are at greater risk of experiencing a skin reaction. Oral ulcers and stomatitis may occur; if severe this will mean a discontinuation of therapy. Oral mucosal involvement is often present in pemphigus. There is a significant level of mortality amongst patients with D-penicillamine-induced pemphigus (Joyce, 1990).

A metallic taste and loss of taste may occur in the first eight weeks of treatment. It may take several months to recover. This can be a particularly distressing symptom for patients and advice may need to be given on food supplementation (Ryan, 1995). Taste disturbance may be a consequence of zinc chelation by the D-penicillamine but zinc therapy does not remove the complaint (Joyce, 1990).

Nausea and Anorexia

If these symptoms occur the patient may need to reduce the dose of D-penicillamine and then increase slowly when the symptoms settle. The use of anti-emetics should also be considered.

Haematological

There can be a gradual or rapid haematological effects at any stage during treatment with D-penicillamine. Thromobocytopenia can be precipitated and serious.

Neutropenia due to D-penicillamine as opposed to RA itself is suggested by a rapid or progressive fall in neutrophils and is the commonest cause of death attributed to this treatment (Kay, 1979). Aplastic anaemia also has a high fatality rate.

Renal

Proteinuria is common. Increased urinary protein excretion can exceed 0.5 g/day in approximately 9% of patients taking this drug (Stein, Schroder and Dillion, 1986). The presence of HLA B8 and DR 4 antigens coupled with the occurrence of previous proteinuria on gold therapy increases the risk of more severe proteinuria leading to nephrotic syndrome (Joyce, 1990).

The majority of patients experiencing severe proteinuria have membranous glomerulonephritis with minimal change neuropathy (Hall *et al.*, 1988). Plasma urea and creatinine may rise intermittently but this does not seem to be related to permanent renal impairment (Hall *et al.*, 1988).

D-penicillamine should be stopped if over 1 gram of proteinuria occurs in a 24-hour period. Even after the drug has been discontinued the proteinuria may persist for up to 21 months.

The appearance of haematuria may indicate rapidly progressive glomerulonephritis — for example, Goodpasture's syndrome or SLE and can be life-threatening requiring steroids and immunosuppressives. However, the presence of haematuria usually does not lead to serious complication and recurrent haematuria is quite common in RA patients without serious renal pathology (Leonard *et al.*, 1987).

Pulmonary

There have been cases of bronchiolitis obliterans reported (Day, 1994). Although this is a rare side effect it may be irreversible and present as dyspnoea late in therapy (Kay, 1986).

Autoimmune

Myasthenia gravis. This rare complication may evolve after years of uneventful therapy and may take over a year to resolve (Kay, 1986).

Auto-antibodies may appear including anti-striated muscle antibody, anti-centromere antibody and anti-glomerular basement membrane antibody. The latter is associated with the life-threatening complication of Goodpasture's syndrome.

Dermatomyositis/Polymyositis

Drug-induced SLE usually resolves after stopping D-penicillamine. Pemphigus (oral involvement common) is dangerous and requires cessation of D-penicillamine, glucocorticosteroids and perhaps plasmapheresis.

D-penicillamine should be stopped if the following occur:

- Severe rash.
- Severe mouth ulcers.
- Autoimmune side effect.
- Platelets $<150 \times 10^9 L$
- Total white cell count $<3.5 \times 10^9$ L
- Neutrophils $<2 \times 10^9$ L
- Proteinuria > 1 gm/24 hours.

SULFASALAZINE EN THERAPY (SALAZOPYRIN)

Sulfasalazine is used in its enteric coated form (EN) as second line treatment for RA, spondyloarthropathies and reactive arthritis. To reduce nausea the drug should be commenced at 500 mg daily increasing by 500 mg daily at weekly intervals to the usual maintenance dose of 1 g twice daily. Incomplete responders sometimes require 1 g three times a day. It may take three to six months for a patient to respond to treatment with sulfasalazine. This preparation ranks with the antimalarials and auranofin as the best tolerated of the DMARDs and is a popular first choice of DMARDs amongst rheumatologists (Kay and Puller, 1992).

Caution

- Moderate renal impairment.
- May impair folate absorption.
- Pregnancy and breastfeeding.

Contraindications

- Hypersensitivity; sulfonamide/co-trimoxazole.

Adverse Effects

These are commonest in the first three months of therapy. Only 20–25% of patients need to stop treatment because of toxicity (Amos *et al.*, 1986) and only about 5% of patients will experience potentially serious side effects (Farr, Scott and Bacon, 1986).

Commonest adverse effects are gastrointestinal and on the central nervous system. They include nausea, vomiting, malaise, anorexia, abdominal pain, dyspepsia, indigestion, headache, light-headedness and dizziness. If a patient experiences nausea the dose should be reduced to the previously tolerated dose and further increase should be attempted slowly. Make sure the patient is taking enteric coated tablets and administrating them on a full stomach. Anti-emetics may be required. With headaches again the dose should be initially reduced and further increases attempted slowly. If headaches are severe the patient may need to discontinue sulfasalazine.

Pyrexia is a rare side effect and can be considered only when other causes of raised temperature have been excluded.

Hypersensitivity

This is relatively common and may manifest itself in a number of ways ranging from skin rash to fatal multi-organ involvement.

Skin

Rashes. If these are mild, treatment can be continued and the rash can be treated symptomatically. Skin rashes will occur within 5% of cases and take the form of a generalized pruritic maculopapular rash, urticaria or photosensitivity (Amos et al., 1986). If the rash occurs within the first two weeks of treatment then desensitization can be tried. Initially given in 1 mg doses sulfasalazine is built up over 25–56 days. Successful desensitization has been achieved in as many as 85% of cases in RA patients (Bax and Amos, 1986). Rarely severe reactions such as Stevens–Johnson syndrome or exfoliative dermatitis can occur. In the case of this happening all drugs should be stopped and urgent dermatological advice should be obtained. Rarely serum sickness occurs.

Pulmonary

Most toxicity is allergic in origin from sulfasalazine. The commonest presentation is eosinophilic pneumonitis; symptoms include dyspnoea with fever, rash, weight loss, pulmonary infiltration on X-ray and reduced pulmonary function tests. Reduction of symptoms occurs following cessation of therapy (Tydd and Dyer, 1976).

Haematological

Leucopenia in 1–5% of cases: It is most likely to occur in the first six months of treatment although it can occur at any time. It is the commonest potential serious side effect associated with sulfasalazine. It indicates the need for continued review particularly as early recognition with dosage reduction or cessation leads to reversal in most cases.

Thrombocytopenia is less frequent than leucopenia.

Agranulocytosis is rare but can develop rapidly and present with intercurrent infection. It has been recorded in association with a transient but marked plasmocytosis.

Mean cell volume (MCV): Sulfasalazine causes the erythrocyte MCV to rise. It inhibits folate uptake in the small bowel; however it would be rare to see folate deficiency at a dose of 2 g daily.

Abnormalities of red cell morphology: Morphological changes are due to oxidant damage resulting in red cell membrane abnormalities leading to low grade haemolysis (Pounder et al., 1973). The changes are reversible on discontinuation of therapy but this action would only be necessary if the haemolysis was causing a problem. Significant methaemoglobin can cause headaches and may require a dosage reduction.

Hepatoxicity

Allergic hepatic responses to sulfonamides are well known; raised hepatic enzyme levels and eosinophilia may cause fever rash and hepatomegaly (Amos *et al.*, 1986).

Granulomatosus hepatitis may occur necessitating discontinuation of therapy. Minor rises in hepatic enzyme levels during treatment occur in about 3% of cases but do not seem to be productive of severe hepatic reactions and treatment may continue (Puller, Hunter and Capell, 1987).

Reversible oligospermia. About 70% of men develop oligospermia and abnormal sperm motility (Birnie, Mcleod and Watkinson, 1981). Therefore this drug should be avoided in men wishing to have a family. This temporary reduction in fertility is reversible on stopping sulfasalazine treatment.

Miscellaneous. Sulfasalazine can cause orange staining of soft contact lenses. The urine can become bright orange. Rarely drug-induced lupus.

Sulfasalazine should be stopped if the following occur:

- Severe rashes.
- Severe headaches.
- Deteriorating liver function.
- Platelets $<150 \times 10^9$ L.
- Total white cell count $<3.5 \times 10^9$ L.
- Neutrophils $<2 \times 10^9$ L.

METHOTREXATE

Treatment Regime

Methotrexate is an antimetabolite cytotoxic agent used in RA, psoriatic arthritis, myositis and vasculitis. It is given either orally, subcutaneously, intramuscularly or intravenously. Weekly doses are usually between 5 mg and 25 mg. Rarely the maximum dose can be 30 mg per week. The initial dose will vary depending on the severity of the condition and patient characteristics such as age, renal function and co-morbid conditions. It is preferable to use only one strength (2.5 mg) of tablets and patients should be reminded of the need to check the dose and strength of the tablets with each prescription. It is co-prescribed with folic acid, which may reduce the likelihood of side effects. Clinical effect is usually evident after two to three months but doses may need to be increased to maintain this effect. A chest X-ray is taken prior to starting treatment as pre-existing lung disease requires special attention. Any patient suspected of alcohol abuse is usually unsuitable for methotrexate therapy. Patients should be advised to limit their alcohol intake to well within national limits.

Cautions

Patients with clinically significant renal impairment.

Contraindications

- Pregnancy and breastfeeding.
- Suspected local or systemic infection.

Drug Interactions

- Phenytoin, co-trimoxozole, trimethorpim-antifolate effect of methotrexate is increased.
- Probenecid, penicillin, azapropazone, NSAIDs-methotrexate excretion is reduced. Clinically significant interaction between NSAID and methotrexate is rare. All patients should be advised to avoid over-the-counter medications including aspirin and ibuprofen without the knowledge of the rheumatology team.

Adverse Effects

Gastrointestinal

These are the most common side effects which include anorexia, nausea, dyspepsia, vomiting, diarrhoea and abdominal pain. It is recommended that the therapy is taken with food. Anti-emetics may be required on the day of methotrexate administration and the following 24−48 hours. If nausea and vomiting are problematic and doubts exist about absorption, methotrexate can be given intramuscularly.

Mouth Ulcers

Mouth soreness can present with or without ulceration (Kremer and Joong, 1986). The use of folic acid to minimize stomatitis has been recommended (Segal, Yaron and Tartakowsky, 1990). Minor ulcers can be treated symptomatically whilst major mouth ulcers may necessitate dose reduction or discontinuation.

Rashes

Minor rashes can be treated symptomatically whereas severe rashes may necessitate discontinuation of methotrexate.

Haematological

Leucopenia is the most common bone marrow toxicity from methotrexate (Kremer and Joong, 1986). This is usually managed by reducing the dosage of methotrexate. Anaemia and thrombocytopenia can also occur. Macrocytosis is a sign of toxicity and may precede bone marrow suppression. Pancytopenia is a rare but potentially fatal complication of methotrexate, which may develop suddenly and without warning signs (Lim, Gaffney and Scott, 2005). It can occur early within one to two months of commencing methotrexate possibly reflecting an idiosyncratic reaction (Lim, Gaffney and Scott, 2005) and more commonly later on in the patient's experience reflecting a cumulative effect (Lim, Gaffney and Scott, 2005).

Hepatoxicity

Hepatoxicity defined as elevation of transaminase occurs within 69–89% of patients (Williams *et al.*, 1985). These increases do not usually correlate with the development of cirrhosis. Liver fibrosis and cirrhosis can occur with normal liver enzymes and imaging findings. Current studies in patients with RA suggest that liver biopsies are not cost-effective for at least the first 10 years of methotrexate use in patients with normal liver function (Jones and Patel, 2001).

Hypersensitivity Reactions and Pneumonitis

Hypersensitivity reactions include rashes, fever and pneumonitis (Cannon *et al.*, 1983). Methotrexate pneumonitis occurs in 1–6% of cases (Fuhrman *et al.*, 2001). It is a potentially fatal hypersensitivity reaction most frequently seen within the first year of treatment (Kinder and Hassell, 2005). Many studies suggest that the incidence of pneumonitis is much higher in patients with pre-existing lung disease (Alarcon *et al.*, 1997; Saravanan and Kelly, 2004). Pulmonary function tests may be a useful investigation to detect pre-existing lung disease as methotrexate pneumonitis tends to occur in 48% of patients with pre-existing lung problems (Grove and Hassell, 2001). If pre-treatment X-ray suggests abnormal shadowing it may be worth considering a high resolution computerized scan and pulmonary function tests. Airway obstruction may not be a contraindication to the use of methotrexate but the presence of interstitial lung disease is.

Renal

Acute renal decompensation and renal failure have been reported although rarely, and appear related to high dose therapy with concomitant NSAIDs with underlying renal disease (Thierry *et al.*, 1989).

Infections

Methotrexate should be stopped immediately if infection is suspected. Significant mortality and morbidity can be associated with viral infections due to herpes zoster/varicella. Patients with a history of contacts with such viral infections need special advice and the consideration of treatment with anti-herpes zoster immunoglobulin.

Folate Supplementation

Folic acid has been shown to reduce the likelihood of derangements of liver function tests (Vn Ede, Laan and Rood, 2001) as well as mucosal and gastrointestinal side effects (Ortiz *et al.*, 2000). No consensus exists amongst specialists as to the optimal dose and timing of folate supplementation (Lim, Gaffney and Scott, 2005) and no studies have proven an unequivalent protective effect of folate supplementation on methotrexate-related haematological toxicity (Lim, Gaffney and Scott, 2005).

Folinic Acid Rescue

In suspected cases of methotrexate overdose or severe haematological toxicity, folinic acid can be given. The initial dose should be at least 20 mg given intra-venously. Subsequent doses of 15 mg orally should be given at six-hourly intervals until the haematological abnormalities are improved.

Surgical Intervention

Research suggests that continuation of methotrexate treatment does not increase the risk of infection or surgical complications in patients with RA (Bridges *et al.*, 1991; Grennan *et al.*, 2001).

Methotrexate should be stopped if the following occur:

- Major mouth ulcers.
- Severe skin rashes.
- Infection is suspected or present.
- Severe sore throat.
- Abnormal bruising.
- Acute pneumonitis.
- Deteriorating liver function – that is, AST, ALT greater than twofold rise.
- MCV .105fl -check serum B12, Folate and TFT.
- Platelets $<150 \times 10^9$ L.
- Total white blood cell count $<3.5 \times 10^9$ L.
- Neutrophils $<2 \times 10^9$ L.

AZATHIOPRINE (IMURAN) THERAPY

Treatment Regime

Azathioprine is an immunosuppressant antimetabolite used in RA, psoriatic arthritis and in vasculitis. It is widely used to suppress transplant rejection. It is given orally in daily doses of up to 3 mg/kg. It can be used in combination with corticosteroids as a 'steroid sparing agent'. It may take three to six months for patients to respond to treatment.

Cautions

- Thiopurine methyl transferase deficiency.
- Older people with renal impairment.
- Localized or systemic infections with hepatitis B and C or a history of TB.

Contraindications

- TPMT deficiency − can be fatal.
- Aminosalicylates − for example, sulfasalazine contributes to bone marrow toxicity.
- Co-trimoxazole and trimethoprim can cause life-threatening haematoxicity (Norgard *et al.*, 2001).
- Pregnancy and breastfeeding.

Adverse Effects

Gastrointestinal

This includes nausea and vomiting; patients may have to reduce the dose and then increase again when symptoms settle. Anti-emetics may be required. It is advisable to take azathioprine on a full stomach.

Mouth Ulcers

Minor ulcers can be treated symptomatically whilst severe ulceration may necessitate stopping azathioprine.

Hepatoxicity

This is rare but if occurs may be severe and require dose reduction or withdrawal.

Haematological

The most important side effect is reversible marrow suppression (Luqmani, Palmer and Bacon, 1990). Macrocytosis is common but is not a sign of toxicity.

Lymphoma

Long-term effects may include the induction of lymphoid tumours (Rosman and Bertino, 1973). In RA the azathioprine-related risk of lymphoma and non-Hodgkin's lymphoma is confounded by an increased relative risk secondary to RA. Overall there appears to be a small added risk of developing malignancy when using azathioprine in RA (Frust and Clements, 1994).

Miscellaneous

Hypersensitive reactions occur early in treatment and may include headaches, confusion and aseptic meningitis.

Drug Interactions

Allopurinol can increase the myelosuppression of azathioprine. Allopurinol can inhibit the anticoagulant effects of warfarin. Azathioprine can reduce the absorption of some antiepileptic drugs.

Azathioprine should be stopped if the following occur:

- Platelets $<150 \times 10^9$ L.
- White cell count $<3.5 \times 10^9$ L.
- Neutrophils $<2 \times 10^9$ L.
- Deteriorating liver function > twofold rise in AST, ALT.
- MCV >105 − check serum folate, vitamin B12 and TSH.
- Abnormal bruising or severe sore throat.

CYCLOPHOSPHAMIDE (ENDOXANA) THERAPY

Treatment Regime

Cyclophosphamide is a cytotoxic alkylating agent used for immunosuppression in SLE, vasculitis, resistant rheumatic arthritis, polyarteritis nodosa, Wegener's granulomatosis, myositis and as a steroid sparing agent. A daily oral dose of 1−2 mg/kg body weight is used, it may be given as pulsed intravenous or oral therapy. Cyclophosphamide reaches its peak of effectiveness after approximately 16 weeks and although remission may be maintained for several years on withdrawal of the drug the majority of patients will experience some recurrence of symptoms. Nonarticular complications of RA such as interstitial lung disease, cutaneous ulcers and peripheral neuropathy may respond well to oral cyclophosphamide. Cyclophosphamide should be used with care in patients with diabetes as it may induce hyper- or hypoglycaemia.

Pre-treatment check:

- Avoid if possible in men and women of childbearing age. Otherwise offer gamete storage and ensure adequate contraception.
- Carry out a full infection screen including chest, urine testing and culture, joint examination, sinuses and perineum.
- Some rheumatology units advise patients on this therapy to minimize or stop alcohol consumption.
- Pre-treatment investigations include chest X-ray and a full blood count, including differential white count and platelets, electrolytes and liver function tests.

Adverse Effects

Mouth Ulcers

Minor ulcers can be treated symptomatically. Severe ulcers may necessitate stopping cyclophosphamide.

Nausea and Vomiting

If gastrointestinal intolerance occurs the patient may require anti-emetic therapy. It is advisable to take this treatment with food.

Alopecia

This is usually mild in dosages less than 100 mg daily.

Infections

Suppression of the immune system exposes patients to the risk of infections. This can be minor — for example, herpes zoster — or major — for example, septicaemia. There is also the increased risk of patients experiencing opportunistic infections.

Haemorrhagic Cystitis

Bladder toxicity is due mainly to the effects of acrolein on the urinary metabolite of cyclophosphamide. As well as causing haemorrhagic cystitis and bladder fibrosis it has been associated with bladder carcinoma. Therefore the occurrence of haemorrhagic cystitis is an indication for cessation of therapy. Haemorrhagic cystitis has been reported in about a third of subjects receiving oral cyclophosphamide daily (Baker *et al.*, 1987). It is rare in patients receiving intermittent high dose intravenous cyclophosphamide therapy (Bacon, 1987), where it is often co-prescribed with Mesna which reacts specifically with the metabolite acrolein preventing urothelial toxicity. Patients should be advised to take at least 3 litres of fluid per day whilst taking cyclophosphamide therapy.

Malignancy

Kinlen *et al.* (1979) reports a relative risk of 12.8 for all cancers combined and a tenfold increase in bladder cancer for patients receiving at least three months of treatment with cyclophosphamide. There appears to be a relationship of total dose and duration of therapy with the incidence of malignancy (Baker *et al.*, 1987). There is also an increased risk of leukaemia (Adamson and Seiber, 1981).

Fertility

The risk of infertility, azoosperma and amenorrhoea with cyclophosphamide increases with higher dosages, longer duration of therapy and increased age in women (Schilsky *et al.*, 1980). Infertility is not always reversible.

Pulmonary Fibrosis

This can occur with therapy.

Haematological

Abnormalities are detected by blood monitoring. Maximum effect on the marrow dose not occur until 5−10 days after dosage. Recovery is seen within 10−14 days. Macrocytosis is not inevitable but is a sign of toxicity and dosage reduction may be necessary.

Drug Interactions

Allopurinol can increase the myelosuppression of cyclophosphamide.
Cyclophosphamide should be stopped if the following occur:

- Severe mouth ulcers.
- Platelets $<150 \times 10^9$ L.
- Total white cell count $<3.5 \times 10^9$ L.
- Neutrophil $<2 \times 10^9$ L.
- Macroscopic haematuria or persistent confirmed macroscopic haematuria (infection excluded).

CICLOSPORIN

Treatment Regime

Ciclosporin A is a fungal metabolite of *Trichoderma polysporum* and *Ciclocarpon leucidium*. Studies have confirmed potent effects of this drug in several arthritic and other cell-mediated chronic inflammatory conditions (Cannon *et al.*, 1990). It may be instituted at doses of 2.5 mg/kg/day given in 2 divided doses every 12 hours. The dose may be cautiously increased 25−50% every 2−4 weeks until a maximum of 4 mg/kg/day is reached assuming there are no adverse reactions. Ciclosporin is used in the treatment of RA and Behçet's disease. Clinical improvements in patients receiving ciclosporin are associated with a reduction in C-reactive protein, d-1-acidglycoprotein and platelet counts but not rheumatoid factor or the ESR (Dougados, Awada and Amor, 1988). When ciclosporin is used in the treatment of rheumatic disease side effects are generally mild and reversible at low doses (Frust and Clements, 1994).

Cautions

- Uncontrolled hypertension.
- Use of potassium sparing diuretics.
- Pregnancy and lactation.
- Grapefruit juice to be avoided for one hour after administration.
- Malignancy such as lymphomas.

Contraindications

- Uncontrolled hypertension.
- Renal and liver failure.
- Severe electrolyte imbalance.
- Suspected systemic infection.

Adverse Effects

Minor reactions – can include nausea and vomiting, tinnitus, tremor, paraesthesia and gum hyperplasia.

Major reactions – Nephroxicity. Ciclosporin should be avoided in patients with pre-existing renal disease. Increases in serum creatinine are common during ciclosporin immunosuppression. Ciclosporin therapy in doses of 10 mg/kg/day for even two months may lead to an irreversible loss of more than 10% of renal function in RA patients. Nephrotoxicity is dose-related (Berg *et al.*, 1989). Long-term influences on renal function are significant even after cessation of the drug especially in view of the potential for apparent persistent impairment of creatinine clearance. A study by Tugwell *et al.* (1990) showed that although serum creatinine rose and creatinine clearance decreased over the period of ciclosporin administration the effects stabilized after four months with no further changes. After discontinuation of therapy serum creatinine fell to within 15% of baseline in all except two patients. Dosage reductions of 25–50% are required if serum creatinine increases above baseline by 30–50% or if hypertension cannot be controlled.

Hypertension

Hypertension has always been a factor predisposing to nephrotoxicity in RA (Shiroky *et al.*, 1989). New onset hypertension has been reported in about one third of RA and psoriatic patients. Hypertension should be managed with beta blockers and ACE inhibitors; potassium sparing diuretics should be avoided because ciclosporin may cause hyperkalemia (Kowal, Carstens and Schinitzer, 1990). If hypertension is present prior to commencing ciclosporin the hypertension should be treated first before ciclosporin is introduced.

Hepatoxicity

This can occur with higher dosages of ciclosporin and present with elevated hepatic enzymes and bilirubin.

Drug Interactions

Diltiazem, ketoconazole, rifampicin and phenytoin may all require adjustment of ciclosporin dose.

St John's Wort decreases ciclosporin activity. Colchicine should be avoided and the dose of diclofenac reduced by 50%.

Ciclosporin should be discontinued if the following occur:

- Elevation of serum creatinine >30% from baseline on two consecutive occasions.
- Potassium rises to above the normal range.
- Raised blood pressure — diastolic 95mm Hg on two consecutive occasions.
- Ciclosporin levels are >300 mg/ml.
- Elevated hepatic enzymes — > twofold increase in AST or ALT or alkaline phosphatase from the upper limit of the normal range.
- Platelets <150.
- Abnormal bruising.

CHLORAMBUCIL

Treatment Regime

Chlorambucil like cyclophosphamide is a bifunctional alkylating agent. It is not a cytotoxic but is metabolized to phenylacetic acid — its principal and most active metabolite. It is given in an oral preparation. The intravenous preparation is unstable because of rapid hydrolysis. Chlorambucil can be commenced in doses of 0.1−0.2 mg/kg/day. Once response or toxicity has occurred it is suggested that a dose of 3−4 mg daily is adopted.

Chlorambucil has been used in patients with RA, vasculitis and connective tissue disorders, inflammatory eye disease and amyloidosis.

Adverse Effects

The advantages of chlorambucil therapy have to be balanced against the risk of inducing adverse effects. The most common toxicities with chlorambucil use are dose-related bone marrow suppression and infertility.

Bone Marrow Suppression

Cumulative bone marrow toxicity occurs regularly and often requires discontinuation of the drug.

Neoplasms

Kahn *et al.* (1979) reported that leukaemias occurred in patients with RA who had received a total dose of at least 1 g of chlorambucil and who had been treated for at least six months. Luqmani, Palmer and Bacon's (1990) review of the literature on patients receiving chlorambucil indicated that tumours occurred in less than 1% of patients. The majority of the malignancies were leukaemias with a particularly high incidence of acute myeloid leukaemia. It is not possible to exclude the part that the disease process itself plays in the likelihood of malignancies and Palmer and Denman (1984) found that patients with connective tissue disorders were more sensitive to the leukaemiogenic effects of chlorambucil than patients with other non-malignant conditions.

Infertility

The risks of infertility, azoospermia and amenorrhoea increase with duration of therapy and high doses. Infertility affects men at a greater rate than women; irreversible azoospermia was regularly reported in men who received greater than 400 mg of chlorambucil. In post-pubertal females both gametogenesis and hormonal function are altered adversely and menopause occurs.

PHENYLBUTAZONE (BUTACOTE)

Treatment Regime

Phenylbutazone is not longer recommended or indeed available in many countries for the treatment of arthritis conditions due to the risk of marrow aplasia. Although it is still used in the United Kingdom, it is available only on hospital prescription for patients with ankylosing spondylitis and other spondyloarthropathies. Phenylbutazone is a NSAID but it may also affect the immune response (Furst, 1988). It is usually prescribed in dosages of 100−200 mg, two to three times a day. It should help with pain and swelling within a week but will take months before an immune response can be assessed.

Adverse Effects

Gastrointestinal

Nausea and vomiting.

Mucocutaneous

Skin rashes, mouth ulcers, stomatitis.

Central Nervous System

Headaches, dizziness and blurred vision.

Pulmonary Toxicity

Care must be taken when prescribing these tablets to patients with asthma or breathing problems as these conditions may be aggravated.

Cardiovascular

Phenylbutazone has fluid retaining properties.

Hepatic

Serious hepatocellular reactions have been reported (Benjamin *et al.*, 1981) and hepatic clearance of drugs is reduced as phenylbutazone inhibits oxidase drug metabolism.

Haematological Abnormalities

A range of haematological abnormalities have been reported. Long-term recipients may develop iron deficiency anaemia due to chronic blood loss from inflammation of the small intestine. Aplastic anaemia has been associated with the slow metabolism of phenylbutazone (Leyland *et al.*, 1974) suggesting that this adverse effect is related to excessive concentrations of the drug. Thrombocytopenia, effects on platelet function, agranulocytosis, pancytopenia and haemolytic anaemia have also been noted but are still rare although can be fatal (O'Brien and Bagley, 1985).

Interactions

Phenylbutazone interacts with oral anticoagulants, lithium, oral hypoglycaemic agents, phenytoin, methotrexate (causing pancytopenia probably due to retention of methotrexate due to inhibition of proximal renal tubular secretion), digoxin, aminoglycosides, probenecid and barbiturates.

DAPSONE

Treatment Regime

Dapsone is best known as an anti-leprotic agent but it also has effects on the immune system and has been used for the treatment of RA and psoriatic arthritis. There is a delay of two to three months before onset of action but when successful it will reduce the ESR. The dosage is 50 mg daily for one week increasing then to 100 mg daily depending on the result of the haemoglobin. Occasionally patients may require 150 mg daily.

Adverse Effects

Minor side effects such as rashes and gastric upset can occur. Haematological —
haemolysis occurs in all patients and gives a drop in haemoglobin of 1–2 g. This
therefore requires monitoring before increases in dosage are considered. Patients
also develop a pallor which is more marked than the drop in the haemoglobin
would produce. It is worth warning patients that they will look pale. Patients of
Mediterranean origin will require a G6PD estimation prior to starting treatment
since massive haemolysis will occur if there is a deficiency in this enzyme. Agranulocytosis has been reported but is rare.

MINOCYCLINE (MINOCIN)

Minocycline is a broad spectrum antibiotic often prescribed in the treatment of
acne. It has also been used in the treatment of RA. Its mode of action is not
known but it is thought to be effective at inhibiting the pro-inflammatory enzyme
metalloproteinase. It does not become fully effective for two to three months. The
dosage is 100–300 mg twice daily.

Adverse Effects

An abnormal metallic taste can occur when first starting the treatment. Dizziness,
nausea and diarrhoea have also been reported. The treatment is best taken with
food.
    Although severe side effects are rare a drug-induced lupus syndrome and hepatitis
can occur that resolves on stopping but necessitates that treatment is monitored
with a full blood count and biochemistry monthly and an anti-nuclear antibody
six-monthly.

Interactions

Minocycline should not be taken at the same time as antacids, calcium and iron
preparations. A two-hour gap is required between administration of minocycline
and these preparations.

Warfarin

If prescribed penicillin, leave off minocycline until the course of penicillin is
completed.

LEFLUNOMIDE

Treatment Regime

Lefluomide is usually prescribed as a daily dose of 10–20 mg. It is common in
the United Kingdom not to use a loading dose of 100 mg daily for three days

although this practice is seen in other European countries (Maddison *et al.*, 2005). Loading doses are associated with an increased incidence of side effects (Erra *et al.*, 2003). On doses of 10 mg it will take over six months to reach a therapeutic level (Maddison *et al.*, 2005). The recommended daily dose is 20 mg. In patients receiving other potentially hepatotoxic drugs, such as methotrexate, or who are renally impaired 10 mg is recommended (Maddison *et al.*, 2005). Alcohol ideally should be avoided.

Caution

- Evidence of Hepatitis B or C infection.
- History of tuberculosis.

Contraindications

- Serious infections.
- Impaired liver function.
- Severe unexplained hypoproteinaemia.
- Renal impairment − moderate to severe.

Adverse Effects

Many adverse effects can be managed by reducing the dosage or by concomitant administration of symptomatic therapy (Maddison *et al.*, 2005). If it is necessary to rapidly remove the drug from a patient's system then a washout with cholestyramine will quickly reduce the plasma levels of the drug.

Washout Procedure

Cholestyramine 8 mg is administered three times daily. Alternatively 50 mg of activated powered charcoal is administered four times daily. Duration of a complete washout is usually 11 days. The duration may be modified depending on clinical or laboratory variables.

Gastrointestinal Symptoms

Data from a US database (Emery *et al.*, 2002) on the use of leflunomide by 40 000 RA patients indicated that gastrointestinal tract-related problems were the commonest reasons for stopping treatment. Problems experienced included diarrhoea, nausea, vomiting, oral mucosal disorders (e.g. aphthous stomatitis, mouth ulceration) and abdominal pain.

The prevalence of nausea is less in lefluomide than in patients taking sulfasalazine or methotrexate but the prevalence of diarrhoea is increased and should be treated, in the first instances, rather than stopping the drug. Daily doses of leflunomide 20 mg are associated with more nausea and diarrhoea than a daily dose of 10 mg.

Skin Reactions

In cases of ulcerative stomatitis, leflunomide administration should be discontinued. Minor rashes can be treated symptomatically but severe rashes will necessitate discontinuation of leflunomide. Severe dermatological toxicity has a higher prevalence than is seen in patients taking sulfasalazine or methotrexate (Maddison et al., 2005). Cases of Stevens−Johnson syndrome or toxic epidermal necrolysis have been reported.

Hypertension

The manufacturers recommend that blood pressure monitoring is carried out on patients taking leflunomide but hypertension does not appear to occur more often with this DMARD in comparison to other DMARDs such as methotrexate, except where loading doses have been used (Maddison et al., 2005).

Respiratory Reactions

Interstitial lung disease has been reported during treatment with leflunomide. Interstitial lung disease is a potentially fatal disorder, which may occur acutely during therapy. Pulmonary symptoms, such as cough and dyspnoea, should be investigated.

Pulmonary infiltration as an acute allergic reaction has been demonstrated in a small number of patients after commencing leflunomide.

Hepatoxicity

Raised liver tests can occur and require monitoring; liver toxicity is more common in methotrexate that with leflunomide (Maddison et al., 2005). Rare cases of severe liver injury (some with fatal outcome) have been reported after drug treatment with leflunomide. Most cases occurred within six months and were associated with other risk factors for hepatotoxicity. Patients should be asked to limit alcohol intake well within normal limits at four to eight units a week.

Haematological Abnormalities

It is recommended that patients on leflunomide have regular full blood counts although there is no data to suggest an increase in blood dyscrasias due to leflunomide (Maddison et al., 2005).

Leflunomide should be stopped if the following occur:

• Major mouth ulcers or skin rashes.
• Respiratory reactions.
• Liver function deteriorates − > twofold rise in AST, ALT.
• Platelets <150.
• Total white blood cell count <3.5.

- Neutrophils <2.
- Weight loss of >10% with no other cause identified.
- Severe persistent headaches.
- Severe sore throat.
- Abnormal bruising.

MYCOPHENOLATE MOFETIL

Treatment Regime

Mycophenolate mofetil is a potent reversible selective inhibitor of purine synthesis. It has been shown to inhibit T cell proliferation and antibody production by B cells. It is used in the treatment of systemic lupus erythematosus, scleroderma and vasculitis and after organ transplantation. Mycophenolate is usually taken in capsule form twice a day on an empty stomach. A typical dose may be 500 mg twice a day for four weeks; then, if tolerated, 1 g twice a day thereafter. Alcohol should only be taken in small amounts as it can affect the liver. Mycophenolate should not be taken with cholestyramine or antacids with magnesium or aluminium hydroxides as absorption may be reduced. If being used with azathioprine, lower doses should be used. Pre-treatment assessment includes FBC, urea and electrolytes, creatinine and liver function tests.

Adverse Effects

The most common side effects are sickness, diarrhoea, vomiting or abdominal pain. These side effects are usually dose-related and resolve on discontinuation of the drug. Severe neutropenia occurs in 0.5% patients receiving 1 g twice daily compared to 0.8% patients receiving azathioprine; it is most commonly seen within the first six months. There is a slight increase in the risk of skin cancer and patients should avoid exposure to strong sunlight and protect their skin with sunblock or sunscreen. Symptoms of allergy include wheezing, shortness of breath, swelling of the face, lips, tongue or throat. Urogenital reactions include sterile haematuria, urinary tract infection and renal tubular necrosis.

Reasons for Stopping Treatment

Mycophenolate should be stopped if the following occur:

- WBC<3.5 x 10/L.
- Neutrophils< 2.0 x 10/L.
- Platelets<150 x 10^9/L.
- Rash or oral ulceration.
- MCV>105fl
- Abnormal bruising or sore throat.
- Gastrointestinal disturbances — withhold until settle then reintroduce at a lower dose.

Table 3.5 Vaccines.

Live vaccines	Inactivated vaccines
Measles	Influenza
Rubella	Typhoid (injected)
BCG	Poliomyelitis (IPV injected)
Mumps	Cholera
Poliomyelitis (OPV)	Diptheria
Yellow fever	Haemophilis influenza type 2
Typhoid (oral)	Hepatitis A
	Hepatitis B
	Meningococcal
	Pertussis
	Pneumococcus
	Tetanus

3.9 VACCINATION

Live vaccines (shown in Table 3.5) should be avoided in patients taking azathio-prine, methotrexate, cyclophosphamide or high doses of corticosteroids. Patients on these medications should be considered for varicella-zoster immunoglobulin after exposure to chicken pox or herpes zoster and should be advised to avoid close contact with patients recently vaccinated with live polio vaccine because of the risk of infections from faecal excretion. Sulfasalazine, D-penicillamine, gold – in general vaccination are safe for patients on these therapies although is probably preferable to avoid live vaccines. Ciclosporin has a poor response to vaccines and patients should ideally have any appropriate vaccinations prior to therapy.

3.10 PREGNANCY

Patients planning a family will require advice and support from various members of the rheumatology team. Pregnancy and related issues such as breastfeeding must be addressed when patients are receiving a DMARD. It is necessary to be absolutely certain about the effects of the DMARD on the fetus as well as on lactation. One of the major concerns of any pregnant woman is the risk of congenital malfor-mation due to drugs and this will cause even greater concern to the woman with rheumatoid arthritis (Richardson, 1992). The most vulnerable period of gestation is during embryonic and fetal development but many congenital abnormalities occur for reasons other than those that are drug-related. Spontaneous and serious malfor-mations occur in 2–3% of all pregnancies and minor malformations occur in a further 6% (Oka and Vainio, 1966).

Women with rheumatoid arthritis often need to achieve disease suppression to increase their chance of conceiving. Adequate control of the disease will enable a woman to feel capable of bearing and raising a child. Decisions regarding the withdrawal of potentially toxic drug therapy need to be made in good time since many drugs can affect the vulnerable stages of embryogenesis. Women should discontinue teratogenic agents such as methotrexate, azathioprine and cyclophosphamide at least six months before attempting conception. Leflunomide, one of the newer DMARDs, has proven teratogenic and fetotoxic effects in animal studies and its active metabolite is detectable in plasma two years after discontinuation of the drug. Consequently the fetus could have *in utero* exposure to leflunomide up to two years after the end of treatment unless an oral cholestyramine regimen, 8 g 3 times daily for 11 days is administered to obtain undetectable plasmatic levels. The manufacturer recommends that for women of childbearing age 'treatment with leflunomide must not be started until pregnancy is excluded and it has been confirmed that reliable contraception is being used'. Ideally all drug therapy should be avoided during pregnancy and lactation. The effects of drug therapy used in rheumatic disease are shown in Table 3.6 (Le Gallez, 1988).

In ankylosing spondylitis 80% of patients may experience a worsening of symptoms or no alteration of their condition during pregnancy (Le Gallez, 1988) and will require advice on coping with pain. This should include relaxation techniques, the application of hot and cold therapy and the use of diversional techniques. In RA 75% of women experience some remission of their condition during pregnancy but often return to disease status comparable with their pre-pregnant state within eight

Table 3.6 Drugs and pregnancy.

Analgesia
    Paracetamol
    Can be taken during pregnancy

NSAIDs
    Aspirin
    Avoid in first trimester, may cause cleft palate
    Avoid during late pregnancy, may cause prolonged gestation and labour and increased blood
    loss at delivery antepartum haemorrhage. May lead to premature closure of the ductus gloriosus

Corticosteroids
    Considered safe when taken in low dosages (5−10 mg daily). If withdrawn within two months of labour steroid cover should be provided

DMARDs
    Sulfasalazine: avoid in late pregnancy − neonatal janudice
    Auranofin, D-penicillamine, mycophenolate mofetil and gold are all contraindicated
    Ciclosporin and sulfasalazine − use with caution
    Hydroxychloroquine can be used in pregnancy but needs to be discussed with the rheumatologist
    Leflunomide, methotrexate, cyclophosphamide and azathioprine are all teratogenic

months of giving birth. Women who develop an exacerbation of their condition post-partum will need to recommence their suppressive drug therapy and individual advice from the rheumatology nurse will be required if the mother is breastfeeding.

CONTRACEPTION

Reliable contraception should be advised for all women receiving disease modifying anti-rheumatic drug therapy and all proposed pregnancies will need discussing on an individual basis with the rheumatology nurse. For those medications known to be teratogenic – for example, methotrexate, azathioprine, leflunomide, chlorambucil and cyclophosphamide – patients must have contraceptive cover and discontinue the drug for six months before trying for a family. In the case of leflunomide the manufacturers recommend that the drug should be discontinued for two years before becoming pregnant. If this waiting time is considered unpractical, prophylactic institution of a washout procedure may be advisable.

3.11   THE ROLE OF THE COMMUNITY TEAM IN DRUG THERAPY

Musculoskeletal disorders are a common cause of long-term disability in the United Kingdom, making up 15% of the workload of GPs (Martin, Meltzer and Eliot, 1998). Shared care is the management of the patient between the hospital team – consisting of the rheumatologists, specialist nurse, occupational therapist and physiotherapist – and the primary healthcare team (see Table 3.7). Drug therapy should be carefully planned between the rheumatologist and the general practitioner. The rheumatologist's main role is to diagnose and establish a treatment plan to

Table 3.7 Members of the shared care team.

- GP
- Patient
- Practice nurse
- Physiotherapist
- Family
- Rheumatologist
- Occupational therapist
- District nurse
- Health visitor
- Orthotist
- Social services
- Podiatrist
- Pharmacist
- Nurse specialist

be followed in primary care or shared between primary and secondary care. The latter is the case with rheumatoid arthritis, as it is a progressive chronic disease. The specialist nurse acts as a resource for the patients, other professionals and for the primary healthcare team. The nurse is required to be a counsellor, educator and adviser on many aspects of rheumatoid arthritis, particularly drug therapy. Physiotherapists provide a whole range of treatments and aim to maintain and improve function, alleviate pain and motivate the patient to carry out regular exercises. The occupational therapist provides help and support with problems of daily living and is often instrumental in enabling the patient to develop coping strategies including pacing of activities, joint protection and self-management interventions including relaxation. The primary healthcare team provide health services outside the hospital. They consist primarily of the general practitioner, the practice nurse, the district nurse and the health visitor, all of whom provide valuable information about the patient's family and home situation. They are often the first point of contact the patient makes. An analysis of the work practice nurses do showed they offered practical treatment, health promotion and disease management (Bryan, 1995). When each team complements the other and, provided there is communication and respect for each other's roles, then good quality treatment should be available for all patients.

According to Bryan (1995) practice nurses are isolated from colleagues and need a forum for the exchange of ideas, the updating of skills and the acquisition of new knowledge. In order to try and fill this need, education and opportunities for updating knowledge are provided by the hospital team in the form of study days, visits to the rheumatology unit and the team visiting the general practice. The practice team will then be able to support and advise patients, recognize when side effects require a change of treatment or when the patient would benefit from an early hospital appointment. The early identification of symptoms of the disease, the side effects of drug therapies, the interpretation of the blood results and their implications, plus the psychological effect of arthritis on the patient and their family are important requisites for managing the condition.

An evaluation of two study mornings for practice nurses delivered by a specialist nurse in the rheumatology department of a general hospital enabled clinical scenarios to be discussed, increasing the clinical knowledge and consequently reducing the number of telephone calls from practice nurses (Sigworth, 2004).

MINIMIZING CONFUSION

Nurses in the primary healthcare team can play an important part in alleviating confusion in the administration of drugs by using medication cards stating how and when patients are to take the prescribed dose (Figure 3.2). Pill dispensers are invaluable for patients with poor memory as they have compartments containing drugs for each day on a weekly basis. To obtain the maximum benefit, medicines should be taken in the correct way at the correct time. Some patients will have failing eyesight and be unable to read the instructions. Many pharmacists will print large labels

Name of tablet	Dosage	How/when to take	Special instructions
Diclofenac (Voltarol)	75 mg twice daily	One after breakfast. One after evening meal.	Always take with food. Report any sickness/ indigestion.
Azathioprine (Imuran)	150 mg daily	Three 50 mg tablets after breakfast.	Take with food. Report any sickness or mouth ulcers.

Figure 3.2 Medication card.

to overcome this. Patients who have poor hand grip often cannot open the child-proof bottles. It is helpful to liaise with the pharmacist who will provide screw tops or ring caps. Patients with reduced manual dexterity frequently can experience difficulties with blister packs. Eye drops also often present a problem. The pharmacist and the occupational therapist can help with the provision of aids to maintain independence. An increased number of tablets taken, and doses involved, often reduces concordance. Patients with poor memory may find drugs to be taken daily of more benefit. Patients with Sjögren's syndrome can find swallowing tablets difficult. It may therefore be more appropriate to prescribe drugs in liquid form.

Many patients do not comply with the drug therapy as they are afraid of the side effects or of being dependent on a drug, particularly analgesia. Confusion often arises as many drugs have three different names, the brand, the pharmaceutical and the generic name.

Low patient adherence to therapeutic regimes is an obstacle to achieving therapeutic goals in arthritis management. Improvement of concordance is a prime goal of much patient education and counselling (Daltroy, 1993). This area will be discussed in greater depth in Chapter 4.

3.12   COMMUNITY DRUG MONITORING

In GP surgeries most of the drug monitoring is carried out by the practice nurse, guided by protocols issued and agreed with the rheumatologist and GP. The Royal College of Nursing rheumatology forum has produced guidelines for nurses involved in

• The administration of intramuscular sodium aurothiomalate (see Appendix 3.B).
• The administration of intramuscular methotrexate.

The objective of these guidelines is to ensure that the patient receives the same standard of care and high quality service, independent of the setting in which they are nursed. The guidelines also provide the nurse with a framework for practice.

Helliwell and O'Hara (1995) found that the percentage of cases in which the standard monitoring protocol had been complied with within the GP practice was 26% for sodium aurthoimalate, 67% for sulfasalazine and 93% for methotrexate. (The discrepancy relating to the monitoring of sodium aurothiomalate concerned an annual chest X-ray requirement).

Havelock (1998), in an audit undertaken of shared care monitoring, found that the majority of patients were being adequately monitored, less than 2% of patients were not being monitored and a significant number of patients were actually receiving more blood tests than had been stated on the agreed protocols.

DOCUMENTATION

Close monitoring of second line drugs ensures their safe use and is a guide to their efficacy. To provide close communication between the general practitioner and the rheumatologist, shared care booklets are often issued to patients from the rheumatology department. The use of a patient-held booklet has been strongly endorsed by the British Society of Rheumatology, the British Health Professionals in Rheumatology and the National Patient Safety Agency. Such booklets can be used to record the blood results serially and monitor the urinalysis (where required) for the presence of blood and protein. This enables the rheumatology specialist to examine the trends of the haematological and biochemical results and the presence of abnormalities in the urine. This therefore helps the rheumatology specialist to decide whether to discontinue the drug or reduce the dose. Each book issued should have the contact number of the rheumatology department with which the patient or a member of the primary healthcare team can make contact for advice and support. Serious side effects can be avoided by the hospital team and the primary healthcare team explaining to the patients the necessity of having regular blood tests and reporting side effects early. In Helliwell and O'Hara's study (1995) there was unanimous agreement by the GPs that shared monitoring cards were helpful. The GPs involved were prepared to keep them updated and were willing to follow suggested protocols. Havelock (1998) also found that this method of documentation worked well within both the primary and secondary care settings.

Computerized patient monitoring systems have been gaining popularity in rheumatology (Lee, Lenert and Kavanaugh, 2004) as they offer automized validation, improved data capture and immediate result availability (Buxton, White and Osoba, 1998; Velikova et al., 1999). Lee, Lenert and Kavanaugh (2004) suggest that patient outcome measures could also be completed by patients via a computer program, which would enable the clinician to receive the information required to access the efficacy of drug therapy at the optimal time and prevent the delay that often occurs as a patient waits for an outpatient appointment. Clinicians could then review and compare results with earlier visits and adjust medications accordingly ensuring patients achieve a therapeutic dose at the optimal time (Lee, Lenert and Kavanaugh, 2004).

GPs' CONCERNS RELATING TO PRACTICE-BASED MONITORING

Anxieties over various aspects of GP-based drug monitoring included:

- Poor facilities for the collection and distribution of blood samples to the hospital laboratory.
- A perceived lack of time to perform domiciliary visits on those patients unable to attend the practice. One could argue that it may be more appropriate for a community practitioner – for example, a district nurse with expanded knowledge in the field of rheumatology – to carry out such visits.
- A lack of clarity regarding the responsibility for prescribing and monitoring drug therapy.

One practice cited by Helliwell and O'Hara (1995) was unwilling to monitor second line therapy due to a perceived lack of time to perform the necessary blood tests and a reluctance to accept the responsibility inherent within this practice.

PATIENTS' EXPERIENCES OF DRUG MONITORING

Arthur and Clifford (2004a) compared the satisfaction of patients attending follow-up monitoring care within primary and secondary care locations. They found that whilst patients from both locations were satisfied with the care they received, those receiving specialist nursing care in the secondary care location were more satisfied. Empathy, specialism, information provision, technical aspects, time and continuity of care were identified as being important for patients attending monitoring clinics (Arthur and Clifford, 2004b), with the specialist nurse able to positively influence patients' perceived ability to cope with their arthritis (Ryan et al., 2006).

3.13 COMMUNITY CLINICS

At the heart of community care is the principle that services should support people in their own home and locality (Wolf, 1997). In certain chronic conditions shared management between the hospital and general practitioner is well established, especially in areas such as diabetics and asthma (Jones et al., 1991; Thorne and Russell, 1973).

The essential features of community clinics are that they are:

- In a location close to the patient's home.
- Performed by a consultant specialist.
- Providing educational opportunities for GPs.
- Improving communication between the hospital and community staff (Helliwell, 1996).

Shared care should include:

- Effective communication between primary and secondary care teams.
- Shared documentation in the form of agreed guidelines.
- Ongoing support, education and training.
- An appreciation of both service commitments and difficulties (Barrett and Thomas, 1992).

3.14 GENERAL PRACTICE

Most GPs will have only a very small case load (often single figures of patients) of those requiring DMARDs. Therefore the practitioner is unlikely to be familiar with all aspects of this therapy including adverse effects. Although the NHS management executive has decreed that the doctor who has clinical responsibility for the patient should undertake the prescribing, there is a clear need for shared management in both the clinician's and the patient's interest. The British Society of Rheumatology (1992) has recommended the referral of all patients with RA to the hospital setting with the subsequent sharing of treatment between the hospital and general practitioner.

GPs feel confident managing the majority of musculoskeletal conditions within their surgery provided they have adequate support with: joint injection techniques, complex cases with poor outcome (including pain syndromes), access to physiotherapy and a multidisciplinary approach to pain control (Roberts, Adebajo and Long, 2002). GPs' knowledge of their patients with RA in the areas of functional disability, social situation and involvement of health and social care professionals was very variable (Memel and Kirwan, 1999), with GPs significantly underestimating the functional disability of their patients. The education and training of GPs may not equate with the needs of musculoskeletal patients. A lack of confidence in managing rheumatological conditions is related to lack of experience and poor teaching (Lanyon, Pope and Croft, 1995). This situation is being addressed through the training of GPs with a specialist interest in rheumatology.

3.15 EVALUATION OF COMMUNITY CLINICS

Community clinics run by a rheumatologist in a GP's surgery demonstrated increased patient satisfaction and greater patient access to a specialist, in comparison with traditional outpatient clinics, but only a slight improvement in health benefits (Bond et al., 2000). Whilst patients' own costs were lower, NHS staffing and treatment costs were more expensive per patient in outreach than outpatient clinics (Bond et al., 2000).

The advantages of community clinics cited by both the GP and the specialist included:

• Improved patient access to the specialist (Bailey, Black and Wilkin, 1994).
• Patient convenience.
• Shorter waiting time for first appointment.
• Fewer non-attenders.
• Improved communication between GP and the specialist.

Patients in Helliwell's (1996) study reported experiencing a greater satisfaction with their consultants than their counterparts attending a hospital-based clinic. Patients attending the community clinic stated that their questions were always answered.

POTENTIAL PROBLEMS WITH CONSULTANT-BASED COMMUNITY CLINICS

• Infrequent follow-up intervals (if the specialist attends every four to six weeks then follow-up consultations are delayed).
• Increase in GP administrative costs and time.
• Many consultants working within the community have a minimal number of support staff, and the time spent travelling will reduce the number of patients seen per session (Barnyl et al., 1990; Bond et al., 2000).
• The opportunity for education as a result of personal contact between the consultant and GP is often infrequent due to GPs engaging in busy surgeries of their own (Helliwell, 1996). In a survey by Bailey, Black and Wilkin (1994) GPs were in attendance at only 5% of outreach clinics.
• Case mix disruptions may occur and the consultant is not available for other clinical practices whilst in the community (Walker, 1994). Although fewer patients were seen in the community clinic with a higher old/new ratio than the hospital-based clinic, Helliwell (1996) found no difference in the case mix data between the two healthcare settings.

3.16 NURSE-LED COMMUNITY CLINICS

In Norfolk a weekly rheumatology nurse practitioner clinic was established in the general practice to provide the following range of services (Mooney, 1996):

• Physical assessment of joints.
• The monitoring of the safety and efficacy of drug treatment.
• Initiation and interpretation of clinical laboratory data.

- Referrals to the multidisciplinary team.
- Liaison between the patient and other healthcare professionals.

The patients were highly satisfied with this service provision. This finding was in accordance with work carried out by Hill (1997). Patients who were allocated to a nurse-led clinic within the outpatient setting were more satisfied with their overall care when compared to a similar group of patients attending the consultant clinic. Mooney (1996) concludes that the reported patient satisfaction could be attributed to the improved continuity of care the patients were receiving, coupled with the length of consultation time the patient spent with the nurse.

The nurse practitioner clinic in the doctor's surgery also had other benefits. These included:

- The provision of disease education for patients and the opportunity to discuss issues with the nurse.
- Less travelling for patients as the clinic was located in a more convenient setting with no parking fees.
- The patients experienced a continuity of care in their management.
- The rheumatology nurse practitioner acted as an advocate between the practice, rheumatologist and patient thereby enhancing and improving communication.
- Early referral could be made to other healthcare professionals.
- If necessary quicker access to a rheumatologist was available and appropriate investigations could be carried out before referral.
- The number of outpatient visits to the hospital rheumatology clinics was reduced.
- The provision of specialist advice could be given in a familiar environment.
- General practitioner visits for rheumatological complaints were reduced (Mooney, 1996).

Dargie and Procter (1993) established a nurse-led arthritis clinic in the health centre in which they worked. One of the primary objectives of this development was to provide an easily accessible service for the assessment, support, education and monitoring of treatment for patients with arthritis and their families. Additional advantages that Mooney (1996) cites included a focus on prevention rather than crisis management. The two individuals involved (a district nurse and a practice nurse) also felt they were able to make full use of their nursing skills which enhanced their own job satisfaction. Potential disadvantages in the provision of this much-needed service were the lack of community services in some areas – for example, physiotherapist and occupational therapist. The extra time commitment required to provide such a service could also be viewed as a disadvantage in economic terms but the pay-off was that patients received a service that was tailored to their individual needs.

The advantage of community clinics to the patient include convenience whilst maintaining a high standard of care from a specialist practitioner. For the hospital one of the benefits is the devolution of some of the care to general practice, creating the scope for more new patients to be seen in the hospital setting (Helliwell and O'Hara, 1995).

3.17 NEW WAYS OF UTILIZING OUTPATIENT APPOINTMENTS

Hewlett *et al.* (2000) evaluated the clinical efficacy, cost and acceptability of a shared care system of patient or GP-initiated review in patients with RA. Patients were randomized to either shared care with their GP (no routine hospital review but rapid access on request) or traditional hospital care (regular planned outpatient review usually three- to four-monthly). Patients (or their GPs) in the shared care group could request review by any member of the rheumatology team via the nurse-run telephone helpline. Patients in the study appeared representative of a hospital-based RA population with moderate inflammatory activity, pain and disability. Patients who declined to take part were older and more affected by their arthritis. Results showed no clinical deterioration and some clinical benefit in the shared care group, which was achieved at a 33.5% cost saving, with both patients and GPs experiencing greater satisfaction and confidence in the system (Hewlett *et al.*, 2000).

3.18 DRUG THERAPY AND OSTEOPOROSIS

As is often the case in the management of many chronic conditions, it is the primary healthcare team who are responsible for the early diagnosis and continuing care of patients with established osteoporosis (Brennan, 1996). Osteoporosis is a silent disease that can affect all age groups. Symptoms are not usually present until a fracture occurs, often as a result of minimum trauma. Bone is a living tissue and is being continually regenerated. Cells, called osteoclasts, destroy bone and eat away areas of bone, whilst other cells, called osteoblasts, are bone builders and follow the osteoclasts filling in and repairing the bone. When this process becomes imbalanced, more bone will be destroyed than is being replaced; then osteoporosis results with bones becoming thinner and more brittle. Peak bone mass is generally achieved between the ages of 25 and 36. Following this peak, bone mass then decreases by 0.3% a year. When women reach the menopause, however, bone is lost more rapidly and may be as much as 5% per year over a 10-year period. Thus 1 in 3 women and 1 in 12 men are likely to sustain a fracture related to osteoporosis by the age of 90 years (Peel and Eastell, 2004).

CLASSIFICATION OF OSTEOPOROSIS

Osteoporosis falls into two categories, primary and secondary. Primary osteoporosis is caused by ageing, the menopause and impaired adult peak bone density.

Secondary osteoporosis accounts for 40% of cases in women and 60% of cases in men. It is caused by:

- Anorexia and bulimia.
- Amenorrhoea for more than six months.
- Premature menopause in women (whether surgical, natural or radiation-induced).

Table 3.8 Foods rich in calcium.

Yoghurt	150 g	225 mg calcium
Skimmed milk	190 ml	235 mg
Semi-skimmed milk	190 ml	231 mg
Silver top milk	190 ml	234 mg
Soya milk	190 ml	25 mg
Cheddar cheese	28 g	202 mg
Edam cheese	28 g	216 mg
Sardines (tinned)	56 g	258 mg
Spinach (boiled)	112 g	179 mg
Baked beans	112 g	59 mg
Bread white − 1 slice	112 g	33 mg
Bread wholemeal − 1 slice	112 g	16 mg

- Excessive exercise − for example, ballerinas and athletes.
- Lifestyle factors − smoking and excessive alcohol.
- Dietary factors − for example, lack of calcium and vitamin D (Table 3.8 shows food groups rich in calcium).
- Gut malabsorption and chronic liver disease.
- Immobilization.
- High dose corticosteroid therapy (over 7.5 mg daily).
- Anticonvulsants.
- Heparin therapy.
- Genetic links.
- Cushing's syndrome.
- Throtoxicosis.
- Primary hyperparathyroidism.
- Hypogonadism.

It is important that the primary healthcare team recognize those individuals who are potentially at risk and discuss with them preventive strategies or management of the condition.

RISK FACTORS FOR OSTEOPOROSIS FRACTURE

Risk factors do not have adequate sensitivity or specificity to identify people at risk and measurement of bone mineral density is needed to quantify an individual's risk of fracture (Peel and Eastell, 2004).

Risk factors for osteoporosis:

- Female sex.
- Increasing age.
- Early menopause (before 45 years).

- Hypogonadism.
- Smoking.
- High alcohol intake.
- Physical inactivity.
- Low body mass index.
- Heredity (Peel and Eastell, 2004).

Risk factors that act independently of bone mineral density (Peel and Eastell, 2004):

- Prevalent low trauma fracture, particularly vertebral fractures.
- Family history, particularly of maternal hip fracture.
- Current smoking habit.
- Low body weight.
- Increasing age.

INVESTIGATIONS FOR OSTEOPOROSIS

- X-rays: radiography has an essential role in identifying fractures. However, standard radiographs cannot be used to diagnose osteoporosis on the basis of apparent osteopenia. The appearance of osteopenia on plain X-rays depends on the dose of X-ray used, volume of soft tissues and other variables, in addition to the bone density itself.
- Dual energy X-ray absorptiometry (DEXA) scanning: this is considered to be the gold standard technique for measuring bone density. Typically scans are taken at the proximal femur and spine. The radiation dose to the patient from this procedure is small, approximately one tenth of a chest X-ray. A T score and a Z score is reported. The T score is the number of standard deviations above/below the peak adult (premenopausal) mean. The Z score is the number of standard deviations above/below the age-matched mean. For every one standard deviation fall in bone density, fracture risk approximately doubles. DEXA scanning is useful for measuring bone density in patients with risk factors in whom results will affect management. This form of scanning may be unreliable in the presence of skeletal deformities − for example, scoliosis or degenerative changes.

3.19 HORMONE REPLACEMENT THERAPY (HRT)

Once considered to be the gold standard in the treatment of osteoporosis, HRT now only has a role in the treatment of menopausal symptoms such as hot flushes or in women who have undergone an early menopause. Due to concerns in the increased risk of breast cancer and cardiovascular events it is no longer thought to be appropriate to use HRT in the management of osteoporosis.

3.20 PAIN MANAGEMENT

Simple analgesics such as paracetamol and non-steroidal anti-inflammatory drugs are sometimes beneficial for chronic pain in osteoporosis. Opiates (e.g. morphine) and calcitonin are sometimes given for the intense pain of a vertebral fracture. If chronic pain is not managed then the patient becomes less active, more helpless and isolated, and self-esteem is greatly reduced. Non-pharmacological management of pain is shown in Table 3.9.

3.21 DRUGS TO REDUCE FRACTURE RISK

BISPHOSPHONATES

Bisphosphonates act to block the action of osteoclasts. They are poorly absorbed from the gut and readily bind to other agents in the gut and must be taken on an empty stomach.

ETIDRONATE

This is the first of the bisphosphonates to be used commonly in osteoporosis. Due to the risk of osteomalacia, 400 mg is taken daily for two weeks every three months, with the option of taking calcium supplements for the remaining weeks. It must be taken with water in the middle of a four-hour fast to ensure adequate absorption.

Contraindications for this drug are severe renal impairment, hypocalcaemia, hypercalcinuria, pregnancy and lactation.

Cyclical etidronate reduces bone loss from the spine and vertebral fracture risk in post-menopausal women with osteoporosis (Peel and Eastell, 2004).

ALENDRONATE SODIUM (FOSAMAX)

It is taken as a single 5−10 mg daily dose. There is now an option to take one 70 mg tablet per week. Patients should swallow a 10 mg tablet when getting out of bed in

Table 3.9 Pain management (non-pharmacological).

- Pacing activities
- Relaxation
- Joint protection techinques
- Aids and adaptation
- Hydrotherapy
- Exercise
- Use of heat − for example, heat pads
- Massage (aromatherapy)
- Diversional therapy
- Counselling
- Transcutaneous electrical nerve stimulation (TENS) machine

the morning half an hour before any food and with a 7oz drink of plain water. It is important that patients should stand or sit for at least 30 minutes after taking the tablet, after which the first beverage, meal or medication of the day may be taken. Antacids can affect the absorption of this drug. Contraindications are patients with significant renal impairment, pregnancy, breastfeeding women, abnormalities of the oesophagus or upper gastrointestinal problems. The side effects include nausea, dyspepsia and diarrhoea. Treatment is continued long term. Alendronate prevents bone loss from vertebral and non-vertebral sites and decreases the risk of spine and hip fractures (Peel and Eastell, 2004).

Risedronate. Risedronate is taken daily as a 5 mg tablet. It should be taken with water 30 minutes before the first drink, food or medication of the day in the middle of a four-hour fast and not before going to bed. Risedronate prevents bone loss from the vertebral and non-vertebral sites and decreases the risk of spine and hip fractures (Peel and Eastell, 2004).

In 2005, NICE issued guidelines on the secondary prevention of osteoporosis and recommended the use of bisphosphonates for post-menopausal women who had already experienced a fracture.

3.22 OTHER DRUG TREATMENTS

Selective estrogen receptor modulators (SERMs). These are synthetic compounds that stimulate oestrogen receptors of bone tissue and work in a similar way to HRT. Oestrogen receptors of breast and endometrial tissue are not engaged and so it is considered that this treatment will not increase the risk of breast or endometrial cancer. Raloxifene is a commonly used SERM. It has been shown to reduce the risk of vertebral fractures but has not been shown to reduce the risk of non-vertebral fractures (Peel and Eastell, 2004). Like HRT raloxifene is associated with small increases in the number of thrombo-embolic events but is associated with a reduction in the number of new cases of breast cancer (Peel and Eastell, 2004).

CALCITONIN

Calcitonin inhibits osteoclast activity slowing the breakdown of bone. It can be given as subcutaneous injections or as a nasal preparation that is associated with fewer side effects. Nausea, vomiting, diarrhoea and dizziness have been reported. Calcitonin has been shown to reduce the risk of vertebral fracture. It has analgesic properties that may be useful in the acute management of vertebral fracture (Peel and Eastell, 2004).

CALCIUM (1000–1200 mg DAILY)

Calcium supplementation may be considered where dietary calcium intake is deficient or in cases of malabsorption. It has a less marked effect on fracture reduction than the other antiresorptive agents but it is usually well tolerated (Peel and Eastell, 2004).

VITAMIN D

Vitamin D is required to facilitate calcium absorption. Most people achieve their vitamin D requirement by the action of sunlight on their skin, in addition to that obtained from food. A French study in nursing homes showed that 800 iu of vitamin D3 and 1.2 g of elemental calcium daily reduces the risk of hip fracture by 43% (Chapuy et al., 1992). There is no evidence that vitamin D and calcium supplementation decreases spine bone loss or the incidence of vertebral fracture. A combination of calcium and vitamin D should be considered in all elderly patients who are housebound or in residential care (Peel and Eastell, 2004).

CALCITRIOL

Calcitriol is an active form of vitamin D which increases calcium absorption from the gut and decreases calcium excretion. It is used when there is active vitamin D deficiency which may be the cause of diminished bone mass. Patients should be monitored for hypercalcaemia whilst taking calcitriol. Calcitriol reduces post-menopausal bone loss and reduces spinal and extra-spinal fractures (excluding the hip).

FORMATION STIMULATING AGENTS

Fluoride

Fluroide dramatically increases bone mass but evidence of fracture prevention is inconclusive and the therapeutic window is narrow. Consequently it is rarely used in the United Kingdom (Peel and Eastell, 2004).

Parathyroid Hormone (PTH)

Intermittent injections of recombinant parathyroid hormone have recently been licensed in the United Kingdom (Peel and Eastell, 2004).

Teriparatide (Forsteo) is almost identical to human parathyroid hormone. It stimulates osteoblast production and is used to reduce vertebral fractures. It is administered as a daily subcutaneous injection.

STRONTIUM RANELATE (PROTELOS)

Is licensed for post-menopausal women with osteoporosis to reduce the risk of vertebral and hip fracture. It works by suppressing the action of osteoclasts and stimulating osteoblasts. It is administered in powder form mixed with water, taken daily in the evening, in the middle of a four-hour fast. Unlike bisphosphonates, strontium ranelate has very few gastrointestinal side effects; nausea and diarrhoea can occur on commencement of treatment but are usually mild and short-lived. There is a slight increased risk of blood clots and it would not be recommended to patients already at risk from thrombolytic events.

3.23   PREVENTION (LIFESTYLE STRATEGIES)

DIET

For optimum bone health a well-balanced diet is recommended with adequate calcium and vitamin D (see Table 3.8). Calcium requirements change throughout life and an adequate intake is particularly important during childhood, adolescence, pregnancy and lactation. Excessive caffeine, salt and fibre can hamper absorption or increase calcium excretion.

SMOKING

Smoking should be discouraged. Smoking alters oestrogen metabolism resulting in a reduction in the biologically active oestrogens which are beneficial to bone health. Women smokers tend to have an earlier menopause. Smokers also tend to have a lower body weight.

ALCOHOL

Alcohol intake should remain moderate. Excessive alcohol intake has a detrimental effect on bone turnover and formation; it can also effect calcium metabolism.

EXERCISE

Weight bearing exercise can increase bone formation, improve muscle strength and coordination. Exercise must be sustained as bone loss will resume once exercise stops. Exercise can also improve coordination and reduce the likelihood of falls. Three sessions of 20-minute exercise weekly are required. Excessive exercise will have a negative effect and increase the risk of osteoporosis due to low body weight and the effects on the hypothalamic-pituitary-gonadelaxis.

FALLS

Nurses have an input in fall prevention by improving awareness, identifying these who might be at risk and addressing risk factors such as poor eyesight, non-supportive footwear, reduced mobility and unsafe situations in the home environment.

CONCLUSION

The primary healthcare team play a valuable preventative role, especially with regard to osteoporosis, emphasizing the importance of a healthy lifestyle from the cradle to the grave. They often have a good relationship with the patients because they see them for a multitude of conditions. The more the practice healthcare team are involved with the hospital care team the better for patients with chronic disease. The efficacy of this arrangement requires continuous audit, with each practice reviewing how it can improve. There are variations in the quality of care of chronic conditions. It is the responsibility of the primary healthcare team, with the support of the rheumatologist and their team, to ensure the continuity of complex care which is offered to the rheumatology patient. What is regarded as routine in the rheumatology clinic may be rare to the GP. It is therefore important that the appropriate information be given to the patient on ward discharge and after clinic appointments, and to the GP with a diagnosis and details of medication and treatment. A network of support and communication between rheumatology services, the rheumatology team, the district nurses, the practice nurses and other community-based services will ensure consistent, clinically effective management of the patient and their rheumatoid disease. It is important that the practice nurse team uses the rheumatology nurse practitioner in a coordinating role as a resource and advisor. Management of arthritis is a long-term partnership between the patient and the primary and secondary healthcare team.

APPENDIX 3.A

Information Sheet (arc 2005)
The Rheumatology Nurse Specialist

WHAT IS IN THIS LEAFLET?

This leaflet contains information about the role of the rheumatology nurse specialist in helping you with your arthritis.

WHAT IS A RHEUMATOLOGY NURSE SPECIALIST?

The rheumatology nurse specialist is a trained nurse who has special experience in looking after the physical, emotional and social needs of patients with arthritis. These nurses have different titles, such as clinical nurse specialist, rheumatology nurse practitioner or liaison rheumatology nurse. Rheumatology nurse specialists work with people with rheumatoid arthritis and with people with other rheumato-logical conditions, such as scleroderma, osteoarthritis, fibromyalgia and lupus.

People with arthritis have many different needs. For this reason, most hospital rheumatology departments have a team of health professionals to look after all aspects of your care. The team itself may vary from hospital to hospital but generally will include a rheumatology nurse specialist, a physiotherapist and an occupational therapist (see arc leaflets A Mind Map on the Rheumatology Department, Physiotherapy and Arthritis and Occupational Therapy and Arthritis).

Some rheumatology nurse specialists have received special training which allows them to act in an 'extended role'. This involves some tasks usually done by doctors, such as carrying out an examination of your joints, reviewing and requesting investigations, performing joint injections and making changes to your treatment as required. The rheumatology nurse specialist will work closely with the consultant rheumatologist and, when necessary, will discuss your care with one of the rheumatology doctors.

HOW CAN YOU BE REFERRED TO A RHEUMATOLOGY NURSE SPECIALIST?

People with arthritis are often referred to a rheumatology nurse specialist when a diagnosis has been made by their consultant rheumatologist and the drug treatment has been agreed on. Some rheumatology departments also offer an open system, where patients can request to see the rheumatology nurse specialist (usually if a problem arises between appointments).

HOW CAN A RHEUMATOLOGY NURSE SPECIALIST HELP YOU?

Helping You Learn About Your Condition

The diagnosis of arthritis or a related condition can lead to a mixture of emotions. These may include anger, bewilderment, fear and anxiety. A detailed explanation about what the diagnosis means can reduce anxiety and fear. The rheumatology nurse specialist will listen to your particular concerns (e.g. 'Can I carry on working?') and provide information and support during periods of adjustment.

The rheumatology nurse specialist will explain what symptoms the arthritis can cause, and will work with you to reduce their impact. This often involves a process known as goal setting. Here problems are identified – for example, pain – and a plan is drawn up to help you manage the problem. This plan may include using a combination of methods, such as painkillers, exercises and pacing techniques. Verbal information will often be supported by written information (such as arc booklets), which enable you to learn at your own pace. The booklets can be shared with family members so that your family can also become involved in your care. If appropriate, the rheumatology nurse specialist can also spend time with your family discussing their concerns.

When you are first diagnosed you will probably see the rheumatology nurse specialist on an individual basis so that you can receive advice and support which is specific to your individual needs. You may have the opportunity of joining a patient education group if there is one in your area. These groups provide you with the option of learning from other people who have arthritis as well as developing new coping skills − for example, relaxation to reduce muscle pain. Most programmes will have input from other members of the rheumatology team, including physio-therapists and occupational therapists.

Helping You Learn About Drug Treatments and Monitoring Needs

Drug treatment plays a key role in the management of rheumatoid arthritis and related conditions. Some drugs − for example, non-steroidal anti-inflammatory drugs (NSAIDS) help reduce pain and stiffness. Other drugs, known as disease modifying anti-rheumatic drugs (DMARDs − see arc leaflet Drugs and Arthritis), dampen down the arthritis itself. These drugs require regular 'monitoring' blood tests and some need regular blood pressure and urine testing. The rheumatology nurse specialist will provide you with information before you start taking any DMARDs so that you are fully involved in your treatment. This may include:

- The benefit of the drug.
- How to take the drug.
- Whether to continue with other tablets.
- What to do if you forget to take a dose.
- Side effects and what to do if they occur.
- Any special instructions − for example, avoid alcohol.
- Monitoring requirements.
- Contact telephone number.

The rheumatology nurse will also arrange for your drug treatment to be monitored in a hospital clinic or at your GP surgery.

Offering Telephone Support

In some rheumatology departments, rheumatology nurse specialists run a telephone advice line to provide you (and health professionals, including GPs) with easy access to a nurse who knows about you, your condition and your treatment.

Involving Other Members of the Rheumatology Team

When the rheumatology nurse specialist assesses you, they might identify a problem which another member of the team may help with. For example, it may be that you are having difficulties opening jars and you would benefit from an assessment by an occupational therapist. The rheumatology nurse specialist will be able to make arrangements for you to be seen by the occupational therapist or other members of the rheumatology team.

Providing Emotional Support

Having arthritis can have a major effect on how you feel about yourself, your mood, your job and your relationships with other people. The rheumatology nurse specialist can provide expert help and support to improve your confidence, mood and relationships.

APPENDIX 3.B

GUIDELINES FOR NURSES ON THE USE OF AND ADMINISTRATION OF SODIUM AUROTHIOMALATE IN RHEUMATOID ARTHRITIS

What is Sodium Aurothiomalate?

Sodium Aurothiomalate (intramuscular gold) belongs to the group of drugs known as slow-acting anti-rheumatic drugs (SAARDs). These drugs suppress clinical and laboratory markers of disease activity and are thought to slow the progression of the disease but the precise mode of action is unknown. Unlike non-steroidal anti-inflammatory drugs (NSAIDs) which produce an immediate therapeutic effect, SAARDs are unlikely to produce any benefit before 12 weeks and often take as long as 24 weeks before improvement is attained.

Indications for Using Sodium Aurothiomalate

Sodium aurothiomalate is used in cases of active rheumatoid arthritis.

Contraindications

Females who are pregnant or are breastfeeding should not be given intramuscular gold. Likewise those who have gross renal or hepatic disease, history of blood dyscrasias, exfoliative dermatitis or systematic lupus erythematosus.

Administration and Dosage of Sodium Aurothiomalate

The drug is given by deep intramuscular injection, followed by gentle massage of the area. An initial test dose of 5−10 mg is usually given and if there are no adverse reactions (skin rash or hypersensitivity), weekly injections of 20−50 mg are administered until a response occurs. Most patients will feel no benefit until they have received a total dose of 500 mg−800 mg. Once in remission and providing they do not experience any side effects, patients are usually maintained on a dose of 50 mg administered monthly, but the physician may vary the dose according to the activity of the disease. If no major improvement has occurred after reaching a total dose of 1000 mg (excluding the test dose) the treatment is usually discontinued, although sometimes weekly injections of 100 mg for five weeks are given.

Adverse Reactions

Side effects occur in approximately 30% of patients and can appear at any time during the course of the treatment, even after the patient has been successfully treated with sodium aurothiomalate for many years. They are mostly mild, but up to 5% experience severe reactions which are potentially fatal.

Skin

Skin reactions are perhaps the most common of the side effects to intramuscular gold and are usually mild, However, if they do develop, the injection should be withheld and their presence should always be reported to the physician as they may be the forerunners to severe gold toxicity. This side effect occurs most commonly after a total cumulative dose of 300—400 mg.

Rashes may be localized or general and range from minor reactions to major skin lesions. They can mimic almost any skin eruption.

Pruritus or 'itching' is quite common and is often first felt between the fingers.

Mucous Membranes

Stomatitis and mouth ulcers can develop in some patients. Pharyngitis should raise the question of leucopenia. Patients sometimes complain of a metallic taste in the mouth which although unpleasant is not a permanent side effect.

Blood

Thrombocytopenia, neutropenia, agranulocytosis and fatal marrow suppression can develop but the latter is rare. Bruising, particularly around the shins, can be the first indication of thrombocytopenia. A fever and sore throat can indicate the presence of agranulocytosis.

Eosinophilia may be an indication of developing toxicity but does not always necessitate stopping gold.

The drug manufacturer recommends that a full blood and platelet count is taken before each injection is given and this should be meticulously adhered to. These results should be recorded sequentially. A sudden fall in platelet or white cell count outside normal limits may be reason for the physician to suspend treatment. A fall on three consecutive occasions, even if within normal limits, should also be reported as the physician may wish to suspend or modify the treatment.

Blood dyscrasias are most likely to happen when between 400 mg and 1000 mg of intramuscular gold has been given but can occur at any time during treatment.

Kidney

Proteinuria develops in about 10% of patients but is severe in less than 2%.

A gradual increase in protein concentration is more significant than a single result and so, if protein is detected, do not give the gold but ask the patient to return a few days later for a retest. If the protein persists, consult the physician and it may be necessary to estimate the amount of protein excreted in 24 hours by a more accurate measure than use of dipsticks.

If blood and protein are present, eliminate the possibility of a urinary infection by collecting a midstream urine specimen; if the MSU is negative, the physician may decide to stop the gold.

Rarer Side Effects

Rarer side effects include peripheral neuritis, alopecia and colitis. A small number of patients may experience flushing, nausea or vertigo after an injection.

THE NURSE'S RESPONSIBILITY WHEN GIVING SODIUM AUROTHIOMALATE

Before beginning the gold injections, you should discuss the treatment with the patient. This should include an explanation of what the treatment is for, how it is to be given, how the treatment will help and what side effects may occur. It is also important to make sure that the patient knows where the treatment and monitoring will take place, and who they should contact if they are unable to attend or if they experience any problems. It is always helpful to provide written information to the patient as a backup to this verbal explanation.

Before Each Injection

- Inspect the skin for rashes and ask if any pruritus has been experienced.
- Ask the patient if they have experienced any soreness of the throat, developed mouth ulcers or loss of taste.
- Ascertain that blood has been taken for a full blood count.
- Check that the prescribing doctor has seen and approved the results of the previous blood tests.
- Inspect the skin for bruising.
- Inquire if the patient has experienced any undue bleeding such as epistaxis or bleeding gums.
- Ask the patient if they are experiencing any flu-like symptoms.
- Record the dose given, haematology and urinalysis results, the presence of any unwanted effects and any action taken on the patient's gold card.

If the monitoring reveals any adverse effects, withhold the gold and report the symptoms to the doctor.

REFERENCES

Adamson, R.H. and Seiber, S.M. (1981) Chemically induced leukaemia in humans. *Environmental Health Perspective*, **39**, 93–103.

Alarcon, G.S., Kremer, J.M., Macaluso, M. *et al.* (1997) Risk factors of methotrexate induced lung injury in patients with rheumatoid arthritis. A multicentre case control study. Methotrexate lung study group. *Annals of Internal Medicine*, **127**, 356–64.

Alarcon, G.S., Tracy, I.C. and Blackburn, W.D. (1989) Methotrexate in rheumatoid arthritis: toxic effect is the major factor in limiting long term treatment. *Arthritis and Rheumatism*, **32**, 671–6.

Amos, R., Pullan, T., Bax, D. *et al.* (1986) Sulphasalazine for rheumatoid arthritis: toxicity in 774 patients monitored for 1–11 years. *British Medical Journal*, **293**, 420–3.

Arluke, A. (1980) Judging drugs: patients' conceptions of therapeutic efficacy in the treatment of arthritis. *Human Organisation*, **39**, 84–7.

Arthur, V. and Clifford, C. (2004a) Rheumatology: a study of patient satisfaction with follow up monitoring care. *Journal of Clinical Nursing*, **13**, 325–31.

Arthur, V. and Clifford, C. (2004b) Rheumatology: the expectations and preferences of patients for their follow up monitoring care: a qualitative study to determine the dimensions of patient satisfaction. *Journal of Clinical Nursing*, **13**, 234–42.

Bacon, P. (1987) Vasculitis – clinical aspects and therapy. *Medical Scandinavian Supplement*, **715**, 157–63.

Bailey, J.J., Black, M.E. and Wilkin, D. (1994) Specialist outreach clinics in general practice. *British Medical Journal*, **308**, 1083–6.

Baker, G.L., Leahl, L.E., Zee, B.C. *et al.* (1987) Malignancy following treatment of rheumatoid arthritis with cyclophosphamide long term case control follow up study. *American Journal of Medicine*, **83**, 1–9.

Barnyl, A., Dieppe, P., Haslock, I. and Shipley, M.E. (1990) What do rheumatologists do? A pilot audit study. *British Journal of Rheumatology*, **29**, 295–8.

Barrett, C.W. and Thomas, J. (1992) Shared care the way forward. *Hospital Update Plus*, **18**, 7–10.

Bax, D. and Amost, R. (1986) Sulphasalazine in rheumatoid arthritis; desensitising the patient with a skin rash. *Annals of the Rheumatic Diseases*, **450**, 139–400.

Benjamin, S.J., Ishale, K.G., Zimmerman, H.J. *et al.* (1981) Phenylbutazone liver injury: a clinical pathologic survey of 23 cases and review of the literature. *Hepatology*, **1**, 255–63.

Benner, P. (1984) *From Novice to Expert. Excellence and Power in Clinical Nursing Practice*, Addison-Wesley Publishing Company, California.

Berg, K.J., Frre, O., Djseland, O. *et al.* (1989) Renal side effects of high and low cyclosporin A doses in patients with rheumatoid arthritis. *Clinical Nephrology*, **31**, 232–8.

Birnie, G., Mcleod, T. and Watkinson, G. (1981) Incidence of sulphasalazine induced male infertility. *Gut*, **22**, 452–5.

Bond, M., Bowling, A., Abery, A. *et al.* (2000) Evaluation of outreach clinics held by specialists in general practice in England. *Journal of Epidemiology of Community Health*, **54**, 149–56.

Bradley, L.A. (1989) Adherence with treatment regimes among adult rheumatoid arthritis patients: current status and future directions. *Arthritis Care and Research*, **2**, 33–9.

Brennan, J. (1996) In practice managing osteoporosis care of the elderly. *Geriatric Medicine*, **26** (6), 1–2.

Bridges, S., Lopez, M. *et al.* (1991) Should Methotrexate be discontinued before elective orthopaedic surgery in patients with rheumatoid arthritis? *Journal of Rheumatology*, **18**, 984–8.

British Society of Rheumatology. (1992) Guidelines and audit measures for the specialist supervisor of patients with rheumatoid arthritis. Joint working group with the Royal College of Physicians. BSR, London.

Bryan, C. (1995) Practice nursing – the study of the role. *Nursing Standard*, **9** (17), 25–9.

Buxton, J., White, M. and Osoba, D. (1998) Patients experience using a computerised program with a touch sensitive video monitor for the assessment of health quality of life. *Quality of Life Research*, **7**, 513–9.

Cannon, W., McCall, S., Cole, B.C. *et al.* (1990) Effects of indomethacin, cyclosporin, cyclophosphamide and placebo on collagen induced arthritis of mice. *Agents and Actions*, **29**, 315–23.

Cannon, G.W., Ward, J.R., Clegg, D.O. *et al.* (1983) Acute lung disease associated with low dose pulse methotrexate therapy in patients with rheumatoid arthritis. *Arthritis and Rheumatism*, **26** (10), 1269–74.

Champion, G., Graham, G. and Zeigler, J. (1990) The gold complexes, in *Slow Acting Anti-Rheumatic Drugs and Immunosuppressives. Ballieres Clinical Rheumatology* (ed. P. Brookes), Balliere Tindall, London, pp. 491–534.

Chapuy, M.C., Arlot, M.E., Duboeuf, F. *et al.* (1992) Vitamin D3 and calcium to prevent hip fractures in elderly women. *New English Journal of Medicine*, **327**, 1637–42.

Clarke, P., Tugwell, P., Bennett, K. and Bombardier, C. (1989) Meta-analysis of injectible gold in rheumatoid arthritis. *Journal of Rheumatology*, **16**, 442.

Clegg, D.O., First, D.E., Toleman, K.G. and Bogue, E. (1989) Acute reversible hepatic failure associated with methotrexate treatment of rheumatoid arthritis. *Journal of Rheumatology*, **16**, 1123–6.

Cook, R. (1996) Urinalysis: ensuring accurate urine testing. *Nursing Standard*, **10** (46), 49–53.

Crisp, A.J., Armstrong, R.D., Grahame, R. *et al.* (1982) Rheumatoid lung disease, pneumothorax and eosinophilia. *Annals of Rheumatic Disease*, **41**, 137.

Daltroy, L.H. (1993) Doctor–patient communication in rheumatological disorders, in *Psychological Aspects of Rheumatic Disease. Balliere's Clinical Rheumatology* (eds S. Newman and M. Shipley), Balliere Tindall, London pp. 221–39.

Dargie, J. and Procter, L. (1993) Arthritis clinics in practice, *Practice Nurse*, 1–14 June, 144–8.

Day, R. (1994) Pharmacologic approaches SAARD I, in *Rheumatology* (eds J. Klippel and P. Dieppe), Mosby Year Book Europe limited, London, Section 3, p. 8.1–10.

Donovan, J. (1991) Patient education and the consultation – the importance of lay beliefs. *Annals of Rheumatic Diseases*, **50**, 418–21.

Donovan, J.L., Blake, P.R. and Fleming, W.G. (1989) The patient is not a blank sheet: lay beliefs and their relevance to patient education. *British Journal of Rheumatology*, **28**, 58–61.

Dougados, M., Awada, H. and Amor, B. (1988) Cyclosporin in rheumatoid arthritis: a double blind placebo controlled study in 32 patients. *Annals of the Rheumatic Diseases*, **47**, 127–33.

Elderman, J., Davis, P. and Owen, E.T. (1983) Prevalence of eosinophilia during gold therapy for rheumatoid arthritis. *Journal of Rheumatology*, **10**, 121–3.

Emery, P., Cannon, G., Holden, W. *et al.* (2002) Results from a cohort of over 40, 000 rheumatoid arthritis patients: adverse event profiles of leflunomide, methotrexate and other DMARDS. *Annals of Rheumatic Disease*, **61 (Suppl. 1)**, 42.

Erra, A., Tomas, C., Barcelo, P., Vilodill, M., Marsal, S. (2003) Is the recommended dose of leflunomide the best regimen to treat rheumatoid arthritis patients? *Rheumatology*, **42**, 1123−4.

Farr, M., Scott, D. and Bacon, P. (1986) Side effect profile of 200 patients with inflammatory arthritis treated with sulphasalazine. *Drugs*, **32 (Suppl.)**, 49−53.

Feinman, J. (1997) Fellow travellers. *Nursing Times*, **93** (42), 44−5.

Fernandes, L., Sullivan, S., McFarlene, J.G. *et al.* (1979) Studies on the frequency and pathogenesis of liver involvement in ra. *Annals of Rheumatic Diseases*, **38**, 501.

Frust, P.E. and Clements, P.J. (1994) Pharmacologic approaches SAARD II, in *Rheumatology* (eds J. Klippel and P. Dieppe), Mosby Year Book Europe limited, London, Section 3, 9.1−10.

Fuhrman, C., Parrot, A., Wislez, M. *et al.* (2001) T cell rates in lymphocytic alveolitis associated with methotrexate induced pneumonitis. *American Journal of Respiratory Critical Care Medicine*, **164**, 1186−91.

Furst, D.E. (1988) The basis for variability of response to anti-rheumatic drugs, in *Anti Rheumatic Drugs. Ballieres Clinical Rheumatology* (ed. P. Brooks) Balliere Tindall, London, 395−424.

Ganley, C.J., Paget, S.A. and Reidenberg, M.M. (1989) Increased renal tubular cell excretion by patients receiving chronic therapy with gold and with non steroidal anti-inflammatory drugs. *Clinical Pharmacology and Therapeutics*, **46**, 51−5.

Gardener, D.L., Duthme, J.R., Macleod, J. *et al.* (1957) Pulmonary and digital arteries. *Scottish Medical Journal*, **2**, 183.

Golding, D. (1981) *Problems in Arthritis and Rheumatism*, FA Davis Company, Philadelphia.

Grennan, D., Gray, J., Loudon, J. and Fear, S. (2001) Methotrextae and early postoperative complications in patients with rheumatoid arthrits undergoing elective orthopaedic surgery. *Annals of Rheumatic Disease*, **60**, 214−7.

Grove, M.L. and Hassell, A.B. (2001) Adverse reactions to DMARD in clinical practice. *Quantitive Journal Medicine*, **94**, 309−19.

Hall, C.L., Jawad, S., Harrison, P.R. *et al.* (1988) Natural course of penicillamine nephropathy. A long term study of 33 patients. *British Medical Journal*, **296**, 1083−6.

Harris, S., Watts, N. and Jackson, R. (1993) Four year study of intermittent cyclic etidronate treatment of post menopausal osteoporosis. *American Journal of Medicine*, **95**, 557−67.

Havelock, M. (1998) Audit of compliance of monitoring of slow-acting anti-rheumatic and cytotoxic agents in rheumatology outpatients. Conference presentation Royal College of Nursing Rheumatology Forum, Bath, March.

Helliwell, P. (1996) Comparison of a community clinic with a hospital out-patient clinic in rheumatology. *British Journal of Rheumatology*, **35**, 385−8.

Helliwell, P. and O'Hara, M. (1995) An audit of DMARD monitoring in rheumatoid arthritis. *British Journal of Rheumatology*, **34**, 673−5.

Henderson, A. (1994) Power and knowledge in nursing practice. *Journal of Advanced Nursing*, **20**, 935−9.

Hernadez, L.A., Rowan, R.M., Kennedy, A.C. *et al.* (1975) Thrombocytosis in RA: a clinical study of 200 patients. *Arthritis and Rheumatism*, **6**, 635.

Hewlett, S., Mitchell, K., Haynes, J. *et al.* (2000) Patient-initiated hospital follow-up for rheumatoid arthritis. *Rheumatology*, **39**, 990−7.

Higgins, C. (1996) Leucocytes and the value of the differential count test. *Nursing Times*, **92** (20), 34−5.

Hill, J. (1992) A nurse practitioner rheumatology clinic. *Nursing Standard*, **7** (11), 35−7.

Hill, J. (1994) An evaluation of the effectiveness safety and acceptability of a nurse practitioner in a rheumatology outpatient clinic. *British Journal of Rheumatology*, **33**, 283−8.

Hill, J. (1997) Patient satisfaction in a nurse led rheumatology clinic. *Journal of Advanced Nursing*, **25** (2), 347−54.

Hopkin, R. (1990) Sans awareness. *Nursing Times*, **86** (30), 50−1.

Jones, K., Lane, D., Holgate, S. and Price, J. (1991) A diagnostic and therapeutic challenge. *Family Practice*, **8**, 97−9.

Jones, K. and Patel, S. (2001) Family physician's guide to monitoring methotrexate. American Acadamy of Family Physicians, www.aafp.org.2001

Joyce, D. (1990) D-Pencillamine, in *Slow Acting Ant Rheumatic Drugs and Immunosuppressives. Ballieres Clinical Rheumatology* (ed. P. Brooks), Baillere Tindall, London, pp. 553−74.

Kahn, M.F., Arlet, J., Block-Mitchel, J. *et al.* (1979) Acute leukaemias after treatment with cytotoxic drugs in rheumatology. *Nouvelle Press Medical*, **8**, 1393−7.

Kaplan, R.L. and Waite, D.H. (1978) Progressive interstitial lung disease from prolonged methotrexate therapy. *Archives of Dermatology*, **114**, 1800−2.

Kay, A. (1979) Myelotoxicity of D-penicillamine. *Annals of the Rheumatic Diseases*, **38**, 232−6.

Kay, A. (1986) European league against rheumatism study of adverse reactions to D-penicillamine. *British Journal of Rheumatology*, **25**, 193−8.

Kay, A. (1989) Monitoring of slow acting remission inducing drugs. *British Journal of Rheumatology*, **28**, 239−41.

Kay, A. and Puller, T. (1992) Variations among rheumatologists in prescribing and monitoring of disease modifying anti-rheumatoid drugs. *British Journal of Rheumatology*, **31**, 477−83.

Kinder, A. and Hassell, A.B. (2005) The treatment of inflammatory arthrits with methotrexate in clinical practice: treatment duration and incidence of adverse drug reactions. *Rheumatology*, **44**, 61−6.

Kinlen, L.J., Sheil, A.G.R., Peto, J. and Doll, R. (1979) Collaborative United Kingdom − Australian study of cancer in patients treated with immunosuppressive drugs. *British Medical Journal*, **2**, 1461−6.

Kleerekoper, M., Peterson, E.L. and Nelson, D.A. (1991) A randomised trial of sodium fluoride as a treatment for post menopausal osteoporosis. *Osteoporosis International*, **1**, 155−61.

Klein, R. (1974) *Notes Towards a Theory of Patient Involvement*, Canadian Public Health Association, Ottawa, Canada.

Kowal, A., Carstens Jr, J.H. and Schinitzer, T.J. (1990) Cyclosporin in rheumatoid arthritis, in *Immunomodulators in the Rheumatic Disease* (eds D.E. Furst and M.E. Wenblatt), Marcel Dekker, New York.

Kremer, J.M. and Joong, K.L. (1986) The safety and efficacy of the use of methotrexate in long term therapy for rheumatoid arthritis. *Arthritis and Rheumatism*, **29**, 822−31.

Lanyon, P., Pope, D. and Croft, P. (1995) Rheumatology education and management skills in general practice: a national study of trainees. *Annals of Rheumatic Disease*, **54**, 735−9.

Le Gallez, P. (1988) Teratogenesis and drugs for rheumatic disease. *Nursing Times*, **81** (27), 41−4.

Lee, S.J., Lenert, L. and Kavanaugh, A. (2004) Internet-based monitoring of patients with rheumatoid arthritis. *Clinical and Experimental Rheumatology*, **22**, S34−8.

Leonard, P.A., Bienz, S.R., Clegg, D.D. and Ward, J.R. (1987) Haematuria in patients with rheumatoid arthritis receiving gold and penicillamine. *Journal of Rheumatology*, **14**, 55−9.

Levine, M.E. (1973) *Introduction to Clinical Nursing*, FA Davis Company, Philadelphia.

Leyland, M.J., Cunningham, J.L., Delamore, I.W. and Price, D.A. (1974) A pharmacokinetic study of phenylbutazone-associated hypoplastic anaemia. *British Journal of Haematology*, **28**, 142−3.

Liang, M.H. (1989) Compliance and quality of life: confessions of a difficult patient. *Arthritis Care and Research*, **2**, 71−4.

Lim, A.Y.N., Gaffney, K. and Scott, D.G.I. (2005) Methotrexate induced pancytopenail: serious and under reported? Our experience of 25 cases in 5 years. *Rheumatology*, **44**, 1051−5.

Lockie, L.M. and Smith, D.M. (1988) Forty seven years experience with gold therapy in 1,019 rheumatoid arthritis patients. *Seminars in Arthritis and Rheumatism*, **14**, 238−46.

Lorig, K., Konkol, L., Gonzalez, V. *et al.* (1987) Arthritis patient education: a review of the literature. *Patient Education and Counselling*, **10**, 207−52.

Luqmani, R.A., Palmer, R.G. and Bacon, P.A. (1990) Slow acting anti-rheumatic drugs and immunosuppressives, in *Ballieres Clinical Rheumatology* (ed. P. Brooks), Balliere Tindall, London, pp. 595−620.

Maddison, P., Kiely, P., Kirkham, B. *et al.* (2005) Leflunomide in rheumatoid arthritis: recommendations through a process of concensus. *Rheumatology*, **44**, 280−6.

Malin, N. and Teasdale, K. (1991) Caring versus empowerment consideration for nursing practice. *Journal of Advanced Nursing*, **16**, 657−62.

Martin, J., Meltzer, H. and Eliot, D. (1998) *The Prevalence of Disability Among Adults*, Office of Population Censuses and Surveys, London.

Matteson, E.L., Cohen, M.D. and Conn, D.L. (1994) Rheumatoid arthritis clinical features and systemic involvement, in *Rheumatology* (eds J. Klippel and P. Dieppe), Mosby Year Book Europe Limited, London, Section 4, 4.1−8.

Memel, D.S. and Kirwan, J.R. (1999) General Practitioners' knowledge of functional and social factors in patients with rheumatoid arthritis. *Health and Social Care in the Community*, **7** (6), 387−93.

Mooney, J. (1996) Audit of rheumatology nurse outreach clinics. *Rheumatology in Practice*, **Winter**, 18−20.

Newman, S., Fitzpatrick, R., Revenson, T. *et al.* (1996) *Understanding Rheumatoid Arthritis*, Routledge, London.

Norgard, B., Czeizel, A.E., Rockenbauer, H. *et al.* (2001) Population based case control study of the safety of sulfasalazine use during pregnancy. *Alimentary Pharmacology Therapy*, **15**, 483−6.

O'Brien, W.M. and Bagley, G.F. (1985) Rare adverse reactions to non-steroidal anti-inflammatory drugs. *Journal of Rheumatology*, **12**, 785−90.

Oka, M. and Vainio, U. (1966) Effects of pregnancy on the prognosis and serology of rheumatoid arthritis. *Rheumatology Scandinavia*, **12** (47), 7.

Oppenheim, J.J., Koacs, E.J. and Matsushima, M. (1986) There is more than one interleukin - 1. *Immunology Today*, **7**, 45−56.

Ortiz, Z., Shea, B., Almazor, M. *et al.* (2000) Folic acid and folinic acid for reducing side effects in patients receiving methotrexate for rheumatoid arthritis. *Cochrane Database Systematic Review*, **2**, CD0000951.

Palmer, R.G. and Denman, A.M. (1984) Malignancies induced by chlorambucil. *Cancer Treatment Reviews*, **11**, 121−9.

Parrish, R.S., Franco, A.E. and Schur, P.H. (1971) Rheumatoid arthritis associated with eosinophilia. *Annals of Internal Medicine*, **75**, 199.

Peel, N., Eastell, R. (2004) Osteoporosis, in *ABC of Rheumatology* (ed. M.L. Snaith), 3rd edn, British Medical Journal Books, London.

Penny, W.J., Knight, R.K., Rees, A.M. *et al.* (1982) Obliterative bronchiolitis in RA. *Annals of Rheumatic Diseases*, **41**, 469.

Phelan, M.J., Byrne, J., Campbell, A. and Lynch, M.F. (1992) A profile of the rheumatology nurse specialist in the United Kingdom. *British Journal of Rheumatology*, **31**, 858−9.

Pincus, T., Olsen, N.J., Russel, J.I. *et al.* (1990) Multicentre study of recombinant human erythropoietin in correction of anaemia in rheumatoid arthritis. *American Journal of Medicine*, **89**, 161−8.

Potts, M.K., Mazzuca, S.A. and Brandt, K.D. (1986) Views of patients and physicians regarding the importance of various aspects of arthritis treatment. Correlations with health status and satisfaction. *Patient Education and Counselling*, **8**, 124−5.

Pounder, R., Craven, E., Henthorn, J. and Bannatyne, J. (1973) Red cell abnormalities associated with sulphasalazine maintenance therapy for ulcerative colitis. *Gut*, **16**, 181−5.

Powell, J. (1991) Reflections and the evaluation of experience prerequisite for therapeutic practice, in *Nursing as Therapy* (ed. R. McMahon), Chapman and Hall, London, pp. 26−42.

Puller, T., Hunter, J. and Capell H.A. (1987) Sulphasalazine and hepatic transaminases. *Annals of the Rheumatic Disease*, **46**, 421−4.

Recker, R.R., Karpf, D.B. and Quan, H. (1995) Three year treatment of osteoporosis with alendronate effects on vertebral fracture incidence. Abstracts of the 77th Annual Meeting of the Endocrine Society, Washington DC.

Reid, I.R., Ames, R.W. and Evans, M.C. (1993) Effects of calcium supplementation on bone loss in postmenopausal women. *New English Journal of Medicine*, **328**, 460−4.

Richardson, A. (1992) Rheumatoid arthritis in pregnancy. *Nursing Standard*, **6** (45), 25−8.

Roberts, C., Adebajo, A.O. and Long, S. (2002) Improving the quality of care of musculoskeletal conditions in primary care. *Rheumatology*, **41**, 503−8.

Rossman, M. and Bertino, J.R. (1973) Azathioprine. *Annals of Internal Medicine*, **79**, 694−700.

Ryan, S. (1995) Nutrition and the rheumatoid patient. *British Journal of Nursing*, **4** (3), 132−6.

Ryan, S. (1996) Living with rheumatoid arthritis: a phenomenological exploration. *Nursing Standard*, **10** (41), 45−8.

Ryan, S. (1997) Nurse led drug monitoring in the rheumatology clinic. *Nursing Standard*, **11** (24), 45−7.

Ryan, S., Hassell, A.B., Lewis, M. and Farrell, A. (2006) A study into the impact of the expert nurse on the patients attending a drug monitor clinic. *Journal of Advanced Nursing*, **53** (3), 277−86.

Ryan, S. and Hill, J. (2004) A survey of practice in nurse led rheumatoid arthritis clinics. *Rheumatology*, **43** (2), 411.

Sambrook, P.N., Browne, C.D., Champion, G.D. *et al.* (1982) Terminations of treatment with gold sodium thiomalate in rheumatoid arthritis. *Journal of Rheumatology*, **9**, 932−4.

Samuels, B., Lee, J.C., Engleman, E.P. *et al.* (1977) Membranous nephropathy in patients with RA: relationship to gold therapy. *Medicine*, **57**, 319.

Saravanan, V. and Kelly, C.A. (2004) Reducing the risk of methotrexate pneumonitis in rheumatoid arthritis. *Rheumatology*, **43**, 143−7.

Schilsky, R.L., Lewis, B.J., Sherins, R.J. and Young, R.C. (1980) Gondal dysfunction in patients receiving chemotherapy for cancer. *Annals of Internal Medicine*, **93**, 109−14.

Segal, R., Yaron, M. and Tartakowsky, B. (1990) Methotrexate: mechanism of action in rheumatoid arthritis. *Seminars in Arthritis and Rheumatism*, **20**, 190−9.

Shiroky, J.B., Yodum, D.E., Wilder, R.L. and Klippel, J.H. (1989) Experimental basis of innovative therapies of rheumatoid arthritis, in *Therapy of Autoimmune Diseases* (eds J.M. Cruse and R.E. Lewis), Karger, Basel.

Sigworth, L. (2004) Practice development: an important component of the clinical nurse specialist role. *Musculoskeletal Care*, **2** (1), 72−3, (letter).

Smith, P. (1992) *The Emotional Labour of Nursing*, Macmillan, Worcerster.

Stein, HB, Schroder, M.L. and Dillion, A.M. (1986) Penicillamine induced proteinuria. Risk factors. *Seminars in Arthritis and Rheumatism*, **15**, 282−7.

Storm, T., Thamsborg, G., Steiniche, T. *et al.* (1990) Effects of intermittent cyclical etidronate therapy on bone mass and fracture rate in women with postmenopausal osteoporosis. *New English Journal of Medicine*, **322**, 1265−71.

Talaro, K. and Talaro, A. (1993) *Foundations in Microbiology*, Dublique IO Brown.

Thierry, F.X., Verner, I., Dueymas, J.M. *et al.* (1989) Acute renal failure after high dose methotrexate therapy. *Nephrology*, **51**, 416−7.

Thompson, P.W., Morgan, C.J. and Fletcher, S. (1992) Rheumatology monitoring clinics, in *The Course and Outcome of Rheumatoid Arthritis. Ballieres Clinical Rheumatolgy* (ed. D.L. Scott), Balliere Tindall, London, pp. 95−116.

Thorne, C., Urowitz, M.B., Wanless, I. *et al.* (1982) Liver disease in Felty's syndrome. *American Journal of Medicine*, **73** (1), 35−40.

Thorne, P. and Russell, R. (1973) Diabetic clinics today and tomorrow; mini clinics in general practice. *British Medical Journal*, **2**, 534−6.

Thwaites, C. (2004) Rheumatology telephone advice lines. *Musculoskeletal Care*, **2** (2), 120−6.

Tones, K. (1991) Health promotion − empowerment and the psychology of control. *Journal of the Institute of Health Education*, **29 (1)**, 17−25.

Tugwell, P., Bombardier, C., Gent, M. *et al.* (1990) Low dose cyclosporin versus placebo in patients with rheumatoid arthritis. *Lancet*, **335**, 1051−5.

Tydd, T. and Dyer, N. (1976) Sulphasalazine lung. *Medical Journal of Australia*, **1**, 570−3.

UKCC (United Kingdom Central Council for Nursing Midwifery and Health Visiting). (1992) *The Scope of Professional Practice*, UKCC, London.

UKCC (United Kingdom Central Council for Nursing Midwifery and Health Visiting). (1993) *Standards for Records and Records Keeping*, UKCC, London.

Velikova, G., Wright, E.P., Smith, A.B. and Cull, A. (1999) Automated collection of quality of life data. A comparison of paper and computer touch screen questionnaire. *Journal of Clinical Oncology*, **17**, 998−1007.

Vn Ede, A.E., Laan, R.F.J.M. and Rood, M.J. (2001) Effects of folic or folinic acid supplementation on toxicity and efficacy of methotrexate in rheumatoid arthritis: a fourty eight week, multi-center, randomised, double-blind, placebo controlled study. *Arthritis Rheumatism*, **44**, 1515−24.

Walker, D. (1994) Outreach clinics: a consultant replies. *Rheumatology Practice*, **1**, 6−8.

Watt, N.B., Harris, S.T. and Genart, H. (1990) Intermittent cyclical etidronate treatment of postmenopausal osteoporosis. *New English Journal of Medicine*, **323**, 73−9.

Wilke, W.S. and Mackenzie, A.H. (1986) Methotrexate therapy in rheumatoid arthritis: current status. *Drugs*, **32**, 103−13.

Williams, J.H., Wilkins, R.F., Sameulson, C.O. Jr *et al.* (1985) Comparison of low dose oral pulse methotrexate and placebo in the treatment of rheumatoid arthritis. A controlled clinical trail. *Arthritis and Rheumatism*, **28**, 721−300.

Wilson Barnett, J. (1984) Key functions in nursing. The Fourth Winifred Raphael Memorial Lecture, Royal College of Nursing, London.

Wolf, R. (1997) Shared care recording in community care. *Nursing Times*, **93** (28), 2−3.

Yan, A. and Davies, P. (1990) Gold induced marrow suppression: a review of 10 cases. *Journal of Rheumatology*, **17**, 47−51.

Zarday, Z., Ueith, F.J., Gleidman, M.L. and Sobeman, R. (1972) Irreversible liver damage after azathioprine. *Journal of the American Medical Association*, **222**, 690−1.

4 Patient Education and Adherence with Drug Therapy

JACKIE HILL

Learning Objectives

After reading this chapter you should be able to:

- Define patient education.
- Underpin practice with appropriate theoretical models.
- Describe the role of the nurse in patient education.
- Select suitable topics and methods of delivering patient education.
- Compile written information sheets.
- Discuss interventions that enhance adherence to medication regimes.
- Assess the effectiveness of a patient education programme.

It may not be immediately obvious why a book about drug therapy should contain a substantial section on patient education. Drug therapy plays a major role in the management of many rheumatic diseases, but therapeutic benefit is achieved only if the patient actually takes the prescribed drugs. Non-adherence, also known as non-compliance, is a common problem associated with a variety of factors, one of which is lack of knowledge. Amongst its other attributes, patient education addresses this knowledge deficit and enables patients to make informed decisions about their management. A partnership approach to decision making between the practitioner and the patient not only empowers the patient, it also encourages them to adhere to their medication regime as they are in part responsible for the choice of treatment.

4.1 DEFINITIONS OF PATIENT EDUCATION

The term patient education has been used for many years, but the process that we know as patient education is not static and has evolved over time. These changes have inevitably led to alterations in the definition of patient education. Pre-1970s definitions concentrated on the transfer of information about the body and its workings from physician to the patient. However, it became apparent that the biomedical model of care, in which a person's health is considered to be the responsibility of health professionals and the public health system, requiring little contribution from the individual patient, has little to offer those with chronic disease (Callahan and Pincus, 1997). This led to a change of emphasis during the 1970s

Drug Therapy in Rheumatology Nursing: Second Edition. Edited by Sarah Ryan.
© 2007 John Wiley & Sons, Ltd.

and the focus on information transfer changed to that of 'self care' (Levin, 1986). As the process progressed definitions incorporated extended information transfer and promoted self-responsibility (Lindroth, Bauman and Daltroy, 1998).

In the United States the task force of the National Arthritis Advisory Board has developed a set of standards for arthritis patient education, which defines it as:

> organized learning experiences designed to facilitate voluntary adoption of behaviours or belief conducive to health. It is a set of planned educational activities that are separate from clinical patient care. The activities of a patient education program must be designed to attain goals the patient has participated in formulating. The primary focus of these activities includes acquisition of information, skills, beliefs and attitudes which impact on health status, quality of life, and possibly healthcare utilization (Burckhardt, 1994).

Lorig (1996) has pointed out that modern definitions of patient education make no mention of improving knowledge. Activities aimed at improving knowledge are *patient teaching* and she thereby makes a distinction between this and patient education. However, in practice, teaching patients and increasing their knowledge of their disease and treatments is an integral part of an effective patient education programme.

Patient education has evolved into a complex process and it is suggested that the simplest working definition is a modified version of that stated by Lorig (1996): 'any set of planned educational activities designed to improve the patient's health behaviours and through this their health status and ultimately their long term outcome' (Hill, 1997).

4.2 USEFUL THEORIES AND MODELS

The mention of theories can deter many nurses, but theory can aid our practice by providing a very helpful insight as to why particular procedures work. A theory can be defined as a set of hypotheses related by logical argument to explain connected phenomena in general terms. Theories do not tell us what to do or how to do things but they can help to guide best practice. Models are based on theories and act as a skeletal framework on which to build. They have practical use as they provide a formal structure that serves as an *aide-mémoire*, thus helping to ensure consistency of practice.

The most successful patient education programmes are those that are underpinned by a combination of theories and models (Lorig, 1996). The most difficult part is choosing that which is most appropriate for the client group!

A number of theories are relevant to patient education, in particular those that originate in the fields of:

- adult education;
- communication;
- sociology;
- psychology.

Each has something to offer and perhaps the most successful programmes are those which incorporate something from each.

One of the underlying aims of patient education is to bring about health-enhancing behaviours and so theories and models that are grounded in behaviour change are particularly appropriate. Many experts working in the field of patient education advocate a working knowledge of the following:

- learned helplessness theory;
- stress and coping theory;
- health belief model;
- self-efficacy theory.

LEARNED HELPLESSNESS THEORY

Seligman (1975) developed the learned helplessness theory in 1975. His research with animals showed that those that received repeated electric shocks subsequently became helpless and unresponsive, however they reacted to them. This work was later adapted to human behaviour, and implies that believing that one has no control over one's life leads to feelings of increased helplessness and depression. An example would be a patient who has rheumatoid arthritis for whom many of the slow acting anti-rheumatic drugs have produced severe side effects or have been non-efficacious. They begin to expect all subsequent drug therapy to fail and so do not feel it worth adhering to their treatment regimes. Repeated failure leads them to doubt their ability to control their disease and so they come to believe that their actions can have no effect on their eventual health status. This leads to a passive state leaving them unwilling or unable to make behavioural changes. Patients who enter this state of 'learned helplessness' show the characteristics of:

- lack of cognition;
- poor motivation;
- inaction.

STRESS AND COPING THEORY

One of the key elements of nursing is to help patients to cope with their illness (Wilson Barnett, 1984). This is particularly relevant when nursing patients with rheumatic diseases, as these are chronic, incurable, potentially disabling and life-altering. It almost inevitable that these patients experience stress and coping deficits and so stress and coping theory is relevant to rheumatological patient education.

Lazarus and Folkman (1984) have described coping as 'a set of cognitive and behavioural responses to events perceived as stressful'. Humans constantly change their cognition and behaviours to enable them to manage specific external and/or internal demands that they see as taxing or exceeding their resources. As new situations arise, their response changes, and coping strategies will only be employed if the person feels that the threat is a danger to them.

Each person perceives a given situation differently; what is a stressor or threat to one person may not worry his or her neighbour. This is evident when patients with RA are offered disease-modifying drugs and are told of the potential side effects. Some patients are keen to try them whatever the hazards, whilst others see the side effects as more problematic than their disease. The patient's appraisal of what comprises a 'stressor' and their individual response to it is an important factor to be borne in mind when delivering a patient education programme. The educational activities must be relevant to the individual patient, or they will not be acted upon.

Executing Stress and Coping Theory

There is an abundance of literature on coping (Lazarus and Folkman, 1984; Newman, 1993, Newbold 1996). Lazarus and Falkman (1984) have identified eight discrete methods:

- confronting;
- distancing;
- self-control;
- seeking social support;
- accepting responsibility;
- escape-avoidance;
- problem solving;
- positive reappraisal.

These and others are discussed in more detail by Lorig (1996, pp. 208–111). Newbold (1996) suggests that patients tend to cope in two distinct ways, using problem-focused and emotion-focused coping strategies.

- *Problem-focused coping strategies* are based on the acquisition of knowledge about the stressor. This encourages the belief that the stressor can be controlled and its effect modified, avoided or minimized.
- *Emotion-focused coping strategies* are based on the elimination of any undesirable feelings which follow on from the experience of the stressor (Auerbach, 1989).

Coping strategies should be an inherent part of patient education programmes, but they need to be tailored to the individual concerned. Their effectiveness should be assessed and, if they are not shown to meet the patient's needs, new strategies should be explored.

HEALTH BELIEF MODEL

This is one of the oldest and most widely used educational models, originally hypothesized by Becker (1974). It postulates that an individual's behaviour is based on a combination of the perception of threat and the expectation of benefit.

Patients will only change their behaviour if they believe that:

- They are susceptible to threat and that the threat has severe consequences; or
- A new behaviour will be beneficial, they are capable of carrying out the behaviour change and the cost does not outweigh the benefits.

The respect, intimacy and reciprocity within the nurse—patient relationship enables the nurse to perceive the patient as a unique individual each with his or her own knowledge, belief values and experience. These three aspects must be incorporated into any system of care, including patient education programmes. People who have rheumatic diseases are usually adults whose own experience is one of their major resources and, in general, they do not accept advice unless it is justifiable and makes sense to them. It is therefore inappropriate to apply didactic learning and teaching models developed to pass knowledge from teacher to child; a more interactive patient—practitioner model is advocated as being the most successful when working with adults.

The patient's perceptions are paramount and must be considered when choosing a model. This was highlighted in a study carried out in 1989 in which only 6 out of 32 patients adhered to the number of drugs prescribed by their GP. The other 26 compared their perceptions of the potential side effects and efficacy with their symptoms, and made their own judgement on the required dosage. The study recommended a shift of emphasis from didactic programmes to more informal methods of patient education (Donovan, Blake and Fleming, 1989).

SELF-EFFICACY THEORY

Self-efficacy refers to a person's confidence in their ability to perform a specific task or achieve a particular objective (Bandura, 1977). Self-efficacy is a dimension of the cognitive part of social learning theory. Social learning theory postulates that the interplay between physiological, social/physical environment and the individual's cognition of their disease results in health-enhancing behaviours (Bandura, 1986).

Those people who exhibit a high degree of self-efficacy believe that what they do can make a positive difference. This is especially important in the context of patient education, as increases in self-efficacy are thought to bring about increases in appropriate health behaviours and health outcomes (Davis, Busch and Lowe, 1994; Lorig and Holman, 1993; Taal et al., 1993).

Patients who demonstrate a high degree of self-efficacy, when confronted with a stressor, are more likely to maintain a positive sense of well-being and so undertake constructive coping strategies. They are also more likely to be motivated and expend large amounts of effort on their task and persist with it. However, self-efficacy is behaviour-specific. For instance a patient may believe that they can control their pain, but have little expectation of controlling their sleep pattern. This is highlighted by Strecher et al. (1986) who points out that self-efficacy is not an independent personality characteristic; the individual's expectation of efficacy will vary according to the task that confronts them. It is therefore inappropriate to characterize individuals as high or low exhibitors of self-efficacy. There is no such thing as an *efficacious person*!

It is important to understand the difference between a person's outcome expectation and their self-efficacy expectation. Taal, Rasker and Wiegman (1996) describe them in the following manner:

- *Outcome expectation* refers to a person's estimate that a recommended behaviour will have a beneficial effect.
- *Self-efficacy expectation* refers to beliefs in one's ability to successfully execute the behaviour required to produce a desired outcome.

For instance, a patient with rheumatoid arthritis may believe that exercise will improve the outcome of their disease, but they may also have serious doubts about their ability to carry out the exercise. In this scenario, it is unlikely that the patient's behaviour will change even though they believe that the exercise would help them.

It is crucial to emphasize that it is the individual's *perception* of their self-efficacy skills rather than their actual capabilities that are important. Bandura (1986) has stated that 'perceived self-efficacy is a significant determinant of human functioning that operates partially independently of underlying skills'.

CHANGING SELF-EFFICACY

Changes in self-efficacy can bring about changes in:

- behaviour;
- cognitive-related states such as anxiety, depression and pain.

This makes it very relevant to patient education programmes designed for those with a rheumatic disease.

It is possible to improve a person's expectation of their self-efficacy and four efficacy-enhancing mechanisms have been described by Bandura (1986). They are:

- mastery of skills;
- modelling;
- social persuasion;
- reinterpretation of physiological state.

MASTERY OF SKILLS

Mastery is successfully achieving proficiency in a skill, and successful mastery is a powerful tool with which to enhance self-efficacy. Failure undermines self-efficacy and so it is essential that the patients perceive skills as attainable. The attainment of new skills is best approached in a 'one step at a time' fashion. For instance, breaking a large task into smaller more manageable tasks, starting with those that the patient is confident of completing, helps to increase the patient's expectations of self-efficacy. An example would be obese patients who want to lose weight but are afraid that they cannot stick to a weight-reducing diet. If they are confident that they can reduce the amount of sugar they take in their tea by half, this would be a reasonable starting point. Once they have successfully accomplished this task, then they can proceed, perhaps by reducing the amount of fat in their diet.

Making written contracts with themselves often encourages patients to make changes in their behaviour patterns (Lorig and Gonzalez, 1992). Although the health professional can gently guide the patient, the most successful contracting is essentially patient-driven.

Performance feedback is an important factor in attaining mastery (Bandura and Cervone, 1983). Positive feedback and suggested changes if poor progress is made can greatly improve skills. Patients are more likely to complete their contract when they are given this kind of encouragement. Feedback needs to be undertaken in a systematic manner and it is suggested that each session could begin with an update of progress.

Contracting and feedback are considered of such importance that Goeppinger and Lorig (1996) suggest that up to 30% of the time allotted to an educational programme should be spent on these subjects.

MODELLING

Patients often compare themselves with others who have the same disease. They make statements such as 'I feel a fraud when I come to the clinic and see all those other patients whose disease is much worse than mine'. This trait can be used to positive advantage within the realms of patient education. Other patients, who have experienced similar problems and overcome them successfully by behavioural changes, can be used as role models. Modelling is particularly useful for group education and can be adapted for use in a number of different ways. For instance the Arthritis Self-Help Programme (Lorig *et al.*, 1985) uses specially trained lay instructors who have some form of arthritis to lead groups, as it is believed that they exhibit a powerful and positive influence. Patients can also be asked to talk to classes and share their experience of their arthritis. Groups led by a health professional can ensure that the members of the class act as a support group and help each other. For example, discussing patient problems within the group allows individuals to contribute from their personal experience, thereby reinforcing the patients' position as 'experts' and helping them towards a feeling of mastery. If the stated problem is new and has not been experienced by other group members, the health professional should offer guidance.

There are however a number of caveats with modelling:

• Do not choose a model that is dissimilar to the group. Goeppinger and Lorig (1996) suggest that the age, sex, ethnic origin and socioeconomic status of the group and the model should be closely matched.

- Do not choose models that exhibit spectacular achievements; this will only make others feel inadequate. It is better to choose someone to whom the group feels they can relate and that they can emulate.

PERSUASION

Persuasion can have a strong influence on self-efficacy. It emanates from many different sources including arousal of fear, social influences and communication. Health professionals commonly use communication as a source of persuasion; gentle verbal persuasion often convinces patients that they are capable of improving their performance. Having reached their goals, patients may be urged to raise their sights and make further advances but it is important not to become overenthusiastic. Goal-setting should be realistic, as patients are more likely to be persuaded that they can reach their target if it is set just slightly higher than their present performance.

REINTERPRETATION OF PHYSIOLOGICAL STATE

People who have a rheumatic disease endure a number of physiological symptoms such as pain, stiffness and fatigue. Patients frequently interpret these symptoms as signs that they are managing their disease poorly and are therefore using ineffective coping mechanisms. This belief is compounded because some efficacious behaviour, such as undertaking an exercise regime, can cause the same symptoms; following exercise, the patient feels more pain, stiffness and fatigue. Patients need to 'know their body' so that they can differentiate between the symptoms of their disease and their reaction to their treatments. The nurse can play a major role in this area by identifying the patient's beliefs and then helping them to reinterpret where necessary.

4.3   PURPOSE OF PATIENT EDUCATION

The principal purpose of patient education is to improve the patient's health status and so ultimately their outcome. However, for some patients this aim is unobtainable, and in these cases preservation of the status quo or slowing of deterioration should be seen as a reasonable alternative.

Improvement in the health status of those with a chronic rheumatic disease is heterogeneous and complicated, making it unlikely that any single treatment will bring about maximal improvement in health status or outcome. For instance, successful DMARD therapy may improve the patient's symptoms and physical well-being but will not replace any loss or reduction of range of motion or muscle bulk. The best outcome is achieved when treatments are combined and the patient self-manages their disease and patient education equips them to make the necessary changes to their behaviours and to adjust their attitudes. This can be difficult as disease activity can vary dramatically from day to day and so it is important that patients can tailor their therapies accordingly (Hill, 1995). To be effective patient education needs to address a variety of different situations. As well as being able to vary their drug usage according to their symptoms, patients must learn to:

- employ positive coping strategies;
- regulate their daily exercise programmes;
- plan their rest and activity periods.

4.4 LIMITATIONS OF PATIENT EDUCATION

Patient education is not a universal panacea. Although the majority of studies have shown that patient education can change behaviour and increase health status, the literature is not entirely consistent (Lorig, Konkol and Gonzalez, 1987). Even when behaviour changes occur they do not automatically lead to changes in health status, any more than increased knowledge automatically leads to changes in behaviours.

Patient education is an enhancer that magnifies the effects of other therapies. The ultimate success or failure in terms of health status and outcome is dependent upon the inherent effectiveness of the treatment employed (Hill, 1997). A patient may take a particular drug unfailingly, but if the drug is therapeutically ineffective, there will be no change in health status.

Effective self-management relies upon the patient's willingness to cooperate and their ability to comply with self-care activities and so patient education

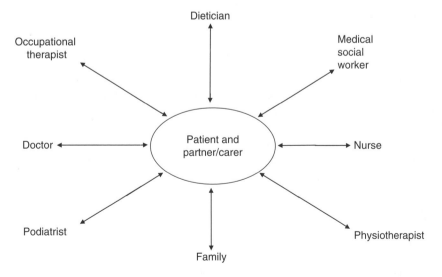

Figure 4.1 The combined multidisciplinary team.

is a combined effort between the multidisciplinary team, the patient and their partner/carer (Figure 4.1). However, not all patients are willing to self-manage even when they have undertaken a patient education programme.

4.5 ROLE OF THE NURSE IN PATIENT EDUCATION

Patient education is one of the key elements of rheumatology nursing (Hill, 1995) and its importance is widely acknowledged (Hill, 2006). Although patient education is not an explicit part of the majority of conceptual or theoretical frameworks used by nurses, Vaughan (1991) suggests that it is implicitly intertwined with many nursing models. The ability to self-care as advocated by Orem (1980) could not be achieved without the sharing of information and belief in self-efficacy. Similarly, Roper, Logan and Tiernay's (1985) ideas of maintaining independence cannot be achieved without the provision of patient education, and it is fundamental to Roy's model of adapting to stresses (1976). Whichever model the nurse decides to use, patient education will be at the core of it.

PATIENT EDUCATION AND SOME FUNDAMENTAL ASPECTS OF NURSING

In whatever setting nurses find themselves, there are a number of underlying beliefs that underpin the care they provide. These are:

• nursing is a therapeutic activity;
• the nurse−patient relationship is reciprocal;
• the nurse−patient relationship is one of 'professional closeness'.

PATIENT EDUCATION AND THERAPEUTIC NURSING

Therapeutic nursing can be described as those nursing activities that result in a movement towards health. McMahon (1991) provides a list of therapeutic activities that can be used as a framework for therapeutic nursing which includes patient teaching as one of its components (Table 4.1). Nurses using this therapeutic model when carrying out the wide-ranging role of administering, advising and monitoring the patient's drug therapy are likely to provide a better outcome for their patients than those who do not.

RECIPROCITY

Reciprocity is the act of mutual exchange and in the context of nursing reflects the belief that the nurse−patient relationship is beneficial to the nurse as well as the patient. Reciprocity is a key concept of nursing and an important aspect to encompass when engaged in the sphere of patient education. If we believe that

Table 4.1 Therapeutic activities in nursing (adapted from McMahon, 1991).

Developing the nurse/patient relationship:
  partnership
  intimacy
  reciprocity

Adapting the environment:
  interpersonal
  physical

Patient education:
  providing information
  promoting self-efficacy
  encouraging behavioural changes
  fostering coping mechanisms

Providing comfort:
  psychological
  physical

Complimentary interventions:
  massage
  aromatherapy

Tested physical treatments:
  leg ulcers
  pressure sores

patients are the experts on how well or ill they feel, their perception and acceptance of pain levels and their knowledge of whether or not a therapy is therapeutic, then we must also acknowledge that we health professionals can learn from the experience of our patients. This reciprocal learning can enhance the process of patient education if both parties act as both teacher and learner throughout their encounters. The incorporation of the patient's unique expertise into the nursing repertoire and the imparting of this knowledge to other patients will help to solve both current and future problems and develop understanding for future practice.

PROFESSIONAL CLOSENESS

Peplau (1969) used the phrase 'professional closeness' over 30 years ago in an attempt to differentiate between the way in which peers learn together and the symbiotic learning that takes place in the nurse–patient relationship. Patients often describe their feelings about their relationship with their nurse by phrases such as 'you are not just my nurse, I feel as though you are a friend'. These feelings stem from the empathy that the nurse exhibits, and this empathy is an important aspect of the educational process. Professional closeness allows the patient to feel safe and share their innermost emotions and fears. Many patients will ask questions of the nurse that they are reluctant to put to doctors; 'Will this drug affect my sex life?' or 'Can it cause impotence?' The skilled nurse can then help patients to learn about themselves and teach them how to deal with their problems. Professional closeness is an important aspect of care, but it can also become a burden to the less-experienced nurse. The imperative is to meet the needs of the patient and the close relationship that develops should not be mistaken for interpersonal closeness where the needs of professional and patient are mutual.

4.6 PLANNING A PATIENT EDUCATION PROGRAMME

Although the emphasis of this book is drug therapy, it is inappropriate to concentrate on this one topic when considering a suitable programme of patient education. Indeed, the findings of Lee and Tan (1979), who studied drug adherence in 108 patients with rheumatoid arthritis, suggest that knowledge of the disease itself has more influence on adherence with drug therapy than knowledge of the medication. It is therefore necessary to contemplate the whole gamut of educational topics and try to bias them towards drug therapy. In addition to the educational content, you will also have to consider:

- the learning environment;
- demographic factors;
- the type of programme;
- teaching aids;
- the length and timing of the programme.

THE LEARNING ENVIRONMENT

The environment in which patient education takes place must be conducive to learning. It should therefore be:

- quiet;
- warm and well ventilated;
- well lit;
- comfortable.

The more disabled patients may use wheelchairs or walking aids, and so easy access is essential. A mixture of seating should be available, as their partners or carers often accompany patients. Raised chairs and perching stools may also be necessary.

Patient education requires people to master new facts and ideas and this is difficult when there are physical distractions such as pain or joint stiffness. Patients in pain will have shortened attention spans so ensure that refreshment is close at hand in case they need to take any drugs whilst attending the session. Sessions longer than 45 minutes should include short breaks that allow patients to exercise, so reducing the risk of inactivity stiffness occurring.

DEMOGRAPHIC CONSIDERATIONS

Patients with rheumatic diseases are of all age groups, come from every social and cultural background and have all levels of educational ability. In fact often the only factor they have in common is that they have a rheumatic disease. When giving one-to-one patient education this is not a problem as the patient education programme can be tailored to the individual. However, if group teaching is anticipated, this lack of homogeneity inevitably raises the question of whether to segregate patients according to disease duration, age, diagnosis and educational ability.

DISEASE DURATION

Many people ask whether it is acceptable to teach newly diagnosed patients along-side those who have had their disease for many years. Those who have only recently been diagnosed are often confused about their illness and can be anxious and depressed. It can be counterproductive to sit them alongside someone who is clearly physically disfigured or whose psychological status is poor. Likewise, the patient with long disease duration may have taken many different drugs during their illness career, some of which may have been ineffective or caused side effects. Many patients are quick to relate any problems to their peer group! This would present an improper picture to a newly diagnosed patient and would surely exacerbate anxiety or depression. However, bear in mind that using other patients as role models can be a powerful stimulus and creates a very positive image of patient education. It's all a question of balance and selection of a suitable role model.

The problem of mixing patients with widely differing disease duration has changed over the last few years as drug therapies such as the new biologics have vastly improved the outcome of patients (White and Bryer, 2006). The management of diseases such as rheumatoid arthritis has also changed dramatically, with DMARDs being introduced at a far earlier stage in the disease process, before physical joint damage has occurred. However, the best solution is to teach newly diagnosed patients in a separate group but to include within the team a patient who has had the disease for some time and is a good role model.

AGE RANGE

The pressure for group patient education sessions to be segregated according to age often comes from the younger age groups who see their problems as being very different from those of the middle-aged and elderly. They worry about their sexual image, marriage and family prospects and employment expectations, and many do not see these topics as being relevant to those older than they are. These fears are understandable and real and as far as is practicable need to be taken into account.

DIAGNOSIS

Teaching patient education programmes to patients with different types of arthritis is possible and works well in the form of the Arthritis Self Help Programme. There are however some topics which are easier to adapt than others. For instance, patients who have RA, osteoarthritis or AS can be taught the elements of pain control such as rest and the application of heat or ice in the same group. When discussing the types of drug therapy that affect pain, some such as analgesics, NSAIDs and intra-articular injections would also be suitable to all. However, DMARDs are not appropriate for those with osteoarthritis, and are of limited use in AS. Specific exercises are another area that can cause confusion. The vigorous exercises recommended for someone with AS are very different from those advocated for a person with RA and so teaching about this topic would be better segregated by diagnosis.

MIXED EDUCATIONAL ABILITY

Successful patient education requires patients to learn a lot about both arthritis and about themselves and some patients find this easier than others. There is substantial evidence of an association between higher levels of education and knowledge of arthritis (Hill et al., 1991; Kaplan and Kozin, 1981; Moll, 1986). Other research has shown that a lower level of formal education is one of the predictors of mortality over a five-year period (Fries et al., 1980; Pincus et al., 1989). It is possible to teach mixed ability classes and there are several techniques that will help:

- assess which participants will need additional help;
- persuade patients to set their own outcome agendas;
- check that participants understand what they have been told and ask them to reiterate;
- encourage those who have difficulty understanding to attend with a partner;
- teach memory aids to those who are forgetful.

THE TYPE OF PROGRAMME

There are a number of types of patient education programme and many have been shown to be successful. They can be delivered either informally, as is the case with opportunity education or more formally as group sessions; in fact many patients receive a mixture of both. The programmes can be taught by either health professionals or lay persons and the sessions can be given on an individual or group basis (Table 4.2). Each method has advantages and disadvantages and each patient will have his or her own preference. Whatever form the programme takes, it is important that the patients are provided with feedback about their performance, being careful to stress the most positive aspects first.

Table 4.2   Types of patient education programme.

Mode of delivery	Taught by	Method
Individual/one-to-one	Single health professional	Formal
Group	Team of health professionals	Formal
Arthritis self management programme	Lay persons and health professionals	Formal
Opportunity education	Health professionals	Informal

4.7   INDIVIDUAL PATIENT EDUCATION

Patient education programmes need to be accessible to the patient. One of the easiest and most convenient routes is when the patient's routine clinic consultation includes a patient education session as part of the normal management package. This is undertaken in some areas of the country and research has shown this approach is both practical and effective (Mahmud *et al.*, 1995).

One-to-one teaching is perhaps the most common way in which specialist nurses deliver patient education regarding drug therapy. This often occurs when patients are referred to nurse-led clinics for monitoring of efficacy and side effects following changes to disease-modifying drugs. One of the most noteworthy aspects of one to one teaching is its flexibility. Although the programme will need to planned, it can be tailored to the specific patient and so include topics that are important to the individual. This method of delivery also allows patient education to proceed at the pace and order of topic dictated by the patient. Before the patient education programme can begin you should:

• explore the patients' preferences about their drug therapy;
• assess their knowledge of drugs;
• establish shared goals;
• discuss any preferred method of information transfer.

PREFERENCES OF DRUG THERAPY

Before starting any drug treatment it is necessary to explore the patient's perceptions and feelings about their drug therapy. Examine some of the practical implications:

Number of Drugs to be Taken

Some patients are happy to take any amount of drugs; others are very wary of any pharmacological intervention. This needs to be explored. If a patient requires a NSAID and is worried about taking 'a lot of drugs', they could be prescribed a medication with a long half life such as piroxicam, which only needs to be taken daily. Drugs with a short half-life, such as ibuprofen, need to be taken three or four times daily to remain in the band of efficacy.

The Size and Formulation of Tablets

Some tablets are rather large and difficult to swallow and for those patients who have problems associated with rheumatic disease, such as Sjögren's syndrome, or oesophageal strictures this can be a major obstacle.

Memory Failure

Some patients find it difficult to remember to take their drugs regularly. This is particularly so in the case of DMARDs as they do not provide immediate effect. Drugs taken daily may be more appropriate for a forgetful patient than those taken less frequently.

Needle Phobia

Needle phobia can pose a real problem and those who suffer from it would feel that injectable gold or methotrexate is an inappropriate option. This is also problematical when patients need careful haematological monitoring if potentially toxic drug therapy has been prescribed.

Side Effects

Side effects are the major question in the minds of many patients. Time spent at an early stage discussing any adverse effects and how to deal with problems can be very advantageous to both the patient and the nurse. Patients value the time spent talking with the nurse and this helps to build up the nurse–patient relationship at an early stage.

All these topics need careful discussion and consideration if patients are to adhere to their treatments.

ASSESS THE PATIENTS' KNOWLEDGE OF DRUGS

The initial interview will enable the nurse to assess what the patients know, or think they know, about drug therapy. This may sound demeaning, but it is not. There is evidence that patients have trouble distinguishing between the types of drug treatment. A study that highlighted this lack of knowledge (Hill *et al.*, 1991) showed there were divergent beliefs about the role of NSAIDs, which are probably the most common of all therapies. Out of a total of 70 patients with rheumatoid arthritis, 15 (21%) believed wrongly that they took many weeks to start working and 11 patients thought they acted as DMARDs and stopped the disease from progressing. Approximately 30% thought NSAIDs such as diclofenac, ibuprofen and indomethacin could induce remission. The majority of patients were taking analgesics; 36% thought these should take with food, and 33% believed that analgesics should only be taken for severe pain. The findings of this study were in keeping with other research (Kay and Punchak, 1988; Mahmud et al., 1995).

Assessing knowledge can be undertaken informally by discussion and questions, or formally, using a questionnaire such as the Patient Knowledge Questionnaire (Hill et al., 1991), or for those with early RA a questionnaire devised by Hennell, Brownsell and Dawson (2004). Obtaining the information by questionnaire has the advantage of producing numerical data that is easier to use as a comparator when assessing the effectiveness of teaching. Having made an assessment of the patient's knowledge base, this will act as a guide as to what knowledge deficits need to be addressed.

ESTABLISHING SHARED GOALS

Following the initial assessment, the next stage is to establish some shared goals. Bear in mind that a skilled nurse can manipulate a patient education session to include her or his own agenda alongside that of the patient. For instance, if the patient prefers to discuss pain and the nurse perceives the need to teach about drug therapy, incorporating an explanation of the effect of analgesics, NSAIDs and DMARDs will serve to meet both ends!

When establishing goals one of the roles of the nurse is to use professional skill to guide the patient and ensure that their goals are realistic. This is only possible if the nurse has adequate pharmacological knowledge. Reaching the goals is important to the ongoing process, and it is at this stage that patients should start to set down a written contract with themselves. The nurse can give further encouragement by following up the visit by a phone call to enquire if they are having any problems with their drugs and achieving their goals. It is also an opportunity to offer practical advice if they are not.

PREFERRED METHOD OF INFORMATION TRANSFER

Patients like everyone else have their preferred methods of learning. Some like written material, some would prefer visual or audio aids such as videos and cassettes and others like face-to-face communication. These methods will be discussed in detail later in the chapter, but the important point is to discuss this issue with the patient. In reality, many patients will be given verbal instruction through discussions, and written material or aids will back this up.

Having established this information, the patient education programme can commence. The format of individualized programmes is flexible, but it is still important to agree some kind of schedule with the patient. When structuring each session, make sure that you leave plenty of time to incorporate feedback of progress at the start of each session and time to set new contracts at the close.

CONTRACTING

Contracting usually consists of three basic steps. The patient decides:

- what activity they wish to accomplish in a given time;
- what their plan of action will be;
- whether the contract is realistic.

THE ACTIVITY TO BE ACCOMPLISHED

This is the first step of the contract and although the nurse initiates the contract, the patients should always choose the activity themselves. It is crucial that the contract is undertaken in a very positive manner and the nurse can help by encouraging the patient to use positive expression such as 'I will take my ibuprofen with food' rather than 'I will *try* to take. . . '

THE PLAN OF ACTION

The plan of action is the key to success. It should state exactly:

- what the patient will do;
- how often they will do it;
- when they will do it.

For instance, patients on penicillamine who keep forgetting to test their urine may make a contract that states that they will test their urine once each week on Saturday morning at 9 a.m. They will do this each week for the four intervening weeks before their next clinic appointment. They may decide to jog their memory by placing a note in a prominent position on Friday evening to remind them to save their urine specimen. Once they get into the weekly habit it becomes a routine part of their life.

CHECKING THAT THE CONTRACT IS REALISTIC

This is the third and final stage of contracting. Once the patient has decided on a particular behaviour they wish to change and made their plan, they should be asked, 'How certain are you that you can achieve your aim?' This should be followed up by a further question. 'If I ask you how certain you are that you can do what you say by giving it a score between 1 to 10, 1 is feeling very unsure and 10 being totally certain, how would you score it?'

Few patients have any difficulty with this scoring concept, but if they do it is worth trying a percentage approach (0–100%). You can be reasonably certain they are confident in their ability if they say between 7 and 10 or 70–100% sure of their abilities. If they perceive difficulties they will score less than 7 (70%), and if this is the case, it is important to explore the reasons for their uncertainty and discuss the problems that they foresee. Counselling skills can be helpful in this situation. Try to get the patients to offer their own solutions, but be prepared to provide help if it is needed.

Once the patient is sure that they have set an achievable objective the contract should be set down in writing. Having completed the contract and asked the patient if they would like to discuss anything else, the session should be closed with an overview of what has occurred during the consultation, and a review of the activities they have agreed to undertake before their next visit.

Having completed the session, it is important to document what has been discussed and agreed to. This will help to provide a clear picture of what has been accomplished and what still remains.

Although one-to-one patient education is labour-intensive and therefore costly, a number of studies have demonstrated that individualized patient education programmes are more effective than rigid routine-type programmes (Lorish, Parker and Brown, 1985; Neuberger et al., 1993; Tucker and Kirwan, 1989). It is therefore suggested that this format be used wherever it is practicable.

4.8   TEACHING IN GROUPS

Many hospitals and community groups have set up structured patient education programmes to be taught to groups of patients, rather than individuals. This method of teaching is becoming very popular, as it can reach greater numbers of patients and is less labour intensive than individualized programmes. However, like any other method it has both positive and negative aspects (Table 4.3). It may be that some skills such as different methods of joint protection, limbering up exercises and relaxation techniques can be taught to groups of patients very effectively. Those patients who have particular problems requiring individual attention need to be given special consideration, and even in a group situation they may require individual time. A generalized overview of the different types of drug therapies can be useful, but those who are embarking on a specific therapy are better catered for in a one to one teaching session.

Table 4.3   Differing aspects of group teaching.

Positive aspects	Negative aspects
Cheap	Wide range of knowledge
Effective way of teaching skills e.g. OT/PT	Different rates of learning
Patients meet others with same disease	Discrepancies in levels of skill
Share experiences and resolutions	Some patients are poor articulators
Social interchange	Difficult to express feelings in a group
Powerful role models	Fear of failure or criticism

It should be remembered that different people join groups for different reasons. Group participation can be a very positive experience from which many people benefit both medically and socially, and there is some evidence that patients learn substantial amounts from each other. Indeed one study found that patients attributed the greatest benefit of attending a group programme was learning from and teaching each other (Campbell *et al.*, 1995).

Unfortunately, there will always be those whose expectations are not met, and the best way to counteract this is to be very specific at the outset about who the programme is aimed at and what it is intended to achieve.

4.9   OPPORTUNITY EDUCATION

Patient education does not have to be undertaken in a formal and predestined manner and every patient encounter should be treated as an opportunity to teach (Daltroy and Liang, 1988). Short, unplanned meetings often take place, for instance:

- at the patient's bedside;
- in outpatient clinics;
- in GP surgeries.

These short encounters can yield positive results in the hands of a skilled practitioner. A patient who is given a new drug can be asked a simple question such as, 'When are you going to take your tablet?' This will highlight any problems, such as whether they realize that it should or should not be taken with food. The ensuing conversation can then be guided in a different direction. For instance, if they are taking a NSAID at lunchtime, it is quite natural to endorse the fact that, to prevent side effects, it should not be taken on an empty stomach. Interactions with other drugs can also quickly be broached.

4.10   THE ARTHRITIS SELF-MANAGEMENT PROGRAMME

Chronic diseases are the greatest cause of disability and escalating medical expenditure in the US (Colvez and Blanchet, 1981), the arthritic diseases being the greatest cause of disability in the elderly (Lorig, Konkol and Gonzalez, 1987). Greater longevity results in a proliferation of certain types of arthritis such as osteoarthritis, and its prevalence magnifies the social and economic consequences. Lorig and her colleagues in the USA developed the Arthritis Self-Management Programme (ASMP) in the late 1970s with the intention of reaching as many patients as possible at an affordable price. It is a community-based programme taught to people with almost any form of arthritis during the same programme of six two-hourly sessions over a period of months (Lorig, 1996). It pioneered the use of lay teachers, many who had arthritis, in preference to health professionals to lead the programmes.

As it has developed and research results have emerged, it has incorporated new ideas and ideologies (Hirano, Laurent and Lorig, 1994; Lorig and Gonzalez, 1992). For instance most programmes are now taught by one health professional and one lay teacher rather than by two lay teachers. As predicted, lay teachers have proved as effective as professionals in their teaching skills and are accepted by both patients and professionals (Lorig *et al.*, 1986).

It is likely that the success of the ASMP owes much to its underlying theoretical basis of self-efficacy, the patient's belief that he or she can affect the consequences of their disease. Perceived self-efficacy, discussed earlier in the chapter, is believed to be a significant determinant of human functioning that operates partially independently of underlying skills.

The topics taught in the ASMP are similar to those of other programmes. However, its authors recognized that imparting knowledge does not necessarily bring about changes in behaviour, but that behaviour changes must occur if patient education is to be of benefit. They therefore developed their programme with an emphasis on:

- problem-solving;
- development of coping skills;
- symptom management;
- utilization of information.

The ASMP has proved to be remarkably effective and is used extensively in the US, Australia, and Europe (Davis, Busch and Lowe, 1994; Lindroth *et al.*, 1989, 1995; Taal, Rasker and Wiegman, 1996; Taal *et al.*, 1993). It is currently being used in the UK by Arthritis Care and is advocated by the government in the form of the Expert Patient Programme. The latter programme is not disease-specific but a generalized chronic disease self-management programme (CDSMP) from which patients appear to gain great benefit. However, recent research by Lorig, Ritter and Plant (2005) has demonstrated that although both programmes provide positive results, the ASMP is more advantageous than the CDSMP for patients with arthritis and so this programme should be used when sufficient resources are available.

4.11 WHAT TO TEACH

Whether the patient education is formally or informally structured, there are a number of core subjects that need to be addressed at some stage. They should include those that patients have cited as wanting more information about (Bishop, Kirwan and Windsor, 1997) as well as those that health professionals think should be taught. A comprehensive programme should include:

- Disease process such as aetiology, symptoms, blood tests.
- Drug therapy: how to use drugs, their effects and side effects.

- Exercise: the effects and how, when and how often to exercise.
- Joint protection techniques: how and when to use splints and lifestyle alterations.
- Fatigue: its causes and how to conserve energy.
- Pain control: pharmacological and other techniques such as relaxation and distraction.
- Coping strategies: self-efficacy, contracting.
- Diet: its effects on health, fatigue.
- Relaxation: what it is, how it works and how to do it.
- Complementary therapies such as acupuncture, aromatherapy and massage.
- Communication: getting the best out of visits to doctors and health professionals.
- Self-help: knowledge of self-efficacy and approaching voluntary organizations.
- Goal-setting: how best to set achievable targets and reach them.

The list looks rather daunting and in the arc survey (Bishop, Kirwan and Windsor, 1997), some doctors expressed their concern that giving too much information about the diseases, drug treatment and its side effects could cause undue anxiety and stress. However, many patients are keen to know more (Ridout, Waters and George, 1986) as is their right, and so patient education programmes must endeavour to meet their aspirations.

TEACHING ABOUT DRUG THERAPY

The inclusion of a session about drug therapy in a patient education programme is one topic almost universally accepted. It is a subject that almost all patients ask questions about, and it is a topic which health professionals feel they should teach!

Rheumatic diseases are both chronic and unpredictable, which means that patients will need to tailor their drug regimes to meet their day-to-day needs. They can do this only if they have adequate knowledge (Hill, 1995). In addition to this unpredictability, patients who have a rheumatic disease usually require drugs from a number of different families either to alleviate their symptoms or, when feasible, to put their disease into remission. It is important that patients are able to distinguish between the different types of drug so that they can identify those drugs in which dosage:

- can be changed;
- can be safely stopped;
- must be continued.

Nurses usually teach patients about their medications verbally. However, the Association of the British Pharmaceutical Industry (ABPI) (1987) has offered guidance about medication information for patients, and they state that written information should be given as a reinforcing instrument. This advice is echoed by patients (Donovan and Blake, 1992) and health professionals alike (Arthur, 1995). There is some research to show that written information increases the patient's knowledge. A study by Hill and Bird (2003) showed significant increases in knowledge after patients had read a drug information leaflet. However, written information alone does not appear to provide sufficient benefit. This was highlighted in a recent literature review of the effectiveness of 'print only' interventions in increasing patient participation in chronic disease management. This study found that the benefits of written information alone were modest. Of the seven studies assessed, significant knowledge improvement occurred in three, adherence improved in two and quality of life declined in one (Harris, Smith and Veale, 2005). A combination of written information and verbal teaching appears to be more effective than either alone (Vignos, Parker and Thompson, 1976).

In addition the ABPI suggest that the written information should also be:

- brief and succinct;
- in a standardized layout;
- included in each medication pack;
- aimed at a reading age of nine years.

WHAT TO INCLUDE

Obviously the type of drugs that patients need to know about will depend on their diagnosis. The more complicated diseases like RA often necessitate the use of an analgesic, a NSAID and a DMARD. They may also require steroids in one of their many forms, oral iron, an additional pain modulator such as amitriptyline and, if they take methotrexate, supplements such as folic acid. This is in addition to drugs that they may be taking for other common health problems such as hypertension or cardiac disease.

Clearly someone taking a plethora of drugs will have a lot to learn and it is best to give information in small, manageable helpings as poor recall of information is an accepted problem. Anderson *et al.* (1979) has shown that verbal information is easily forgotten and that patients only recall about 40% of the information presented to them. It is therefore best:

- not to overwhelm patients with facts as they only remember the first four or five;
- to present the most important points first as they recall best what is said first;
- discuss the patient's priorities, as they will remember what they believe important;
- provide written back-up.

However, each drug needs to be discussed fully and the teaching sessions should include:

- the name of the drug;
- its purpose;
- how long it takes to work;
- dosage instructions;
- the timing of administration;
- how it should be taken;

- the duration of therapy;
- possible common side effects;
- what to do if side effects occur;
- interactions with other drugs;
- special precautions;
- a contact in case the patient has a problem.

This is rather a long list and bearing in mind the recall problems the most commonsense approach is to talk through a drug information leaflet such as the one shown in Appendix 4.A.

It is essential to ensure that patients understand that they have certain responsibilities when taking drugs that have the potential to cause life-threatening adverse effects. However, the point of the exercise is to inform rather than frighten and so it is imperative to ensure that patients feel supported by the nurse and feel free to contact them if they have a problem.

When teaching about drug therapy, ask questions to check that the patient understands what they are being told. For instance in the case of methotrexate:

- 'What day do you think that you will take it on?'
- 'What do you think the best time of day to take it will be?'
- 'When will you take your folic acid?'
- 'Which day will you be able to go to have your blood taken?'

These questions will give an indication as to whether the patient understands the implications. It is also a good idea to phone the patient after they have taken their first or second dose to see if they have remembered and to check that they have made arrangements for their safety bloods if they are being checked by the GP.

RISKS AND ADVERSE EFFECTS

One question that nurses ask is how much to tell the patient about risks and side effects. A survey undertaken in 1975 by Ascione and Raven (cited in Meichenbaum and Turk, 1987) showed that 75% of physicians did not wish patients to be told about the potential side effects of prescribed medication. The reason for this appeared to be the fear that patients would not adhere to their medications if they knew that they held risks. Today the climate has changed and the publication of the *Patient's Charter* and *The Health of the Nation* gives patients the right to information, which enables them to make an informed choice.

It would be impossible and counterproductive to tell patients about all the possible side effects to each drug that they take. The most reasonable approach is to discuss the most common adverse reactions, making sure that you are reassuring and teaching them how to prevent problems occurring. In the case of unpreventable adverse problems, such as thrombocytopenia, reassurance as to the effectiveness of surveillance and the reversion to the normal state after cessation of the drugs should be emphasized.

Another effective strategy is to stress the positive effects of the drug therapy, bearing in mind not to promise the earth! Remember the nurse can be a powerful persuader whose role includes giving advice, instruction and suggestions.

4.12 TEACHING AIDS

There are a number of techniques that will help to reinforce patient education. These include:

- written material;
- videos;
- audiocassettes;
- computer programmes.

Written Material

This has already been alluded to, but the importance of written information cannot be overemphasized. Drug information leaflets are invaluable, and patients themselves are aware of this (Donovan and Blake, 1992). There is also research evidence to show their worth in the community (Gibbs, Waters and George, 1989) and in the outpatients clinic (Hill and Bird, 2003). The results from these studies show that following receipt of an information leaflet, patients improved their knowledge of how to take their medications and their side effects. There is a wealth of written information already available, and organizations such as Arthritis Care and the Arthritis Research Campaign (arc) produce some excellent literature. However, many rheumatology departments still prefer to produce their own drug information leaflets, mainly because prescribing and monitoring practice varies from area to area. Producing this material is an art in itself and thought needs to be given to the:

- purpose of the material;
- intended recipient;
- cost of the exercise;
- quality of the finished product.

The Purpose of the Material

The purpose of a drug information leaflet is to inform and empower the patient, and enable them to share their information with their family and carers. As verbal information is easily forgotten, a hard copy acts as an *aide-mémoire* that can be kept and referred to as the occasion arises. Although patients find this information useful, it should be remembered that knowing and doing are different things. One can know that an analgesic drug can help to modulate pain, but this is not always enough of an inducement to take it! Informing patients by providing a drug information leaflet will not necessarily increase their adherence to their drug regimen. However, if this activity is a component of a patient education programme it will certainly help.

The Intended Recipients

One of the most important factors to consider when writing information is the readership. The majority of the population is not familiar with medical terminology and it is difficult to write patient literature without using it! However, it is possible providing the following guidelines are used (Boyd, 1987):

- keep the sentence structure simple;
- use one- or two-syllable words;
- paragraphs should be short;
- use lay language like 'feel sick' **not** 'nausea', or 'poor clotting' **not** 'thrombocytopenia'.

Always be as positive as possible, using positive rather than negative language. For instance 'do remember' is better than 'don't forget'. Personalizing the information also helps so, use words like I, we, us throughout the document. The format is also important. Most authors now use a question-and-answer format, such as that shown in the methotrexate leaflet in Appendix 4.A. Lastly and very importantly, include information that the patient wants to know as well as information that you feel they ought to know. Nurses should draw upon their experience with their patients to amass this information, but it may also be appropriate to undertake some interviews with patients of different ages and who have had their disease for differing lengths of time.

Reading Levels

The information presented should be written at a level that is understandable to the patient. People with rheumatic disease are not a homogeneous population; they come from a wide range of social and educational backgrounds. If the information is to be accessible to the majority of patients, it must be readable by those with poorer reading skills. This was highlighted in a recent research project in which 12 out of 100 patients surveyed in a rheumatology outpatient clinic were shown to have a reading ability of children aged $7^3/_4 - 13$ years (Hill and Bird, 2003). Although 88% the patients interviewed did not have problems with their reading, these 12% would have had difficulty with much of the information already in the public domain. Some nurses have expressed their doubts that pitching the material at those with lower reading skills will seem demeaning to those with higher abilities. Doak, Doak and Lorig (1996) are reassuring on this matter and state that both research and experience shows that adults find easy to read material is:

- preferable;
- easier to remember;
- faster to learn.

Assessing the Readability of Information

Once the information has been written, it is a good idea to assess its readability. The readability of a document refers to the reader's ability to decipher the text (Meade and Smith, 1991). There are a number of formulae that can be applied to the text that estimate the level of difficulty. The ease of reading depends upon the structure of sentences and the length of the words used. Reading formulae are therefore based upon the number of words in each sentence and the number of syllables in each word. Commonly used ones include:

- Flesch Reading Index (Flesch, 1948);
- Dale−Chall Formula (Dale and Chall, 1948);
- SMOG Grading (McLaughlin, 1969);
- Fry Formula (Fry, 1968).

There is little to choose between these formulae, so use the one most easily available to you. The more popular word processor packages have readability formulae installed in them, for instance Word for Windows has the Flesch Index. This formula was used to assess the methotrexate information leaflet (Appendix 4.A.) and showed it to be in the 'fairly easy' to read category. It is not necessary to test the readability of every word and sentence within a lengthy document. Indeed there is often considerable variation within most writings. It is usually sufficient to select two or three different sections of text. The Reference section at the end of this chapter lists sources of additional and more in-depth information on readability assessment.

Reading formulae are useful tools but they do not negate the need for good writing, and accurate information. However even well-written, easily read material is likely to end up in the waste bin if its layout is poor. The patient needs to be encouraged to read it and the use of an attractive, clear typeface will help. Consideration should also be given to those who have some difficulty with their eyesight and a minimum type size of 12 point is recommended. A cluttered and busy design is off-putting. It is much better to leave plenty of white space between lines and $1\frac{1}{2}$ or double spacing looks attractive.

Avoid using capital letters for headings, because it is more difficult to read. If you want something to stand out try using a different *style*, **bold** or larger type.

The Cost of the Exercise

Obviously cost has to be a consideration. Even a short drug information leaflet can be costly if you take into account the amount of time and effort put into preparing and producing it. If large numbers are required over a long period of time, it is important to make sure that you secure adequate funding into the future. Take into account that medications and any monitoring requirements may change and drug information needs to be reviewed frequently and updated as required.

The Quality of the Finished Product

The information available from agencies such as Arthritis Care and arc is of excellent quality in both content and appearance. It does not make sense to reinvent the wheel! It is only worth expending the time and energy needed to produce new written material if existing material is not suitable for the needs of your clients. It is always worth taking the time to review the material already published before embarking on the complicated task of producing your own.

VIDEOS AND CDs

Videotapes are largely extinct now and CDs are the modern replacement. They are an excellent adjunct to face-to-face teaching particularly for the teaching of skills such as exercise. Videos or CDs can be used at home or shown to groups and are excellent for those who have difficulty reading. They can also be used to demonstrate to patients or their relatives how to give injections. Some patients, particularly those who are in paid employment, find it difficult to attend a surgery to have gold or methotrexate injections. Being able to undertake this themselves not only saves them time; it enhances their feeling of independence. At present new drugs that require subcutaneous administration are being tested in clinic trials. There is no reason why patients cannot be taught to self-administer, and CDs demonstrating injection techniques are invaluable teaching aids.

AUDIOCASSETTES

Audiocassettes are an excellent method of providing information for patients who cannot read or are blind or partially sighted. They are in commonly used to teach relaxation techniques or distraction therapy. They are cheap, easily available and easy to use.

COMPUTER PROGRAMS

Computer-assisted learning has enormous potential, but even today not everyone has a computer. A suitably programmed computer can not only present information and demonstrate skills, it can also answer questions posed by patients. Some research undertaken in the USA showed that patients who used a computer to access a patient education program enjoyed it. They also gained more knowledge, improved their outlook on life, were more hopeful of a good prognosis and changed their behaviours when compared to a control group (Wetstone *et al.*, 1985). This type of program has also been advocated for use in the UK (Luker and Caress, 1989) as it allows the patient to access information in whatever order and time that they require it. This freedom of choice empowers the patient rather than the educator and will be seen by some nurses as a positive move towards self-care, but by others as a threat to their authority.

4.13   THE OPTIMUM TIMING OF PATIENT EDUCATION

The greatest reduction in disability may be achieved by early intensive intervention (DeVellis and Blalock, 1993) but there is a dichotomy within the realms of rheumatology about the ultimate time to commence patient education. There are occasions when sharing information at the wrong time can make the situation worse rather than better for the patient. For instance, the nurse may feel that the patient needs to know about drug therapy when the treatment begins. However this may be detrimental if the patient is in a state of grief or bereavement reaction that sometimes follows the confirmation of their diagnosis (Westbrook and Viney, 1982). Indeed Donovan, Blake and Fleming (1989) suggest that patient education at this stage can exacerbate a state of depression in the newly diagnosed patient. It may be better to use counselling sessions until the patient has accepted their illness and then proceed to patient information-giving (Hill, 1997). To be able to do this successfully, nurses need to develop the skills to enable them to be sensitive to the cues given out by the patient. The nurse then needs to know when the patient is ready to move on from the gathering information stage to the point where they are ready to make positive behaviour changes. The reason that this is important is that the results from research comparing the effects of information-giving, counselling and behavioural therapy show that only the latter demonstrate significant effects (Reimsma, Kirwan and Rasker, 2002). However, assessing readiness for change takes great skill as well as knowledge and understanding. This expertise takes a number of years to acquire and Benner (1984) has identified the acquisition of this kind of competence as that which transforms the nurse from a novice to an expert practitioner.

READINESS FOR CHANGE

Prochaska and DiClemente (1992) have ascertained that there are five stages of change:

- *Precontemplation* − when the patient is not seriously considering changing their behaviour. At this stage and the following contemplation stage, patients will need information about their disease and therapies as this will aid their decisions.
- *Contemplation* − the patient weighs up the apparent benefits and cost of behavioural change against the status quo.
- *Preparation* − once the decision to make a behavioural change has occurred, the patient develops their plan of action.
- *Making the change* − the patient actively develops skills and habits that enable them to undertake the behaviour regularly.
- *Maintenance* − this is the final stage in which the patient develops strategies to maintain long-term behaviour change.

Identifying which of the above stages the patient has reached can be an import factor in determining their participation in patient educational programmes (Keefe *et al.*, 2000).

There are a range of other approaches that the practitioner can use to facilitate positive behaviour changes and these are discussed at length in an excellent article by Hammond (2003).

4.14 PATIENT EDUCATION AND ADHERENCE

There is an extensive literature on patient adherence. Most is in agreement that many patients do not adhere to their medication regime as it is prescribed (Hill, 2005a). This is thought by many to be a major problem and has been cited as perhaps the most important cause of treatment failure (Henry, 1985). In 1984 a literature review estimated that at least 50% of patients with RA were non-adherent with their therapies, irrespective of the nature of the intervention (Belcon, Hayes and Tugwell, 1984). Other authors have estimated medication adherence to range from 30−70% (Donovan and Blake, 1992; Feinberg, 1988). Pullar et al. (1988) found incomplete adherence in 42% of patients prescribed high doses of penicillamine as their disease-modifying drug. Whichever report one reads there is agreement that adherence is a problem, particularly in chronic diseases. The World Health Organization (WHO) has recognized this and has stated that 'poor adherence to treatment of chronic diseases is a worldwide problem of striking magnitude' and cites adherence to long-term therapy for chronic illnesses in developed countries averaging just 50% (World Health Organization, 2003). It is interesting that adherence does not appear to be linked to severity of symptoms. An RA study undertaken by Viller et al. (1999) in different countries demonstrated this.

Different authors have tried to shed light on the reasons for this high rate of non-adherence. A study of newly diagnosed patients with juvenile RA attending a clinic-based, nurse-administered educational−behavioural intervention of adherence with NSAID was conducted over 13 months by Rapoff et al. (2002). The experimental group and their parents saw a 10-minute video about adherent enhancing strategies. The patients also received a booklet for back-up. Strategies included:

- pairing medication taking with an established behaviour such as brushing teeth;
- writing down when they took their medication;
- positive reinforcement such as praising and rewarding;
- discipline such as using time out for intentional non-adherence.

The control group and their parents viewed a videotape which described their disease, symptoms and treatments. The nurse answered any questions and provided written information. Results demonstrated that the experimental group were significantly more likely to adhere to their NSAIDs than the control group over time.

Other research has shown that some of the reasons for intentional non-adherence are:

- complexity of treatment regimens;
- dose frequency;

- lack of belief in the medication;
- lack of family support.

However patients are not always non-adherent by intention. Some simply forget to take their drugs or are too busy or away from their usual environment. In 1989, Lorish *et al.* surveyed 200 patients with RA and identified 16 reasons for both intentional and unintentional missed doses. The majority of intentional non-adherence was attributed to side effects of the medication; changes in usual activity accounted for the majority of unintentional non-adherence.

Many health professionals believe that adherence is influenced by factors such as lack of information about the disease process and its ensuing consequences, and the purpose and possible outcomes of treatment. Katz (1982) has stated 'one of the major factors contributing to unintentional non-adherence may be the patient's lack of understanding as to the nature of the treatment program'. There are a few studies that have explored the association between patient education and adherence with medication. Lee and Tan (1979) studied drug adherence in 108 patients, who were asked whether the physician had given an adequate explanation of the nature of their disease and the reasons for taking their prescribed medication. In all, 53% of the adherent patients thought that they had been given an adequate explanation of their disease compared with 31% of the non-adherent patients. This was a significant difference between the two groups (p<0.05). Of those who thought they had received a sufficient explanation of their medication, the proportion that actually took their drugs compared to those who did not was similar. This research seems to indicate that knowledge of the disease has more influence on adherence than knowledge of medication alone. However, this study relied solely on the patient's perception of adequacy of explanation and there was no attempt to measure knowledge in an objective fashion. Owen *et al.* (1985) studied 178 patients with rheumatoid arthritis and noted that poor comprehension of the purpose of prescribed medications was an important factor in non-adherence. They concluded that to obtain optimal benefit from medication, patients must be taught about their drugs.

Hill *et al.* (2001) has shown that patient education significantly enhances patient adherence with drug therapy and increases their knowledge of their drugs, their disease and their treatments. Patients who received patient education also perceived their disease as having less impact on their lives than controls who were on the same disease-modifying drug therapy but did not receive patient education.

The definitive answer to changing non-adherence is for the most part elusive; this is a very complex problem, but reviews by Haynes *et al.* (2000), McDonald, Garg and Haynes (2002), Hill (2005b) at least point the way.

CONCLUSION

Patient education plays an important and effective role in the treatment of rheumatic diseases, and nurses have a significant role to play in educating their patients. One of the aims of nursing is to assist patients to manage their own lives and live as fully and independently as possible. Delivering patient education programmes to our patients certainly goes some way to achieving this goal. However, patient education should not be seen as a separate function, but rather as an integral part of the practice of therapeutic nursing.

Patient education is an effective method of enhancing what we think of as conventional therapy for rheumatic disease. There is abundant literature to show that patient education programmes increase knowledge – Gerber *et al.* (1987), Hill *et al.* (1994), Lorig, Konkol and Gonzalez (1987), Hirano, Laurent and Lorig (1994), to name but a few. Recent work by Kirwan *et al.* (2005) showed that patients in this study also gained knowledge and reported personal benefit, but only improved self-efficacy for pain and only for a short time. Some of these findings were concordant with the Cochrane review undertaken by Reimsma, Kirwan and Rasker (2002), which demonstrated short-term benefits that were not maintained over time.

Patient education also changes behaviour patterns – for example, increasing the practice of exercises, joint protection and relaxation – and improves health status measures such as pain, stiffness and functional ability (Hawley, 1995; Lorig, Konkol and Gonzalez, 1987).

The question of adherence with drug therapy is very important, but it should be remembered that patients may have good reasons why they do not take their drugs, and they have every right not to do so. The essence of patient education is empowerment that gives patients choice. Nurses should accept that if they have educated their patients to the point where they feel sufficiently knowledgeable to make informed choices, be it to take their drugs or not, they have served them well.

APPENDIX 4.A METHOTREXATE INFORMATION SHEET

What is Methotrexate?

Methotrexate is one of a group of drugs known as disease-modifying drugs. It is used to treat several types of arthritis, including rheumatoid arthritis. It usually comes as a tablet but it can be given by injection.

How does it work?

It is thought to slow down disease activity. It can also make your immune system (your body's defence system) less effective and so it is always used with care.

It is not a painkiller, and so you should continue taking your usual anti-inflammatory tablets and painkillers.

How long will it take to work?

Methotrexate builds up slowly in the body so it does not work straightaway. You may start to feel better after only 3 weeks, but it could take 12 weeks or even longer.

What dose will I take?

When you first start on methotrexate you will begin on a very small dose. This will be increased slowly until you reach your normal dose as follows:

- 2.5 mg a week for one week;
- 5.0 mg a week for one week;
- 7.5 mg a week for one week;
- 10 mg a week as your normal dose.

A few people need a higher dose than 10mg a week and it can be taken in doses up to 25mg a week in some cases.

When should I take the tablets?

You will only take methotrexate once a week. You can take it at any time of the day but you should always try to take it on the same day each week. Because you only take it once a week it is easy to forget. Most people find it best to get into a routine of always taking it at the same time on the same day; before breakfast on Friday, for example.

Take methotrexate with a full glass of water on an **empty** stomach. If it gives you indigestion take it with a little food such as a cream cracker.

How long can I stay on the tablets?

If you have no bad side effects you can stay on it for as long as it is helping. Some people have been taking it for many years.

Are there any side effects?

Only a few people get side effects. They usually occur when you first start taking the tablets. They are **usually mild** and get better in a few hours. They are:

- feeling sick;
- indigestion;
- diarrhoea;
- skin rash;
- headaches;
- mouth ulcers.

More important side effects are:

- large bruises caused by changes in the clotting cells (platelets) in the blood;
- sore throat and fever caused by changes in the white cells that fight infections;
- sudden breathlessness or cough.

WHAT SHOULD I DO IF I GET SIDE EFFECTS?

If you get side effects tell the doctor or nurse **straightaway**.

Do I need special tests because of my tablets?

Yes. Before you begin your methotrexate you should have a chest X-ray.

When you first start on methotrexate your blood must be tested every two weeks for the first eight weeks and then once a month. You will need these tests all the time that you are on methotrexate. They check that your blood can clot properly and that your white cells can fight infections.

If your GP checks your blood, phone the surgery and ask if your blood tests are normal. If there are any problems you may have to stop taking the tablets for a while until your blood gets back to normal.

Can I take other medicines with my tablets?

Some medicines do not mix well with methotrexate. These include:

- trimethoprim;
- sulfonamides;
- probenecid;
- diuretics (water tablets);
- some anti-inflammatory tablets including aspirin.

Always remind your doctor that you are taking methotrexate if she or he prescribes other medicines for you. You should also tell the chemist if you buy 'over the counter' medicine.

Is there anything else that I must be careful of?

If you have never had chicken pox and come into contact with someone who has chicken pox or shingles, you must tell your doctor immediately.

If you catch chicken pox or shingles tell your doctor immediately.

You should not have a vaccination that uses a 'live vaccine' (polio or German measles are the most common). Flu vaccines are safe. To be certain, tell the doctor or nurse that you are on methotrexate before you have a vaccination.

Avoid alcohol, but the very occasional moderate drink on a special occasion will do you no real harm.

Is Methotrexate safe in pregnancy?

Methotrexate can harm an unborn baby. Do not use it if you are pregnant. If you get pregnant while you are taking methotrexate, tell your doctor as soon as you know. If you are planning to have a baby, discuss it with your doctor or nurse. You should stop taking methotrexate six months before you plan to have a baby. This applies to men as well as women.

You should not breastfeed while you are on methotrexate.

Methotrexate can reduce sperm count in men.

Remember to keep all medicines out of the reach of children.

REFERENCES

Anderson, J.L., Dodman, S., Copelman, M. and Fleming, A. (1979) Patient information recall in a rheumatology clinic. *Rheumatology and Rehabilitation*, **18**, 18−22.

Arthur, V.A.M. (1995) Written patient information: a review of the literature. *Journal of Advanced Nursing*, **21**, 1081−6.

Association of the British Pharmaceutical Industry. (1987) Information to Patients on Medicines. Policy Document, October.

Auerbach, S.M. (1989) Stress management and coping research in the health care setting: an overview and methodological commentary. *Journal of Consulting and Clinical Psychology*, **57** (3), 388−95.

Bandura, A. (1977) Self-efficacy: toward a unifying theory of behavioural change. *Psychological Review*, **84**, 191−215.

Bandura, A. (1986) *Social Foundations of Thought and Action: A Social Cognitive Theory*, Prentice-Hall, New Jersey.

Bandura, A. and Cervone, D. (1983) Self-evaluative and self-efficacy mechanisms governing the motivational effects of goal systems. *Journal of Personality and Social Psychology*, **45**, 1017−28.

Becker, M. (1974) The health belief model and personal health behaviour. *Health Education Monographs*, **2**, 236.

Belcon M.C., Hayes, R.B. and Tugwell, P. (1984) A critical review of compliance studies in rheumatoid arthritis. *British Journal of Rheumatology*, **27**, 1227−33.

Benner, P. (1984) *From Novice to Expert − Excellence and Power in Clinical Nursing Practice*, Addison Wesley Publishing Company, California.

Bishop, P., Kirwan, J. and Windsor, K. (1997) The ARC Patient Literature Project − Brief Report. The Arthritis and Rheumatism Council for Research, Chesterfield.

Boyd, M.D. (1987) A guide to writing effective education materials. *Nursing Management*, **18** (7), 56−7.

Burckhardt, C.S. (1994) Arthritis and musculoskeletal patient education standards. *Arthritis Care and Research*, **7**, 1−4.

Callahan, L. and Pincus, T. (1997) Education, self-care, and outcomes of rheumatic disease: further challenges to the 'biomedical model'. *Arthritis Care and Research*, **10** (5), 283−8.

Campbell, B.F., Sengupta, S., Santos, C. and Lorig, K.R. (1995) Balanced incomplete block design: descriptions, case study, and implications for practice. *Health Education Quarterly*, **22**, 201−10.

Colvez, A. and Blanchet, M. (1981) Disability trends in the United States population 1966−1976: analysis of reported causes. *American Journal of Public Health*, **71**, 464−71.

Dale, E. and Chall, J.S. (1948) A formula for predicting readability. *Educational Research Bulletin*, **27**, 11−20.

Daltroy, L.H. and Liang, M.H. (1988) Patient education in the rheumatic diseases: a research agenda. *Arthritis Care and Research*, **1**, 161−9.

Davis, P., Busch, A. and Lowe, J. (1994) Evaluation of a rheumatoid arthritis education program: impact on knowledge and self-efficacy. *Patient Education and Counseling*, **24**, 55−61.

DeVellis, R.F. and Blalock, S.J. (1993) Psychological and educational interventions to reduce arthritis disability. *Baillière's Clinical Rheumatology*, **7**, 397−416.

Doak, C., Doak, L. and Lorig, K. (1996) Selecting, preparing, and using materials, in *Patient Education − A Practical Approach*, 2nd edn (ed. K. Lorig), Sage Education, Thousand Oaks, CA, section 4, 117−29.

Donovan, J.L. and Blake, D. (1992) Patient compliance: deviance or reasoned decision making? *Social Science Medicine*, **34**, 507−13.

Donovan, J.L., Blake, D.R. and Fleming, G. (1989) The patient is not a blank sheet: lay beliefs and their relevance to patient education. *British Journal of Rheumatology*, **28**, 58−61.

Feinberg, J. (1988) The effect of patient-practitioner interaction on compliance: a review of the literature and application in rheumatoid arthritis. *Patient Education and Counseling*, **11**, 171−87.

Flesch, R. (1948) A new readability yardstick. *Journal of Applied Psychology*, **32**, 221−33.

Fries, J.F., Spitz, P., Kraines, R.G. and Holman, H.R. (1980) Measurement of patient outcome in arthritis. *Arthritis and Rheumatism*, **23**, 137−45.

Fry, E. (1968) A readability formula that saves time. *Journal of Reading*, **2**, 513−16.

Gerber, L., Furst, G., Shulman, B. *et al.* (1987) Patient education program to teach energy conservation behaviours to patients with rheumatoid arthritis. *Archives of Physical Medicine and Rehabilitation*, **68**, 442−5.

Gibbs, S., Waters, W.E. and George, C.F. (1989) The benefits of prescription information leaflets (1). *British Journal of Clinical Pharmacology*, **27**, 723−39.

Goeppinger, J. and Lorig, K. (1996) What we know about what works: one rationale, two models, three theories, in *Patient Education: A Practical Approach* (ed. K. Lorig), Sage, Thousand Oaks, CA, Chapter 9, p. 202.

Hammond, A. (2003) Patient education in arthritis: helping people change. *Musculoskeletal Care*, **1** (2), 84−97.

Harris, M., Smith, B. and Veale, A. (2005) Printed patient education interventions to facilitate shared management of chronic disease: a literature review. *Internal Medicine Journal*, **35** (12), 711−16.

Hawley, D. (1995) Psycho-educational interventions in the treatment of arthritis. *Baillière's Clinical Rheumatology*, **9**, 803−2.

Haynes, R.B., Montague, P., Oliver, T. *et al.* (2000) Interventions for helping patients follow prescriptions for medications. The Cochrane Library (Issue 1).

Hennell, S.L., Brownsell, C. and Dawson, J.K. (2004) Development, validation and use of a patient knowledge questionnaire (PKQ) for patients with early rheumatoid arthritis. *Rheumatology*, **34** (4), 467−71.

Henry, J.A. (1985) Compliance. *British Journal of Rheumatology*, **24**, 309−12.

Hill, J. (1995) Patient education in rheumatic disease. *Nursing Standard*, **9**, 25−8.

Hill, J. (1997) A practical guide to patient education and information giving, in *Clinical Rheumatology − Early Rheumatoid Arthritis* (eds A.D. Woolfe and P.L.C.M. Van Riel), Baillière Tindall, London, pp.109−27.

Hill, J. (2005a) Adherence with drug therapy in the rheumatic diseases. Part one: a review of adherence rates. *Musculoskeletal Care*, **3**.

Hill, J. (2005b) Adherence with drug therapy in the rheumatic diseases. Part two: measuring and improving adherence. *Musculoskeletal Care*, **3**, 143−56.

Hill, J. (2006) Patient education, in *Rheumatology Nursing: A Creative Approach*, 2nd edn (ed. J. Hill), John Wiley & Sons, Ltd, Chichester, pp. 435−58.

Hill, J. and Bird, H. (2003) The development and evaluation of a drug information leaflet for patients with rheumatoid arthritis. *Rheumatology*, **42**, 66−70.

Hill, J., Bird, H.A., Harmer, R. *et al.* (1994) An evaluation of the effectiveness, safety and acceptability of a nurse practitioner in a rheumatology outpatient clinic. *British Journal of Rheumatology*, **33**, 283−8.

Hill, J., Bird, H.A., Hopkins, R. *et al.* (1991) The development and use of a patient knowledge questionnaire in rheumatoid arthritis. *British Journal of Rheumatology*, **30**, 45−9.

Hill, J., Bird, H. and Johnson, S. (2001) Effect of patient education on adherence to drug treatment for rheumatoid arthritis: a randomised controlled trial. *Annals Rheumatic Disease*, **60**, 869−75.

Hirano, P.C., Laurent, D.D. and Lorig, K. (1994) Arthritis patient education studies, 1987−1991: a review of the literature. *Patient Education and Counseling*, **24**, 9−54.

Kaplan, S. and Kozin, F. (1981) A controlled study of group counselling in rheumatoid arthritis. *Journal of Rheumatology*, **8**, 91−9.

Katz, W.A. (1982) Compliance. *Seminars in Arthritis and Rheumatism*, **12**, 132−5.

Kay, E.A. and Punchak, S.S. (1988) Patient understanding of the causes and medical treatment of rheumatoid arthritis. *British Journal of Rheumatology*, **27**, 396−8.

Keefe, F.J., Lefebvre, J.C., Kerns, R.D. *et al.* (2000) Understanding the adoption of arthritis self-management: stages of change profiles among arthritis patients. *Pain*, **87**, 303−13.

Kirwan, J., Hewlett, S., Cockshott, Z. and Barrett, J. (2005) Clinical and psychological outcomes of patient education in rheumatoid arthritis. *Musculoskeletal Care*, **3** (1), 1−16.

Lazarus, R.S. and Folkman, S. (1984) *Stress Appraisal and Coping*, Springer, New York.

Lee, P. and Tan, L.J.P. (1979) Drug compliance in out-patients with rheumatoid arthritis. *Australian and New Zealand Journal of Medicine*, **9**, 274−7.

Levin, L. (1986) The lay resource in health and health care. *Health Promotion*, **1** (3), 285−91.

Lindroth, Y., Bauman, A., Barnes, C. *et al.* (1989) A controlled evaluation of arthritis education. *British Journal of Rheumatology*, **28**, 7−12.

Lindroth, Y., Bauman, A., Brookes, P.M. and Priestley, D. (1995) A 5 year follow-up of a controlled trial of an arthritis education programme. *British Journal of Rheumatology*, **34**, 647−52.

Lindroth, Y., Bauman, A., and Daltroy, L.H. (1998) Health promotion and patient education for people with arthritis, in *Rheumatology*, 2nd edn (eds J.H. Klippel and P.A. Dieppe), London, Mosby, section 3, 3.1−8.

Lorig, K. (1996) *Patient Education − A Practical Approach*, Sage, Thousand Oaks, CA.

Lorig, K., Feigenbaum, P., Regan, C. *et al.* (1986) A comparison of lay-taught and professional-taught arthritis self-management courses. *The Journal of Rheumatology*, **13**, 763−7.

Lorig, K. and Gonzalez, V. (1992) The integration of theory with practice: a twelve year case study. *Health Education Quarterly*, **19**, 355−68.

Lorig, K. and Holman, H. (1993) Arthritis self management: a twelve year review. *Health Education Quarterly*, **20**, 17−28.

Lorig, K., Konkol, L. and Gonzalez, V. (1987) Arthritis patient education: a review of the literature. *Patient Education and Counseling*, **10**, 207–52.

Lorig, K., Lubeck, D., Kraines, R.G. *et al.* (1985) Outcomes of self-help education for patients with arthritis. *Arthritis and Rheumatism*, **28**, 680–5.

Lorig, K., Ritter, P.L. and Plant, K. (2005) A disease specific self-help program compared to a generalized chronic disease self-help program for arthritis patients. *Arthritis and Rheumatism*, **53** (6), 950–7.

Lorish, C.D., Parker, J. and Brown, S. (1985) Effective patient education: a quasi-experimental study comparing an individualized strategy with a routinized strategy. *Arthritis and Rheumatism*, **28**, 1289–97.

Lorish, C.D., Richards, B. and Brown, S. (1989) Missed medication doses in rheumatoid arthritis patients: intention and unintended reasons. *Arthritis Care and Research*, **2**, 3–9.

Luker, K. and Caress, A. (1989) Rethinking patient education. *Journal of Advanced Nursing*, **14**, 711–8.

Mahmud, T., Comer, M., Roberts, K. *et al.* (1995) Clinical implications of patients' knowledge. *Clinical Rheumatology*, **14**, 627–300.

McDonald, H.P., Garg, A.X. and Haynes, B.R. (2002) Interventions to enhance patient adherence in medication prescriptions. *Journal American Medical Association*, **288** (22), 2868–79.

McLaughlin, H. (1969) SMOG grading – a new readability formula. *Journal of Reading*, **12**, 639–46.

McMahon, R. (1991) Therapeutic nursing: theory, issues and practice, in *Nursing as Therapy* (eds R. McMahon and A. Pearson), Chapman & Hall, London, p.5.

McMahon, R. and Pearson, A. (1991) *Nursing as Therapy*, Chapman & Hall, London.

Meade, C.D. and Smith, C.F. (1991) Readability formulas: caution and criteria. *Patient Education and Counseling*, **17**, 153–8.

Meichenbaum, D. and Turk, D.C. (1987) *Facilitating Adherence to Treatment*, Plenum Press, New York.

Moll, J.M.H. (1986) Doctor-patient communication in rheumatology studies of visual and verbal perception using educational booklets and other graphic materials. *Annals of the Rheumatic Diseases*, **45**, 198–209.

Neuberger, G.B., Smith, K.V., Black, S.O. and Hassanein, R. (1993) Promoting self-care in clients with arthritis. *Arthritis Care and Research*, **6**, 141–8.

Newbold, D. (1996) Coping with rheumatoid arthritis. How can specialist nurses influence it and promote better outcomes? *Journal of Clinical Nursing*, **5**, 373–80.

Newman, S. (1993) Coping with rheumatoid arthritis. *Annals of the Rheumatic Diseases*, **52**, 553–4.

Orem, D. (1980) *Nursing – Concepts of Practice*, 2nd edn, McGraw-Hill, New York.

Owen, S.G., Friesen, W.T., Roberts, M.S. and Flux, W. (1985) Determinants of compliance in rheumatoid arthritic patients assessed in their own home environment. *British Journal of Rheumatology*, **24**, 313–20.

Peplau, H. (1969) Professional closeness. *Nursing Forum*, **8** (4), 342–60.

Pincus, T., Callahan, L.F., Brookes, R.H. *et al.* (1989) Self-report questionnaire scores in rheumatoid arthritis compared to traditional physical, radiographic, and laboratory measures. *Annals of Internal Medicine*, **110**, 259–66.

Prochaska, J.O. and DiClemente, C.C. (1992) Stages of change in the modification of problem behaviours, in *Progress on Behaviour Modification* (eds M. Hersen, R.M. Eisler and P.M. Miller), Sycamore Press, Campaign, IL.

Pullar, T., Peaker, S., Martin, M.F.R. *et al.* (1988) The use of a pharmacological indicator to investigate compliance with a poor response to anti-rheumatic therapy. *British Journal of Rheumatology*, **27**, 381−4.

Rapoff, M.A., Belmont, J., Lindsley, C. *et al.* (2002) Prevention of non-adherence to non-steroidal anti-inflammatory medications for newly diagnosed patients with juvenile rheumatoid arthritis. *Health Psychology*, **21** (6), 620−3.

Reimsma, R., Kirwan, J. and Rasker, J.J. (2002) Patient education for patients with rheumatoid arthritis. *Cochrane Database of Systematic Reviews*, **3**, CD003688.

Ridout, S., Waters, W.E. and George, C.F. (1986) Knowledge of and attitudes to medicines in the Southampton community. *British Journal of British Pharmacology*, **21**, 701−12.

Roper, N., Logan, W. and Tiernay, A. (1985) *The Elements of Nursing*, 2nd edn, Churchill Livingstone, Edinburgh.

Roy, C. (1976) *Introduction to Nursing − An Adaptation Model*, Prentice Hall, New Jersey.

Seligman, M. (1975) *Helplessness: On Depression, Development and Death*, W H Freeman, San Fransisco.

Strecher, V.J., Becker, M., Devills, B. and Rosenstock, I. (1986) The role of self-efficacy in achieving health behaviour change. *Health Education Quarterly*, **13** (1), 73−91.

Taal, E., Rasker, J.J., Sevdel, E.R. and Weigman, O. (1993) Health status, adherence with recommendations, self-efficacy and social support in patients with rheumatoid arthritis. *Patient Education and Counseling*, **20**, 63−76.

Taal, E., Rasker, J.J. and Wiegman, O. (1996) Patient education and self-management in the rheumatic diseases: a self-efficacy approach. *Arthritis Care and Research*, **9** (3), 229−38.

Tucker, M. and Kirwan, J.R. (1989) Does patient education in rheumatoid arthritis have therapeutic potential? *Annals of the Rheumatic Disease*, **50**, 422−8.

Vaughan, B. (1991) Patient education in therapeutic nursing, in *Nursing as Therapy* (eds R. McMahon and A. Pearson), Chapman & Hall, London.

Vignos, P.J., Parker, W.T. and Thompson, H.M. (1976) Evaluation of a clinic education programme for patients with RA. *Journal of Rheumatology*, **3**, 155−65.

Viller, F., Guillemin, F., Briançon, S. *et al.* (1999) Compliance to drug treatment of patients with rheumatoid arthritis: a three year longitudinal study. *Journal of Rheumatology*, **26**, 2114−22.

Westbrook, M. and Viney, L. (1982) Psychological reactions to the onset of chronic illness. *Social Science and Medicine*, **16**, 899−905.

Wetstone, S.L., Sheehan J., Votaw R.G. *et al.* (1985) Evaluation of a computer based education lesson for patients with rheumatoid arthritis. *The Journal of Rheumatology*, **12**, 907−12.

White, J. and Bryer, D. (2006) Medications in the rheumatic diseases, in *Rheumatology Nursing − A Creative Approach* (ed. J. Hill), John Wiley & Sons Ltd, Chichester, pp. 337−72.

Wilson Barnett, J. (1984) *Key Functions in Nursing: The Fourth Winifred Raphael Memorial Lecture*, RCN, London.

World Health Organization. (2003) *Adherence to Long-Term Therapies. Evidence for Action*, World Health Organization, Geneva.

Index

Drug Therapy in Rheumatology Nursing: Second Edition. Edited by Sarah Ryan.
© 2007 John Wiley & Sons, Ltd.

Coventry University Library